T0191785

Common Pediatric Knee Injuries

Nailah Coleman
Editor

Common Pediatric Knee Injuries

Best Practices in Evaluation and Management

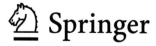 Springer

Editor
Nailah Coleman
Children's National Hospital
Washington, DC
USA

ISBN 978-3-030-55872-7   ISBN 978-3-030-55870-3   (eBook)
https://doi.org/10.1007/978-3-030-55870-3

This Springer imprint is published by the registered company Springer Nature Switzerland AG
The registered company address is: Gewerbestrasse 11, 6330 Cham, Switzerland

Preface

Why

When most people ask me the most common injury I see in clinic, the answer is almost always knee injuries. I am often asked to help evaluate the injured knee of a child or adolescent for a colleague in clinic. When the publisher asked if I would be interested in writing a proposal for a book, I thought this was a great opportunity to provide additional and useful information to my colleagues. We both agreed that pediatricians would appreciate a practical and quick guide on managing pediatric knee injuries and sought to create one.

What Is It About and How It Is Structured

This book is designed as a practical and quick reference guide on the evaluation and management of common pediatric knee injuries. It would be most useful for those who provide clinical care to children and adolescents, including pediatricians, family practitioners, pediatric nurse practitioners, sports medicine physicians, and trainees in these fields. It focuses on the important findings during the evaluation and on appropriate considerations for the management of common knee injuries.

For our readers, we have arranged the book in three general parts, as follows: General Knee Evaluation and Management Strategies, Discussion of Specific Knee Injuries (with important pointers and a chapter summary and table), and Injury Prevention Strategies.

We hope our readers find this book concise and practical, an easy reference for common and concerning pediatric knee issues. It contains cases to aid understanding as well as helpful pearls and pitfalls along with a chapter summary for a quick glance for each condition.

How to Use This Book

Readers can use this book as a study guide or as a quick reference for a specific concern. It can be used with teaching and learning groups, for which the chapter summaries, tables, and cases may be particularly helpful.

Send Off

As one who found show and tell in kindergarten to be an excellent way of sharing my understanding and passion with others, I hope our readers enjoy and learn from this book and are able to use it to help with their teaching of trainees and their care of patients and families.

Washington, DC, USA   Nailah Coleman

Contents

Contributors

Chelsea Backer Family Health Center, MedStar Franklin Square Medical Center, Rosedale, MD, USA

Anthony I. Beutler Department of Family Medicine, Uniformed Services University, Bethesda, MD, USA

Susannah Briskin Rainbow Babies and Children's Hospital, Solon, OH, USA

Shelley Street Callender Department of Pediatrics, Navicent Health System, Mercer University School of Medicine, Macon, GA, USA

Nailah Coleman The Goldberg Center for Community Pediatric Health, Children's National Hospital, Washington, DC, USA

Valerie E. Cothran Primary Care Sports Medicine, University of Maryland, Department of Family and Community Medicine, Baltimore, MD, USA

Larry M. Cowles Department of Family Medicine, Uniformed Services University, Bethesda, MD, USA

Marshall J. Crowther Department of Athletics Health & Sports Performance, University of Mississippi Student Health Services, University, MS, USA

Steven Cuff Department of Pediatric Sports Medicine, Nationwide Children's Hospital; The Ohio State University College of Medicine, Westerville, OH, USA

Svetlana Dani University of Maryland, College Park, MD, USA

Kayla E. Daniel Division of Sports Medicine, Nationwide Children's Hospital, Dublin, OH, USA

Kelly Davis Children's Hospital of Orange County, Orange, CA, USA

Calvin J. Duffaut Family Medicine & Orthopaedics, Division of Sports Medicine, UCLA, Santa Monica, CA, USA

Anastasia N. Fischer Division of Sports Medicine, Nationwide Children's Hospital, Dublin, OH, USA

Department of Pediatrics, The Ohio State University College of Medicine, Columbus, OH, USA

L. Kaleb Friend Orthopedic Surgery and Sports Medicine, Children's National Hospital, George Washington University, Washington, DC, USA

Peter Gerbino Community Hospital of the Monterey, Peninsula, Monterey, CA, USA

Miranda Gordon-Zigel University of Maryland, Department of Family and Community Medicine, Baltimore, MD, USA

Atul Gupta Department of Physical Medicine and Rehabilitation, Virginia Mason Medical Center, Seattle, WA, USA

Jacquelyn Hale Sports Medicine Clinic, 559th Medical Group, JBSA-Lackland, TX, USA

Jessica Heyer Orthopedic Surgery, George Washington University Hospital, Washington, DC, USA

Ingrid K. Ichesco Pediatrics, Sports Medicine, University of Michigan, Ann Arbor, MI, USA

Rajat K. Jain Northwestern University Health Service, Evanston, IL, USA

Lindsay W. Jones Orthopaedics, MedStar Union Memorial Hospital, Ellicott City, MD, USA

Korey Kasper Sports Medicine Clinic, 559th Medical Group, JBSA-Lackland, TX, USA

Steven Koch Sports Medicine Clinic, 559th Medical Group, JBSA-Lackland, TX, USA

Stephanie Lamb Sports Medicine Clinic, 559th Medical Group, JBSA-Lackland, TX, USA

Jessica R. Leschied Henry Ford Health System, Detroit, MI, USA

Jeffrey M. Mjaanes Northwestern University, Evanston, IL, USA

Jonathan Napolitano Sports Medicine, Nationwide Children's Hospital, Westerville, OH, USA

Nathaniel S. Nye Sports Medicine Clinic, Fort Belvoir Community Hospital, Ft. Belvoir, VA, USA

Fort Belvoir Community Hospital, Ft. Belvoir, VA, USA

Thomas L. Pommering Departments of Pediatrics and Family Medicine, Nationwide Children's Hospital, The Ohio State University College of Medicine, Columbus, OH, USA

Joseph M. Powers Sports Medicine, Northside Hospital, Orthopedic Institute, Atlanta, GA, USA

Reno Ravindran Sports Medicine, Nationwide Children's Hospital and The Ohio State University College of Medicine, Dublin, OH, USA

Tracy Ray Sports Medicine, Piedmont Healthcare, Watkinsville, GA, USA

Katherine Rizzone Orthopaedics and Pediatrics, University of Rochester, Rochester, NY, USA

Matthew Sedgley MedStar Union Memorial Hospital, Westminster, MD, USA

Mary Solomon Rainbow Babies and Children's Hospital, Solon, OH, USA

Clinton J. Ulmer University of Texas Health Science Center at San Antonio, San Antonio, TX, USA

Kiyoshi Yamazaki Non-Operative Sports Medicine Physician, HealthFit Clinic, Centura Castle Rock Adventist Hospital, Castle Rock, CO, USA

Kyle Yost Department of Family and Community Medicine, University of Maryland, Baltimore, MD, USA

Chapter 1
General Mechanisms of Injury and Associated Problems

Mary Solomon, Susannah Briskin, and Ingrid K. Ichesco

Introduction

The knee joint is commonly injured or becomes painful in the growing child. As younger patients participate in longer and more intense levels of athletic training and competition, the incidence of acute and chronic knee pain increases. Children undergo significant growth at the knee as they progress through childhood and into adolescence. Children experience different injury patterns, specific to the stages of bony development, which are different from those of an adult. Common acute and chronic injury patterns include the following: sprains; strains; contusions; fractures; and tension, shear, and compression injuries. This chapter describes common knee injury patterns, specific to the child and adolescent.

Acute Injuries

It is important to recognize common signs and symptoms associated with acute knee injuries. Unfortunately, severe pain and the presence of soft-tissue swelling or a joint effusion may limit physical exam tests, such as range of motion or ligament stability testing. Functional testing may also be limited, due to pain with weight-bearing or restrictions in motion. The patient's emotional development or increased stress level, due to injury, may also inhibit a thorough examination. Obtaining an

---

M. Solomon (✉) · S. Briskin
Solon, OH, USA
e-mail: Mary.Solomon@uhhospitals.org; Susannah.Briskin@uhhospitals.org

I. K. Ichesco
Ann Arbor, MI, USA
e-mail: ingridkr@med.umich.edu

© Springer Nature Switzerland AG 2021
N. Coleman (ed.), *Common Pediatric Knee Injuries*,
https://doi.org/10.1007/978-3-030-55870-3_1

accurate history may serve as the main clue to the underlying diagnosis, particularly if a clear mechanism of injury can be identified. Common acute knee injuries include sprains, strains, contusions, and fractures.

Sprain

Ligament injuries, known as sprains, most commonly occur with a rapid change in velocity. The pediatric knee may sustain an abrupt stop when running or a quick shift in direction that results in a ligament sprain. All sprains, regardless of the joint, are graded in the following manner: grade 1—stretch, 2—partial tear, and 3—complete tear. Because ligaments in children are functionally stronger than their bones, the pediatric athlete is more likely to sustain a fracture rather than a sprain. Sprains may occur with either contact (i.e. valgus stress to the knee) or non-contact mechanisms (i.e. ankle inversion). When a sprain does occur, an acute pop may be felt or heard by the patient. Subsequent swelling is usually rapid for ligament tears within the joint, such as the cruciate ligaments; however, sprains of ligaments outside the joint, such as the medial collateral ligament, may not cause swelling at all. The patient will usually report being unable to continue the same level of activity after suffering a sprain. The pain or sense of instability is often severe enough to sideline the individual until he/she seeks medical evaluation.

Strain

A strain is a stretch injury of the muscle or tendon. A strain typically occurs because the muscle has been stretched beyond its limits or the muscle has contracted with too much force. Eccentric contraction injury occurs during the phase of muscle lengthening. A concentric contraction injury, in contrast, occurs as the muscle shortens. As muscles generate greater forces during eccentric contraction, that is when the muscles are more commonly injured. The linebacker who rapidly stops at the line of scrimmage may sustain an eccentric quadriceps muscle strain. Muscle strains, diagnosed clinically with pain in the muscle, present with graded severity, as well. The hamstring is the most common muscle strain of the lower extremity [1]. A grade 1 strain is a minor tear of the muscle and results from injury or stretch to a small amount of muscle fibers within the muscle. Grade 1 strains present with mild pain, mild loss of strength, and no palpable defect on exam. A grade 2 strain involves severe damage to the muscle, due to overstretching and tearing of many of the muscle fibers. Moderate pain results from bleeding into the muscle and surrounding structures. Obvious loss of strength and a palpable defect are identified on exam with grade 2 muscle strains. Grade 3 muscle strains are due to tear of most of the muscle fibers or complete rupture of the muscle. Grade 3 strains cause severe pain, complete loss of strength, and a palpable muscle defect [2].

Injury to a tendon can be the result of either acute trauma or chronic overuse. Acute tendon injury, also classified as a strain, is the result of a sudden stress on a muscle group, due to an intense contraction. A chronic tendon injury is classified as tendinosis and is due to repetitive use of the same muscle–tendon group.

Although acute muscle and tendon injuries occur in the pediatric athlete, these injuries are less common in youth than in adults. The myotendinous junction, where the muscle connects to the tendon, is a common site of weakness in the skeletally mature individual and, hence, more susceptible to injury. In contrast, youth experience a relative weakness of the growing portion of the bone, where the tendon attaches (aka at the apophysis). Although technically considered a growth plate, the apophysis gives the bone contour and does not contribute to vertical growth; it is simply a tendon attachment spot. Age and skeletal maturity influence the site of injury, with skeletally mature patients experiencing tendon ruptures more commonly than those who have not completed ossification [3]. Active bone growth precedes muscle and tendon lengthening (in accommodation); therefore, the myotendinous unit is stretched in response to accelerated bone growth. This relative limitation in muscle and tendon flexibility predisposes the developing athlete to injury of the apophysis, and less commonly, of the attached muscle or tendon [4].

Contusion

A muscle contusion results from direct trauma to the muscle. The quadriceps muscle is the muscle around the knee joint at greatest risk for contusions. Injury occurs from a blunt force to the muscle, such as a helmet-to-thigh tackle in football. Pain and subsequent swelling and bruising develop with a significant contusion. The patient may have pain and limited knee motion, when the muscle flexibility is tested during the physical exam. An area of hemorrhage may look enlarged and/or feel soft and compressible. It may be palpable within the muscle, if significant direct trauma occurred. Myositis ossificans is a delayed finding that may develop at the site of a hemorrhage muscle injury that ossified [1]. Ongoing monitoring for this complication is imperative, particularly when a large hematoma forms within a muscle.

Fracture

Physeal injuries are common fracture patterns in children, because the physis (i.e. growth plate) is relatively weak prior to ossification. The classification system of Salter and Harris is used to describe fractures associated with the physis. The distal femur is the most common site at the knee to suffer a Salter–Harris fracture. Thankfully, fractures at the knee joint are rare in children. When they do occur, patients typically present with the acute onset of pain and swelling. Patients may be unable to bear weight, and pain will localize to the distal femur in most cases.

Avulsion fractures, also common during pediatric knee development, occur when a contracting tendon pulls off a piece of bone and/or cartilage at the apophysis. Avulsion fractures may result from extreme stress, such as from a sudden or powerful muscle contraction [3]. An avulsion fracture may occur at the inferior pole of the patella or at the tibial tubercle. The pathology of specific avulsion fractures is further discussed in a dedicated chapter of this book. Avulsion injuries and tension injuries can oftentimes be distinguished from normal variation, based on the clinical presentation and the presence of fragmentation on radiographs [3]. Comparison films with the unaffected side and advanced imaging, such as MRI, are sometimes needed to determine if such a fracture has occurred.

Chronic Injuries

It is equally important to recognize common patterns of chronic knee injury, as these injuries may be frequently unsuspected. Escalated intensity, frequency, and duration of sports training, combined with a younger age of sports specialization, have resulted in an increased incidence of overuse injuries in children. Overuse injuries occur when repetitive microtrauma to tissue overwhelms the body's innate ability for self-repair. When forces are too great in strength, frequency, and/or duration, then a chronic injury may develop. These injuries typically present initially as inflammatory processes of the bone, cartilage, and/or muscle–tendon or tendon–bone junctions. The pediatric musculoskeletal system is particularly susceptible to overuse injuries, and the epiphyseal cartilage is often the most susceptible. Vascular, grossly traumatic, and microtraumatic factors also contribute to the evolution of an overuse injury [5]. Examples include a sudden onset of Osgood–Schlatter, when a direct blow to the tibial tubercle occurs through a fall or a knee-to-knee contact injury. Microtrauma can also occur to the tibial tubercle through the repetitive pulling stress the patellar tendon causes with repetitive running and/or jumping. Most overuse injuries involve the lower extremity, especially the knee. Common types of chronic injury result from tension/traction, shear, or compression forces.

Tension/Traction

Tension injuries result from a muscle repeatedly exerting force across the associated tendon, where it inserts at the apophysis or bone. Tension/traction injuries of the apophysis will typically present during periods of maturation of cartilage cells within the apophysis and are, thus, unique to the growing skeleton. During the growth of the knee, the tendon remains relatively short, in comparison to the long bones of the knee (femur and tibia). Decreased flexibility increases traction at the apophyseal insertion of the tendon and may also contribute to apophyseal injury, as noted above [4]. The growing cartilage of the apophysis is considerably weaker, relative to the tendon, and, when it is repeatedly subject to a pulling force, traction apophysitis can occur, resulting in microavulsions and potential inflammation [5]. The accumulation of microavulsions along the apophyseal physis occurs in the setting of failure to repair damage from chronic stresses [1].

A thorough musculoskeletal exam can identify the inappropriate biomechanical forces causing stress at the associated apophysis. The exam should focus on evaluating flexibility, strength imbalances, proximal core and hip strength, and functional ability. Tension/traction injuries of the knee result in painful motion and function; weakness of the muscle group, due to pain with contraction; swelling at the apophysis; and occasional limping. Common knee joint traction injuries, such as Osgood–Schlatter's and Sinding–Larsen–Johansson diseases, are further discussed in their respective chapters in this book.

Distinguishing repetitive chronic avulsion injury and tension injury can be challenging. Obtaining a historical description of pain quality and onset, determining the exacerbating and remitting factors, and assessing recent changes in growth velocity and/or participation volume may help guide the physician. Symptoms, such as loss of range of motion or swelling at the site of injury, may require further imaging to assist in making the correct diagnosis and to guide appropriate management.

Shear

Chronic injury caused by shearing forces (forces moving in opposite directions) across the knee is also more common with the growing participation in competitive sports among youth [1]. Articular cartilage coats the weight-bearing surfaces of bone, and the underlying bone is called the subchondral bone. Although somewhat controversial, repeated shear forces delivered across the subchondral bone and the articular cartilage may lead to a stress reaction or microtrauma [1]. Stress reaction and stress fracture within the subchondral bone then develop in the setting of ischemia, due to loss or lack of vascularization. Osteochondritis dissecans (aka osteochondral defect, OCD) results from the delamination, or separation of the articular cartilage from the underlying bone, and fragmentation of the subchondral bone at the articular surface [1]. The medial condyle of the femur is a common site in the children, adolescents, and young adults. A more in-depth discussion of OCD is found within a dedicated chapter of this book.

Compression

Stress fractures are overuse injuries that occur from repetitive compression or tensile stress on the bone [4]. Stress fractures are distinctive from acute fractures that result from a single traumatic event. Stress fractures occur, when extrinsic forces are applied at a rate greater than the bone is able to adapt. When activity and stress on the bone increase, the rate of osteoclastic resorption can exceed that of osteoblastic remodeling. The process of increased activity overwhelms the body, and a "stress response" or "stress fracture" results, leading to the insidious onset of localized, low-grade pain.

Stress fractures around the knee joint are uncommon; however, the distal femur and proximal tibia are at risk. Stress fracture pain worsens with impact activity and can cause significant pain with weight bearing. Rarely does swelling occur. A history of localized pain in a weight-bearing bone that worsens with activity, exercise, or training and then progresses to focal pain at rest is suggestive of a stress fracture. Obtaining x-rays and/or an MRI may assist in making the proper diagnosis.

Chapter Summary

Acute injuries, such as sprains, strains, and contusions, are common in young active people. The lower extremity is especially prone to overuse injuries that can lead to more chronic pain. Analyzing and correcting training techniques, level of competition, lifestyle habits, and sports equipment and avoiding early specialization in sport may prevent a variety of injuries. Children who train for competition should be encouraged to acknowledge and treat pain rather than ignore and push through injuries.

Many injury patterns are specific to the unique anatomy and physiology of the developing musculoskeletal system. Common knee injuries sustained by young athletes are influenced by the biomechanical forces of the supporting ligaments and bones of the pediatric knee joint. Forces acting on the relatively weak physes and apophyses of the knee result in patterns of bone and soft-tissue injuries. Knowledge of the developing anatomy and its normal anatomical and physiologic variants is essential to perform a proper evaluation, make an accurate diagnosis, and formulate an appropriate management plan for common acute and chronic injury patterns.

References

1. Davis KW. Imaging pediatric sports injuries: lower extremity. RadiolClin N Am. 2010;48:1213–35.
2. Gregory A. Sports lingo: musculoskeletal terms. In: Koutures C, Wong V, editors. Pediatric sports medicine essentials for the office evaluation. Thororfare: Slack Inc; 2014. p. 2–8.
3. Maloney E, Stanescu A, Ngo A, Parisi M, Iyer R. The pediatric Patella: Normal development, anatomical variants and malformations, stability, imaging, and injury patterns. Semin Musculoskelet Radiol. 2018;22:81–94.
4. Browne GJ, Barnett PL. Common sports-related musculoskeletal injuries presenting to the emergency department. J Paediatr Child Health. 2016;52(2):231–6.
5. Launay F. Sports-related overuse injuries in children. Orthop Traumatol Surg Res. 2015;101(1):S139–47.

Chapter 2
History

Jeffrey M. Mjaanes

Introduction

Knee pain is a common reason for seeking medical attention, and in children and adolescents, joint pain is commonly caused by either acute or chronic injury. Between 1999 and 2008, 6.6 million youth with knee injuries presented to emergency rooms in the United States, and the two age groups with the highest incidence rates were older adolescents aged 15–24 and children aged 5–14 [1]. Knee injuries in children and adolescents may result from chronic, repetitive overuse or may be caused by an acute, often traumatic mechanism; occasionally, injuries may also result from a combination of acute and chronic factors. Historical details, such as the onset and nature of the pain, presence of associated symptoms, as well as elements from the past medical, family, and sport histories, can help illuminate the cause of knee pain.

Description of Pain

Obtaining a comprehensive history of the knee pain is essential in focusing the differential diagnosis. Important characteristics of the pain include timing (onset and duration), location, nature, and severity of the pain, as well as the mechanism of injury. In terms of timing, onset of knee pain can be either acute or insidious. Traumatic injuries tend to be acute in onset, while overuse injuries tend to be insidious, occurring gradually over time. The clinician should attempt to quantify the duration of pain or, if intermittent, how long the episodes last (Table 2.1).

J. M. Mjaanes (✉)
Northwestern University, Evanston, IL, USA
e-mail: Jmjaanes@northwestern.edu

© Springer Nature Switzerland AG 2021
N. Coleman (ed.), *Common Pediatric Knee Injuries*,
https://doi.org/10.1007/978-3-030-55870-3_2

Table 2.1 Key elements of the medical history of knee pain

History elements	Characteristic	Examples

Pain description	Timing:
	  Onset
	  Duration
		Acute, insidious

	Location	Anterior, posterior, medial, lateral, etc.
	Quality	Sharp, dull, achy, burning, etc.
	Severity	Mild, moderate, severe VAS 0–10
	Aggravating/mitigating factors	Activity, rest, etc.
	Attempted initial treatments	Ice, medications, rehabilitation, etc.
Associated symptoms	Swelling/effusion	Acute, large amount Gradual onset
	Mechanical symptoms	Popping/crepitus Locking Instability
	Other	Erythema, warmth, nocturnal pain, etc.
Past medical history		Prior knee pain Prior knee surgery Hip issues
Family history		Autoimmune, musculoskeletal conditions
Social/ sport history		Sport, position Amount/intensity of participation

The exact location, or lack thereof, of the pain can be helpful in making the diagnosis. One should inquire whether the pain is anterior, posterior, medial, or lateral. Common etiologies of anterior knee pain include patellofemoral pain syndrome, patellar instability (subluxation, dislocation), Osgood–Schlatter or Sinding–Larsen–Johansson apophysitis, pre-patellar bursitis, and patellar tendinitis. Patellofemoral pain is often vague, poorly localized anterior knee pain, while Osgood–Schlatter, for example, localizes directly to the tibial tuberosity. Relatively common causes of posterior knee pain include muscle tendon injuries to the popliteus, hamstring, or calf muscles; ligamentous injuries to the posterior cruciate ligament (PCL); and meniscal injury [2]. Less common causes of posterior knee pain include popliteal cysts, nerve or artery entrapment, and multi-structural entities, such as posterolateral corner injuries. Medial and lateral knee pain can be commonly caused by injury to the medial collateral ligament (MCL) or lateral collateral ligament (LCL), respectively, or meniscal pathology. Distal iliotibial band pain also commonly localizes to the lateral knee. Fractures, growth plate (physeal) injuries, and soft-tissue contusions often occur just above or just below the knee joint itself.

Clinicians should inquire as to the quality and severity of the pain. Common descriptors of pain include sharp, dull, achy, throbbing, and burning. Rating severity can be as simple as mild, moderate, or severe, or more commonly a pain scale, such as the visual analog scale (VAS), may be employed. If the pain was acute and activity-related, the clinician should ask whether the patient was able to bear weight and/or continue participating afterward or if the athlete was forced to stop the activity. Inability to bear weight or continue the activity should raise suspicion for a significant injury, such as a ligament rupture, growth plate or bone fracture, or unstable meniscal tear. Clinicians should also ask about factors that worsen or mitigate the pain, as well as any attempted treatments or therapies and their effectiveness.

In acute injuries, eliciting the precise mechanism of injury, if possible, is often invaluable in the diagnostic process. In addition to patient or witness description of the injury mechanism, video evidence, if available, can prove to be quite useful, as well. Many ligament injuries occur as a result of direct trauma to the knee, when the ipsilateral foot is planted. A direct blow to the lateral leg produces valgus stress and often results in an MCL sprain, while a direct blow to the medial knee conversely results in an injury to the LCL [3]. PCL injuries are classically caused by a posteriorly directed force to the proximal tibia, the so-called "dashboard injury," due to the relatively high incidence seen in front seat passengers involved in motor vehicle accidents. Direct blows to the posterolateral or posteromedial knee in high-velocity sports, such as in football or rugby, can result in injuries to multiple structures, such as posterolateral corner injuries or the "unhappy triad" of MCL, ACL, and meniscal injury.

Acute injuries may also occur without direct trauma to the knee. Noncontact mechanisms can be important contributors to ligament and meniscal injuries. Sudden stops or changes in direction lead to deceleration moments and, when combined with valgus loading, may result in anterior cruciate ligament tears, especially in female athletes and skeletally immature children. Twisting or pivoting on a fixed foot can also result in meniscal injuries. In addition to the "dashboard mechanism," PCL ruptures can also occur from hyperextension of the knee. Acute hyperextension can also produce ACL injuries, anterior tibial plateau contusions or fractures, and impingement of the anterior infra-patellar fat pad.

The lack of any trauma or obvious mechanism of injury in an acutely painful knee may also be a reason for concern. Consideration should be given to other potential etiologies, such as infection or autoimmune conditions. As biomechanics change with age and skeletal maturity, occasionally undiscovered structural issues, such as a discoid meniscus, may result in an acutely painful knee. Finally, prior injuries, such as a small meniscal tear or chondromalacia, may result in an acute-on-chronic picture as exacerbations of pain and swelling may occur secondary to use.

Associated Symptoms

The presence of other symptoms in the knee joint, as well as more systemic symptoms, may help to narrow the differential diagnosis further. Important considerations for the knee include the presence or absence of swelling and mechanical symptoms.

Both the timing and quantity of joint swelling provide important clues. Rapid onset of a moderate-to-large amount of fluid within 1–2 hours after an incident often signifies the presence of blood in the joint (hemarthrosis). Hemorrhage into the joint typically occurs in conjunction with a significant injury to bone (contusion or fracture) and/or disruption of a major ligament, such as the ACL or patellofemoral ligament (i.e. a patellar dislocation). Slower onset, over the course of 24–48 hours, of a small-to-moderate amount of fluid is more consistent with a meniscal or cartilage injury or a less severe ligament sprain. With recurrent effusions, clinicians may consider meniscal, chondral, or autoimmune etiologies.

Medical providers should inquire about the presence of mechanical symptoms, such as popping, locking, or instability. Patients often complain about painless popping or cracking in joints, including the knee. Fortunately, most intra-articular crepitus is benign and does not indicate major structural pathology; however, popping that is painful or is accompanied by an effusion should be investigated more cautiously. Additionally, many cases of popping around the knee joint are extra-articular in origin, especially in younger patients. Movement of the distal iliotibial band as it approaches its insertion on Gerdy's tubercle can cause popping and occasionally mild localized swelling. A symptomatic medial plica (synovial fold) can also cause local pain, swelling, and popping near the anteromedial joint line. Both are fairly benign conditions and are relatively easily managed.

It is important for the clinician to differentiate the type of benign crepitus noted above from true mechanical locking, as patients may use the terms interchangeably. Mechanical locking indicates a mechanical block to extension, or less commonly flexion, of the knee, due to the abnormal interposition of a structure, such as a loose body or unstable meniscal flap, between the tibial plateau and the femoral condyle. This locking is not only painful but also potentially dangerous for the patient and should be treated in an expeditious manner.

Another common point of confusion related to symptom terminology is "giving way" versus true, mechanical instability. Mechanical instability refers to a structural deficiency in the knee, resulting in true instability of the joint. Frequent causes of true mechanical instability are an ACL rupture or patellar dislocation; however, more frequently, many patients complain of their knee "feeling like it's going to give out" but lack any intra-articular, structural abnormality. Often the cause of their insecurity is actually arthrogenic muscle inhibition (AMI), or failure of activation of the quadriceps muscle. This essentially represents a pain reflex and commonly occurs in patients recovering from ACL reconstruction or other knee surgeries but is also seen in patients with anterior knee pain, such as patellofemoral syndrome and patellar tendinitis [4]. One helpful means of clinically differentiating these two entities may be to inquire about the context of the sensation; while AMI typically occurs when navigating stairs or standing from a seated position, true ligamentous instability often occurs when stopping suddenly or changing directions and is often accompanied by a sense of movement within the joint.

Patients may experience additional symptoms in the knee or elsewhere in the body. The presence of erythema, warmth, and significant pain in the joint should alert the provider to the possibility of infection, such as septic arthritis, or other acute arthropathy (i.e. gout, pseudogout, gonococcal disease, etc.). Nighttime pain, in addition to constitutional symptoms, such as weight loss, night sweats, and fatigue, might indicate neoplasia. Other possible symptoms seen with malignancy could include fever, anorexia, and general malaise. The presence of swelling, pain, or erythema in other joints likely indicates a more systemic, autoimmune process, such as systemic lupus erythematosus, rheumatoid arthritis, or juvenile idiopathic arthritis; often these conditions have other extra-articular manifestations, as well, such as rashes, gastrointestinal bleeding, and ocular changes.

Past Medical History and Family History

Patients should be asked about their own medical history as it relates to the knee. A prior history of knee pain or swelling or previous knee surgeries is important to note. One should always ask about issues in the contralateral knee; athletes who have had an ACL reconstruction in one knee are at higher risk to suffer an ACL injury in the contralateral knee [5]. Additionally, prior or concurrent issues in the hips may directly cause or contribute to pain in the knee and should be noted.

In terms of family history, one should inquire about the existence of first-degree relatives with autoimmune conditions. Even some conditions, like pes planus and genu valgum, may have hereditary causes, and a detailed family history may illuminate these possibilities.

Social and Sport History

An understanding of an athlete's sport and his or her level of play is advantageous, when attempting to evaluate knee pain or injury. For example, in high school females, the highest risk sports for ACL rupture are soccer, basketball, softball, and volleyball. For high school males, the highest risk sport is football [6]. Some evidence exists that even certain positions or styles of play may cause a higher risk than others. For example, defending in soccer is associated with a higher risk of ACL rupture, especially in females [7].

Level of play is also important to understand. It is not uncommon now to have young athletes involved in one sport year-round, on multiple teams. The almost constant, repetitive load on their bodies can lead to overuse injuries involving primary growth plates, apophyses, tendons, and bone. A recent study in pediatric athletes demonstrated that single-sport specialized athletes in individual sports report higher training volumes and greater rates of overuse injuries than single-sport specialized athletes in team sports [8]. Abrupt changes in training, especially significant increases in intensity or duration of play over a short period of time, or sudden alterations in footwear or playing surface can also be precipitants for injury [9]. Inquiring about level and intensity of play, including number of hours per week and weeks per year, and any sudden changes in training may provide clues as to the degree of risk for overuse injury and may allow for providing enhanced guidance on injury prevention.

Chapter Summary

Young patients may have difficulty describing their presenting complaint, and the task of obtaining a detailed description of knee pain can be challenging for the provider. By utilizing a standard approach with respect to documenting the history of the complaint, clinicians can avoid missing crucial details that may provide clues to the diagnosis. The history should concentrate on key characteristics of the pain, the mechanism of injury in cases of acute complaints, the presence or absence of any associated symptoms, pertinent details of the patient's past medical history, the family history, and sport participation. Constructing a comprehensive, detailed history of the knee pain will allow the clinician to narrow their differential diagnosis and focus their physical exam.

References

1. Gage BE, McIlvain NM, Collins CL, Fields SK, Comstock RD. Epidemiology of 6.6 million knee injuries presenting to United States emergency departments from 1999 through 2008. Acad Emerg Med. 2012;19:378–85.
2. Wolf M. Knee pain in children: part 1: evaluation. Pediatr Rev. 2016;37(1).
3. Calmbach WL, Hutchens M. Evaluation of patients presenting with knee pain: part I. history, physical examination, radiographs, and laboratory tests. Am Fam Physician. 2003;68(5):907–12.
4. Hart JM, Pietrosimone B, Hertel J, Ingersoll CD. Quadriceps activation following knee injuries: a systematic review. J Athl Train. 2010;45(1):87–97.
5. Wright RW, Dunn WR, Amendola A, et al. Risk of tearing the intact anterior cruciate ligament in the contralateral knee and rupturing the anterior cruciate ligament graft during the first 2 years after anterior cruciate ligament reconstruction: a prospective MOON cohort study. Am J Sports Med. 2007;35(7):1131–4.
6. Joseph AM, Collins CL, Henke NM, Yard EE, Fields SK, Comstock RD. A multisport epidemiologic comparison of anterior cruciate ligament injuries in high school athletics. J Athl Training. 2013;48(6):810–7.
7. Brophy RH, Stepan JG, Silvers HJ, Mandelbaum BR. Defending puts the anterior cruciate ligament at risk during soccer: a gender-based analysis. Sports Health. 2015;7(3):244–9.
8. Pasulka J, Jayanthi N, McCann A, Dugas LR, LaBella C. Specialization patterns across various youth sports and relationship to injury risk. Phys Sports Med. 2017;45(3):344–52.
9. Patel DR, Villalobos A. Evaluation and management of knee pain in young athletes: overuse injuries of the knee. Translat Pediat. 2017;6(3):190–8.

Chapter 3
Exam

Jeffrey M. Mjaanes

Introduction

After formulating a list of potential diagnoses based on a detailed history, the clinician uses the physical examination to confirm or discard possible etiologies. If one consistently approaches the examination in a methodical manner, the process becomes almost second nature. While the exact sequence of the exam may vary from clinician to clinician, if the examiner uses a similar approach each time, details are less likely to be overlooked. The exam typically begins with inspection for visual clues, is followed by an evaluation of range of motion and strength, and is concluded with special testing of specific structures.

Visual Clues

Inspection actually begins the moment the patient enters the exam room with regard to the patient's general disposition, pain, and comfort level. The clinician should also assess the patient's ambulation for antalgic gait, limping, or an inability to bear weight on the extremity, which would likely indicate a serious injury. The examiner should also note the presence of erythema or significant swelling, which may indicate infection or autoimmune arthritis. With swelling, the fluid may be intra-articular, which can be difficult to assess visually unless the amount is significant, or extra-articular, which may be easier to visualize. Focal extra-articular swelling directly over the patella, for example, may indicate pre-patellar bursitis, which can

J. M. Mjaanes (✉)
Northwestern University, Evanston, IL, USA
e-mail: Jmjaanes@northwestern.edu

© Springer Nature Switzerland AG 2021
N. Coleman (ed.), *Common Pediatric Knee Injuries*,
https://doi.org/10.1007/978-3-030-55870-3_3

be a fairly common occurrence after a direct fall or trauma to the anterior knee, while localized swelling or prominence over the tibial tuberosity is a typical finding in Osgood–Schlatter apophysitis [1].

The clinician should inspect both knees for muscular symmetry. The presence of unilateral atrophy of the quadriceps muscle suggests chronic pathology with the extension mechanism or significant disuse of the affected knee. If there appears to be a difference, precise circumferential measurement of the quadriceps can be entertained.

The clinician should also visually inspect for signs indicative of anatomical or biomechanical factors, which may contribute to knee pain or pathology. Significant genu valgum or genu varum may play a role in knee pain. Fortunately, most valgus or varum deformities are congenital and mild; however, significant unilateral genu valgum or varum should raise the suspicion of growth arrest or deformation of a physis, or primary growth plate, in the distal femur or proximal tibia. As anterior knee pain syndromes are common, clinical attention to the patella is recommended. A patella that sits higher, or more superior, than expected is referred to as patella alta, while one that sits more caudal is called patella baja; either can contribute to patellar pain. Patellar mal-tracking refers to abnormal gliding of the patella in the trochlear groove, while moving the knee between flexion and extension. On exam this can be seen by lateral displacement of the patella, when the patient is seated and asked to extend the knee actively ("J-sign"—patellar motion transcribes a "J" as it moves).

Mobility Clues

Range of motion can be assessed actively, passively, or against resistance. Active range of motion refers to the degree to which a patient can voluntarily move a joint. Passive motion refers to movement of the joint solely by the examiner, with no effort by the patient. Normal range of motion for the adult knee is generally considered to be 0 degrees of extension and 135–140 degrees of flexion. Commonly many individuals have slightly increased passive extension of the knee by a few degrees; however, excessive, unilateral extension is referred to as genu recurvatum and may represent prior injury. Always examine both knees, starting with the unaffected knee first. Inability to extend one knee fully, especially when there is a history of locking or catching, should alert the clinician to the possibility of an unstable meniscus tear or a loose body, such as an osteochondral fragment. Inability to flex the knee past 90–100 degrees or significant pain with flexion could indicate a meniscal tear, quadriceps injury, or large intra-articular effusion. Pain with active or resisted motion, but no pain with passive motion of the same muscle, suggests tendinitis or apophysitis.

When assessing motion, one can also evaluate motor strength. To measure quadriceps strength, the clinician typically has the seated patient extend the knee against resistance. To gauge hamstring strength, the ideal patient position is prone and then the patient flexes the knee against resistance applied by the examiner. Universally,

Table 3.1 Strength grading scale

Grade	Significance
0	No contraction (complete paralysis)
1	Slight contractility without any movement
2	Active movement, with gravity eliminated
3	Active movement, against gravity, but tolerates no resistance
4	Active movement, against gravity and resistance
5	Active movement, against gravity, plus full resistance / Normal power

strength is evaluated on a graded scale from 0 to 5 (Table 3.1). Again, comparison to the unaffected knee is helpful.

This table was used with permission of the Medical Research Council, with minimal alterations.

In addition to simple resisted strength testing, the clinician may consider performing a functional evaluation for a more global assessment of true joint performance. Simple maneuvers, such as having the patient perform a double or single leg squat, duck walk (walking in a partially squatted position for several steps), or jogging in the clinic hallway can provide clues to the regular function of the quadriceps and hamstrings, in addition to pelvic stabilizers and lower leg muscles. The ability to complete these motions satisfactorily without pain, particularly the duck walk, is reassuring to the examiner and decreases the likelihood that the patient has a large effusion, ligamentous tear, significant tendinopathy, or meniscal tear [2].

Exam Maneuvers

Palpation

Palpation is a simple yet effective tool for examining the knee. In order to palpate successfully, the clinician must become familiar with the detailed anatomy of the knee joint. Although one should also consider palpating in a methodical fashion so as not to overlook any critical anatomical areas, clinicians will often palpate the expected area of pain last. Important areas to palpate in the young athlete include the apophyses, the medial and lateral joint lines, as well as the distal femur and proximal tibia (Table 3.2). Most of these structures are more easily palpable with the patient supine and the knee flexed to 90 degrees.

Palpation may also be helpful in the evaluation of swelling, particularly with differentiating an intra-articular effusion from extra-articular fluid. Intra-articular effusions typically result from internal derangement, such as injury to the articular cartilage, menisci, or ligaments. If the fluid accumulates quickly, the swelling likely represents hemarthrosis and may be evidence of a fracture or significant bone contusion, such as that seen in a patellar dislocation or rupture of the anterior cruciate ligament (ACL). The presence of intra-articular swelling can often be appreciated

Table 3.2 Important landmarks for pediatric knee palpation

Anatomic Landmark	Potential significance
Tibial tuberosity	Osgood–Schlatter (tibial tuberosity apophysitis)
Inferior pole patella	Sinding–Larsen–Johansson (inferior patellar apophysitis) or patellar tendinitis
Superolateral patella	Bipartite patella
Medial joint line	Medial meniscus, medial collateral ligament
Lateral joint line	Lateral meniscus
Medial or lateral distal femur or proximal tibia	Physeal injury (i.e. Salter–Harris fracture)
Medial or lateral patellar facet	Patellofemoral pain syndrome
Fibular head	Lateral collateral ligament, biceps femoris tendinitis
Gerdy's tubercle, distal iliotibial band	Iliotibial band syndrome

Fig. 3.1 Palpation of intra-articular effusion. With the superiorly placed hand, the fluid is compressed from the suprapatellar pouch toward the inferiorly placed hand which palpates the fluid wave

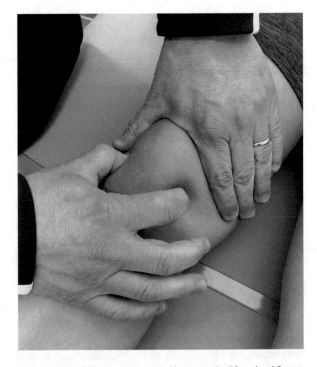

both on visual inspection and palpation in the supra-patellar pouch. If a significant amount of fluid is present, the patient will often "lose" the normal indentations seen alongside the patella when the knee is fully extended. Fluid here can also be detected using a "milking maneuver" by first gently milking the fluid from the medial side of the patella with the palm of the hand and then applying gentle compression to the superolateral aspect—this will elicit a fluid wave, which is often visible and/or palpable along the medial side of the patella (see Fig. 3.1). Comparison to the contralateral knee is important.

Extra-articular collections of fluid may result from simple contusions, bursitis, or tearing of the quadriceps muscle–tendon unit. Pre-patellar bursitis can result from direct trauma to the anterior knee, seen commonly in wrestlers, and may present as focal swelling and tenderness of the anterior aspect of the patella. Pes anserine bursitis results in local swelling and tenderness over the insertion of the gracilis, sartorius, and semitendinosus on the anteromedial knee.

Ligament Testing

Ligamentous injuries can occur in young athletes and, therefore, familiarization with common testing techniques of the major ligaments is essential.

Medial Collateral Ligament

Medial collateral ligament (MCL) injuries typically occur from a direct blow to the lateral aspect of the knee resulting in stretching or, possibly, failure of the ligament. Typically, there will be localized swelling and tenderness over the ligament as it crosses the medial joint line or over its more proximal aspect. The valgus stress test is used to evaluate the integrity of the MCL. To perform the valgus stress test, the knee should be held and passively flexed to approximately 20–30 degrees, and then a medially directed force is applied with the palm of the hand on the lateral aspect of the knee. A mild sprain may result in medial-sided pain with this maneuver; a severe sprain or complete tear will result in palpable opening or "gapping" along the medial side. The test should be repeated at 0 degrees of flexion (see Fig. 3.2). Normally there should be no gapping at 0 degrees; the presence of joint opening in full extension indicates a more severe injury, likely a concomitant injury to a cruciate ligament.

Lateral Collateral Ligament

The lateral collateral ligament (LCL) is often injured with a direct blow to the medial knee or a non-contact extension/varus overload mechanism. The patient will likely have localized tenderness and swelling laterally. To evaluate the LCL, the varus stress test is performed similarly to the valgus stress test but with the hand position reversed and a laterally directed force applied to the medial aspect of the knee, forcing the knee into varus. Again, the clinician assesses for the presence of lateral pain or laxity. After performing the varus stress test at 20–30 degrees of flexion, the examiner should repeat the test at 0 degrees of flexion (see Fig. 3.3). Gapping at both 20–30 degrees and 0 degrees suggests a more severe injury, such as a concurrent tear of the anterior or posterior cruciate ligament (PCL) or other stabilizing structures.

Fig. 3.2 Valgus stress test. The patient is relaxed, and the knee is in 20–30 degrees of flexion. The examiner places one hand along the lateral side of the knee joint and applies a valgus stress to the knee. The examiner assesses for laxity of the medial collateral ligament. The test is then repeated at 0 degrees of flexion

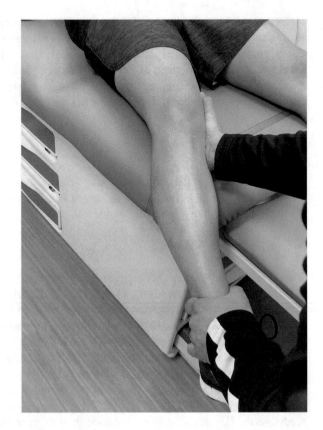

Anterior Cruciate Ligament

Unfortunately, anterior cruciate ligament (ACL) injuries are relatively common among young athletes and represent a significant cause of morbidity. Classically, the method taught to evaluate the ACL is the Anterior Drawer Test. To perform this test, the patient is in a supine position, the hip is flexed to 45 degrees, and the knee is flexed to 90 degrees. The examiner grasps the knee on both the medial and lateral aspects just below the joint line, placing the thumbs over the anterior tibial plateaus. With the foot stabilized, the examiner pulls the tibia anteriorly (see Fig. 3.4). The test is considered positive if there is the lack of a solid palpable endpoint, when compared to the uninjured knee [3]. Unfortunately, the results of the Anterior Drawer Test can be affected by hamstring spasm and guarding; therefore, the test carries a relatively low sensitivity and specificity, reported as 18–92% and 78–98%, respectively [4]. A more sensitive and specific means to examine the integrity of the ACL is Lachman's test. To perform Lachman's test, the patient is supine and relaxed. The examiner grasps the knee with one hand above the knee joint and places the other hand below the knee joint with thumbs on the anterior aspects. The more superior hand controls and positions the leg to approximately 15–25 degrees of flexion;

Fig. 3.3 Varus stress test. Similar to the valgus stress test, the patient is relaxed with the knee flexed to 20–30 degrees. The examiner places one hand along the medial side of the joint and applies a varus stress to the knee, assessing for laxity, or opening, of the lateral collateral ligament. The edge of the exam table can be used as a fulcrum, as seen in the picture here

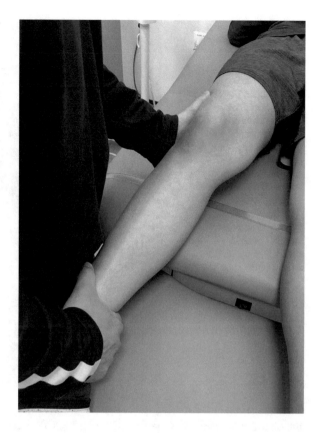

this hand remains still for the exam (see Fig. 3.5). The other hand is then used to pull the tibia anteriorly. Typical anterior translation is less than 5 mm often with a firm endpoint noted; a significant side-side difference is considered abnormal. Sensitivity and specificity of Lachman's test have been reported as 63–93% and 55–99% respectively [4]. The presence or absence of an endpoint may be the most reflective of the state of the ACL [5]. The examiner may note difficulty obtaining either of these tests in the sub-acutely injured knee and may experience more accurate results, if the exam is performed either immediately post-injury or, conversely, after the swelling and pain have subsided.

Posterior Cruciate Ligament

Injury to the posterior cruciate ligament (PCL) is less commonly seen in the young athlete but can occur from either hyperextension or when the tibia is suddenly forced in a posterior direction with respect to the femur. The Posterior Sag Sign and Posterior Drawer Test can be used to assess the integrity of the PCL. For these tests, the patient is supine and relaxed with the knee flexed to 90 degrees and feet resting

Fig. 3.4 Anterior drawer test. The patient is supine and relaxed with hips flexed to 45 degree and the knee flexed to 90 degree. The examiner places both thumbs on the anterior tibial plateaus and stabilizes the patient's foot with their body or an assistant. Then the examiner exerts an anteriorly directed force. The knee with an intact ACL will demonstrate minimal translation; however, an ACL-deficient knee will show increased anterior translation with no solid endpoint

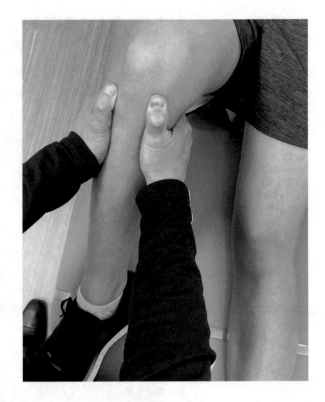

flat on the exam table. For the Posterior Sag Sign, the examiner visually inspects the knee joints from the side and notes the position of the tibial plateaus with respect to the femoral condyles. This "sag" can also be appreciated on palpation as typically the anterior aspect of the medial tibial plateau will sit 5–10 mm anterior to the anterior aspect of the medial femoral condyle; however, in the PCL-deficient knee, gravity will allow the tibia to "fall back," and the plateau will appear to sit more posterior, when compared to that of the contralateral knee. The normal step-off will be absent. For the Posterior Drawer Test, similarly to the Anterior Drawer Test, the examiner approaches the patient from the front and places the thumbs over the anterior tibial plateaus and the fingers behind the flexed knee medially and laterally. Then the examiner applies a posteriorly directed force against the tibia and should note increased posterior translation, typically more than 10–12 degrees in the PCL-deficient knee, compared to the uninjured joint (see Fig. 3.6).

Patellofemoral Instability

Instability at the patellofemoral joint can be a significant cause of morbidity in the young athlete. Injury to the medial patellofemoral ligament can lead to patellar subluxation or frank dislocation. If the clinician encounters a patient with an acutely

Fig. 3.5 Lachman test. The examiner grasps the knee with the one hand above the knee joint and places the other hand below the knee joint with thumbs on the anterior aspects. The more superior hand controls and positions the leg to approximately 15–25 degrees of flexion; this hand remains still for the exam. The inferior hand is then used to pull the tibia anteriorly. In a patient with an intact ACL, a firm endpoint should be noted

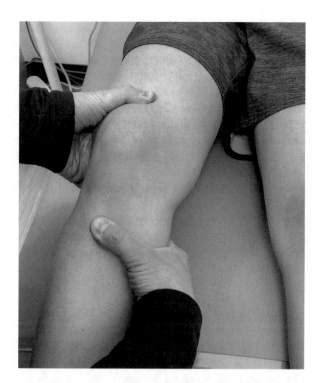

Fig. 3.6 Posterior drawer test. Similar to its anterior counterpart, in the posterior drawer test, the patient is supine and relaxed with the knee flexed to 90 degrees and foot resting flat on the exam table. The examiner places the thumbs over the anterior tibial plateaus and the fingers behind the knee medially and laterally. Then the examiner applies a posteriorly directed force against the tibia and should note increased posterior translation, typically more than 10–12 degrees in the PCL-deficient knee, compared to the uninjured joint

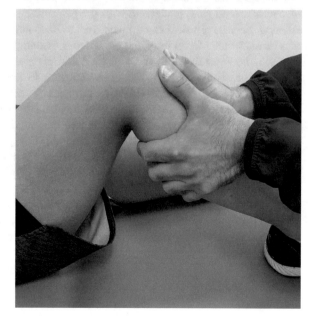

dislocated kneecap, the knee will usually be semi-flexed and the patella in an obviously abnormal position laterally. To reduce, the clinician can simply extend the knee slowly, while applying a slight medially directed pressure along the lateral border of the patella; the kneecap should return to its normal anatomic position by the time the joint is fully extended. Following a patellar dislocation, the patient will usually have a large, swollen knee with tenderness along the medial aspect of the patella and the lateral femoral condyle, due to bone contusions with resulting hemarthrosis. Sub-acutely and chronically, the clinician can test for instability by performing the patellar apprehension test. To perform the test, the patient should be supine on the exam table with the legs fully extended and relaxed. The clinician places the index finger or thumb along the medial border of the patella and applies slight laterally directed pressure. In the case of patella instability, often the patient will abruptly instruct the clinician to stop the maneuver as this recreates the sensation of instability. If compared to the contralateral knee, the clinician will also typically note increased lateral translation of the patella with respect to the trochlear groove.

Meniscal Injury

Meniscal cartilage is susceptible to injury. Tears can occur in the medial or lateral meniscus; however, in both cases the majority of tears occur in the body and posterior horns. Most meniscal tears will present with pain localizable on either the medial or lateral side, tenderness over the respective joint line, and intra-articular effusion. Several physical exam maneuvers exist to aid in confirming the presence of a meniscal tear. In all tests, the objective is essentially to compress the affected meniscus between the tibia and femur. McMurray's test is performed in a supine patient by passively internally rotating and flexing the knee to test the lateral meniscus and externally rotating and flexing the knee to test the medial meniscus (see Fig. 3.7). Classically, a test is described as positive, when the examiner feels a "click" during the maneuver; however, more commonly elicitation of pain along either joint line, when flexing the knee during McMurray's, is considered a positive result. The sensitivity of McMurray's test ranges from 16 to 88% in the medical literature, while the specificity ranges from 20 to 98% [6]. The Thessaly test is performed actively by the patient, who stands on one leg with the knee in approximately 20 degrees of flexion and then rotates medially and laterally upon the leg. Elicitation of pain, which localizes to the respective joint line, is described as a positive test. The sensitivity and specificity of Thessaly's test have been described as 62–66% and 39–55%, respectively [7].

Fig. 3.7 The McMurray test. The examiner places the finger and thumb of one hand along the joint lines and grasps the foot with the other hand. The knee is then brought into maximum flexion with the foot externally rotated to compress the posterior portion of the medial meniscus. Then the examiner extends the knee, internally rotates the foot, and repeats the flexion maneuver to compress the posterior horn of the lateral meniscus. Classically, the test is positive if a "click" is palpable over the injured meniscus, but commonly many clinicians consider elicitation of pain as a positive test

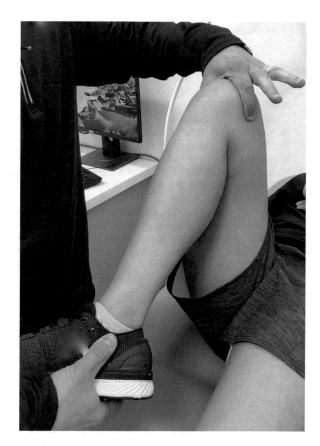

Chapter Summary

Learning and practicing a methodical approach to examining the knee will aid the clinician in narrowing the differential diagnosis. Examination often begins with inspection and observation for visual clues, followed by assessment of range of motion and strength. Palpation for swelling and areas of tenderness is often helpful. Specific exam maneuvers can then be employed to evaluate for injuries to the major ligaments or menisci. One important point to recall is that not all knee pain originates in the joint itself. The clinician who encounters a patient with reported knee pain, but a completely unremarkable exam, would be well served to examine the hip and/or lumbar spine for any potential sources of referred pain.

References

1. Patel DR, Villalobos A. Evaluation and management of knee pain in young athletes: overuse injuries of the knee. Translat Pediat. 2017;6(3):190–8.
2. Schraeder TL, Terek RM, Smith CC. Clinical evaluation of the knee. N Engl J Med. 2010;363(4):e5.
3. Calmbach WL, Hutchens M. Evaluation of patients presenting with knee pain: part I. history, physical examination, radiographs, and laboratory tests. Am Fam Physician. 2003;68(5):907–12.
4. Ostrowski JA. Accuracy of 3 diagnostic tests for anterior cruciate ligament tears. J Athl Train. 2006;41(1):120–1.
5. Mulligan EP, McGuffie DQ, Coyner K, Khazzam M. The reliability and diagnostic accuracy of assessing the translation endpoint during the Lachman test. Inter J Sports Phys Therapy. 2015;10(1):52–61.
6. Hing W, White S, Duncan R, Marshall R. Validity of the McMurray's test and modified versions of the test: a systematic literature review. J Manual Manipulat Therapy. 2009;17(1):22–35.
7. Blyth M, Anthony I, Francq B, Brooksbank K, et al. Diagnostic accuracy of the Thessaly test, standardised clinical history and other clinical examination tests (Apley's, McMurray's and joint line tenderness) for meniscal tears in comparison with magnetic resonance imaging diagnosis. Health Technol Assess. 2015;19(62):1–62.

Chapter 4
Testing – What to Do and When

Ingrid K. Ichesco, Mary Solomon, Susannah Briskin, and Jessica R. Leschied

Diagnostic Imaging

Radiography

Plain radiographs are used as the initial imaging modality in the evaluation of knee pain, due to their wide availability, ease of acquisition for the patient, and low cost. Indications to obtain radiographic imaging include knee effusion, inability to bear weight, decreased range of motion, deformity, and acute injury with concern for fracture. Radiographs should also be obtained in cases of acute and chronic knee pain to evaluate for other potential disorders, such as osteochondral abnormalities, benign or malignant bone tumors, infection, and inflammatory arthritis, and to assess skeletal maturity. Patients with night-time pain, fevers, inability to bear weight, malaise, weight loss, and a history of cancer should also undergo radiographs to initiate evaluation for more worrisome etiologies.

Obtaining multiple views of the knee with radiographs allows for a more thorough evaluation. Oftentimes, AP and lateral views are included in a standard knee x-ray order; however, additional views, including tunnel/notch view & sunrise/merchant views, may prove to be helpful (Fig. 4.1). Figure 4.2 demonstrates the appropriate patient position for obtaining optimal radiographic views of the knee. AP and

I. K. Ichesco (✉)
Ann Arbor, MI, USA
e-mail: ingridkr@med.umich.edu

M. Solomon · S. Briskin
Solon, OH, USA
e-mail: Mary.Solomon@uhhospitals.org; Susannah.Briskin@uhhospitals.org

J. R. Leschied
Detroit, MI, USA
e-mail: jessicale@rad.hfh.edu

© Springer Nature Switzerland AG 2021
N. Coleman (ed.), *Common Pediatric Knee Injuries*,
https://doi.org/10.1007/978-3-030-55870-3_4

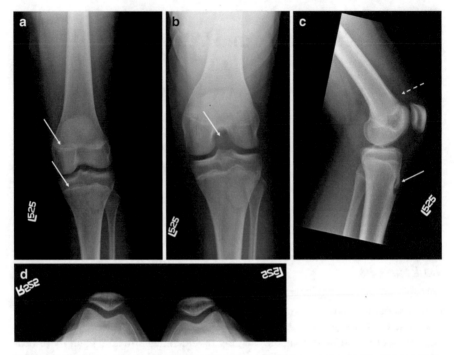

Fig. 4.1 A four-view radiographic knee series in a young adolescent female. (**a**) AP view highlighting normal growth plates (solid arrows) in the femur and tibia. (**b**) Notch view, which is useful for identifying osteochondral abnormalities of the femoral condyles. The white arrow indicates the intercondylar "notch." (**c**) Normal lateral view should be performed with the knee in approximately 30 degrees of flexion to assess for a suprapatellar joint effusion (dashed arrow). Solid arrow identifies the normal tibial tubercle apophysis. (**d**) Bilateral merchant (i.e., skyline or sunrise) views demonstrating normal patellofemoral alignment

lateral views evaluate for fracture of the femur and tibial plateau, tibial tubercle apophysis, tibial eminence, and physeal injuries. The patellar views, such as the merchant or sunrise view, evaluate for patellofemoral morphology and for patellar fracture, bipartite patella, and patellar osteochondral abnormalities. The tunnel or notch view allows for visualization of the weight-bearing aspect of the femoral condyles, which is a common location for osteochondral abnormalities, also referred to as osteochondritis dissecans (OCD) [1]. The lateral aspect of the medial femoral condyle is the most common location for an OCD in the knee. When indicated, a contralateral or comparison view offers additional information to evaluate for asymmetry of the growth plates and growth centers (physes or apophyses). In the pediatric knee, areas of growth are present in the distal femur, proximal tibia, proximal fibula, tibial tubercle, and inferior pole of the patella. Physes and apophyses ossify at different ages. A contralateral view of the unaffected knee evaluates for asymmetry and may increase the reader's confidence level to diagnose a normal finding versus injury, avulsion fracture, or other pathology.

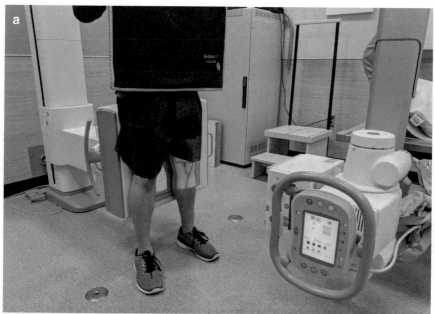

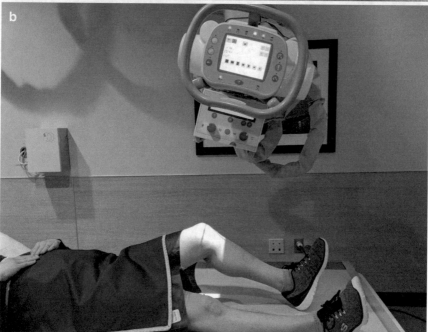

Fig. 4.2 Proper patient positioning for a four-view radiographic knee series. (**a**) AP view. (**b**) Notch view. (**c**) Lateral view. (**d**) Merchant view

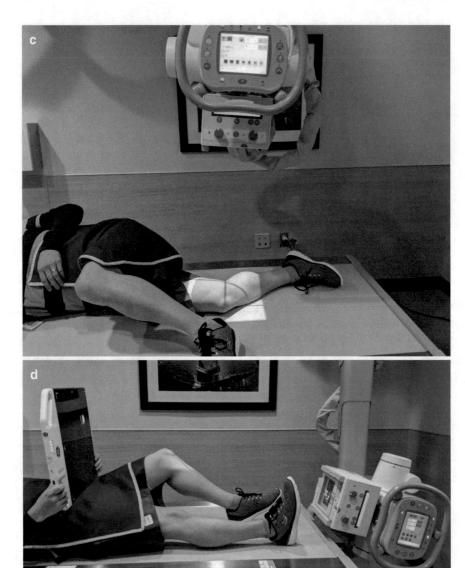

Fig. 4.2 (continued)

Magnetic Resonance Imaging

Magnetic resonance imaging (MRI) studies are able to evaluate soft tissue structures, in addition to osseous structures, in multiple planes (Fig. 4.3). MRI is generally safe, as there is no ionizing radiation associated with obtaining images, and, for
the purpose of imaging musculoskeletal injury, it does not usually require

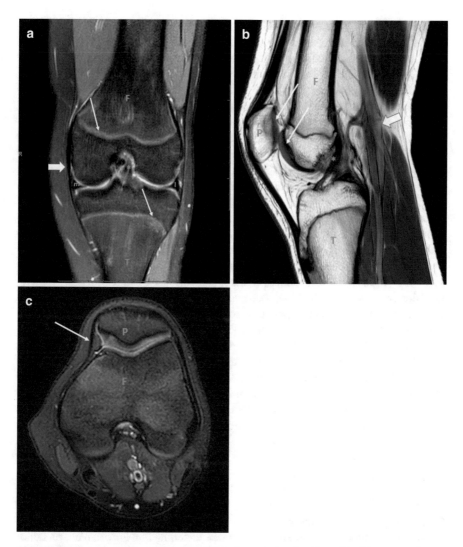

Fig. 4.3 This is reviewing normal anatomy of the knee as visualized by MRI. This shows different views and which structures are visible on each. Figure 4.3a is a coronal PD image with fat saturation in a 13-year-old girl. This plane demonstrates the normal medial (m) and lateral menisci (l), anterior cruciate ligament (*), normal low signal medial collateral ligament (thick arrow), normal fat-suppressed marrow signal in the femur (F) and tibia (T) with normal bright signal growth plates highlighted (thin arrows). Figure 4.3b is a midline sagittal PD image in the same patient. The dark signal anterior cruciate ligament (*) can be evaluated for integrity in all three planes. The slightly hyperintense cartilage of the patella and femur is indicated by the thin arrows and the neurovascular bundle travels in the popliteal fossa (thick arrow). Figure 4.3c, an axial PD fat-suppressed image through the femoral condyles in the same patient, allows for evaluation of the patella (P) and femur (F) morphology and the medial patellofemoral ligament (thin arrow)

gadolinium contrast material administration. MRI may be obtained when radiographs are normal and/or further work up is needed to evaluate for soft tissue injury, such as a ligament, tendon, cartilage, and/or meniscus tear; occult fracture; or OCD. MRI is becoming the gold standard for evaluation of stress injuries and can be useful to diagnose a stress reaction (intermediate stress injury), because it can demonstrate intramedullary bone edema, cortical signal changes, and periosteal reaction not visualized on radiography, allowing for appropriate clinical management prior to progression of the injury to a complete fracture. MRI takes longer than other imaging modalities to perform; thus, sedation of young or uncooperative patients may be necessary. MRI is also noisy and takes place within a confined space, which may cause symptoms of claustrophobia, requiring anxiolytics. Absolute contraindications to MRI include some magnetic implantable sternal hardware, insulin pumps, intraocular metallic foreign bodies, and temporary transvenous pacing wires. If there is a concern about MRI safety, consultation with a pediatric radiologist is suggested.

Indications for obtaining an MRI include osteochondral injuries, occult fracture, soft tissue injury (muscle, tendon, ligament, meniscus, cartilage), stress fracture, infection (osteomyelitis, abscess), bone contusion, avascular necrosis, and bone and soft tissue masses [2]. A knee joint effusion warrants an MRI to evaluate for intraarticular pathology in the setting of injury [3]. Layers within the joint fluid of an effusion, particularly a lipid layer (lipohemarthrosis) is concerning for a fracture [3]. If a lipohemarthrosis is present on radiographs in a first-time lateral patellar dislocation, an MRI is warranted to evaluate for osteochondral injuries [4]. MRI will also demonstrate a classic contusion pattern in the medial patella and lateral femoral condyle in up to 73% of patients with an acute patellar dislocation, and more than one-third of patients will have an osteochondral fracture [5]. MRI can also help with visualization of a medial patellofemoral ligament and medial patellar retinaculum injury. The medial patellofemoral ligament can be torn (partially or completely) in up to 78% of patellar dislocations [5].

About 3% of all children undergoing knee MRI will have a physeal fracture. In this case, MRI can evaluate for widening of the physis, periphyseal edema, fracture lines, and periosteal disruption, injuries that may cause premature closure of the physis [5]. Chronic repetitive stress may cause widening of a growth plate on radiographs and demonstrate signal equivalent to the physis extending into the metaphysis. This can lead to growth disruption and premature growth plate closure, as well. Zbojniewicz & Laor identified a particular finding on adolescents undergoing MRI for evaluation of knee pain, which consisted of a "focal bone marrow edema pattern centered at the physis of the distal femur, proximal tibia, or proximal fibula and extending into both the adjacent metaphysis and epiphysis" [6]. These findings have been suggested to correlate with early physeal closure and are termed FOPE zones (focal periphyseal edema). These physiologic changes do not warrant follow-up imaging [6] but may be associated with pain in the absence of other pathology (Fig. 4.4).

Fig. 4.4 Coronal PD fat-suppressed image in a 14-year-old boy with knee pain demonstrates flame-shaped areas of edema-like signal around the tibial growth plate (dashed arrows), consistent with focal periphyseal edema (FOPE zones). Note also the deep medial collateral ligament injury (solid arrow)

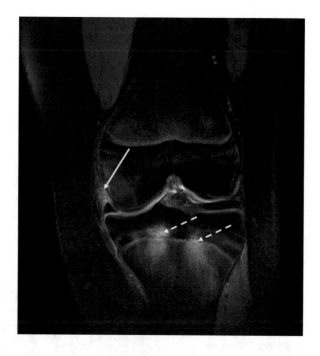

MRI can also help differentiate suspected osteochondral abnormalities (OCD) that are identified on radiographs from normal ossification patterns of the femoral condyles. A normal ossification center will lack surrounding edema, have intact overlying cartilage, and may be bilateral. They are also located in the non-weight-bearing location of the femoral condyle [5]. MRI is more sensitive for OCD than radiographs and provides information about diagnosis, stability, surveillance, and treatment response of lesions, which may affect management [7]. An MRI can also be helpful in identifying a discoid meniscus [5], which is found in about 5% of the population. A discoid meniscus is thick, long, without the normal semilunar shape, and more common on the lateral side [3]. A discoid meniscus is at greater risk for tearing. Pediatric menisci have increased vascularity, which may be confusing when trying to evaluate for a meniscal tear, particularly in children under 12 years old [5, 8].

MRI is useful in evaluating bone marrow signal changes, both normal patterns of marrow conversion and pathologic processes. Diffuse bone marrow replacement should raise concern for potential hematologic malignancy [3]. MRI will show the classic serpentine signal abnormalities that are seen with bone marrow infarcts in sickle cell disease, malignancy, and steroid treatment [3]. In juvenile idiopathic arthritis, an MRI can evaluate for synovial thickening and pannus formation, which enhances with gadolinium contrast material [3]. It is increasingly becoming the preferred method for radiologic evaluation of juvenile idiopathic arthritis; however, it is not as readily available as other imaging modalities. MRI can also identify bone marrow edema, cartilage loss, enthesitis, tenosynovitis, and bone erosions, which are additional findings in inflammatory arthritis [9]. The utility of diffusion-weighted imaging is under investigation for musculoskeletal pathology, but it may be an alternative to contrast-enhanced MRI with the advantage of being relatively fast and without the need for intravenous gadolinium contrast material [10].

Computed Tomography

Computed tomography (CT) has limited indications due to ionizing radiation exposure and the exquisite tissue contrast resolution of MRI. CT is the best modality to evaluate osseous structures in detail. It can provide detail on complex or intraarticular fractures (Fig. 4.5), premature physeal fusion in the setting of Salter-Harris fractures, as well as follow up for specific fracture healing (e.g., Scaphoid fracture).

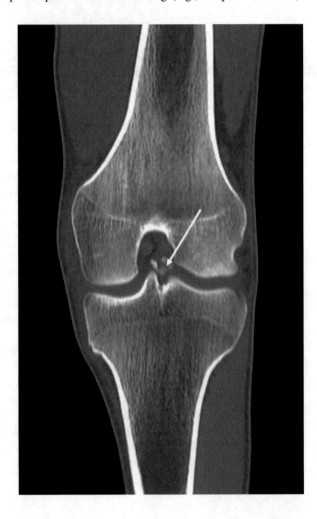

Fig. 4.5 Coronal CT image on a 20-year-old man, following trauma, demonstrates a comminuted avulsion fracture of the tibial eminence (solid arrow), considered an ACL tear equivalent

With the technical advances of other imaging modalities, CT is used less often because of its associated ionizing radiation exposure but may still be a good choice in the setting of trauma because of its ability to be done quickly [2].

Ultrasound

Ultrasound (US) is becoming more popular and readily available. The ability to image the musculoskeletal system dynamically is unique to ultrasound. The lack of ionizing radiation exposure is also particularly important in the pediatric population. US allows visualization of a joint effusion and Baker cyst, as well as soft tissue structures, including tendons, muscles, ligaments, peripheral nerves, and soft-tissue foreign bodies [2]. Ultrasound can also evaluate joints and is becoming more commonplace for diagnosis and surveillance of rheumatologic conditions, as well as for acute hemarthrosis in hemophilic and bleeding disorder populations. In Pediatric Rheumatology, ultrasound is increasingly being used because of its ability to assist with diagnosis, image-guided medication administration, and treatment response monitoring. Ultrasound can detect synovial thickening and effusion in the setting of juvenile idiopathic arthritis, and power or color Doppler can be used to identify active (hypervascular) versus chronic or "burnt out" (hypovascular) pannus. Caution should be taken in interpretation of Doppler findings due to differences in normal vasculature based on age and physical activity level [9]. In patients with hemophilia and bleeding disorders, both MRI and US can be helpful in evaluating for hemarthrosis, with the advantage of US being used as an easily accessible screening tool to detect interval change with point of care use [11, 12]. For musculoskeletal injury, US is somewhat limited in its ability to detect internal derangement due to the depth of the cruciate ligaments and its limited sensitivity to detect meniscal tears; however, for more superficial structures, such as the quadriceps and patellar tendons, medial and lateral collateral ligaments, distal iliotibial band, the pes anserine tendons, and the distal hamstrings tendons, US is helpful in experienced hands.

Bone Scintigraphy

A "bone scan" (bone scintigraphy) is a nuclear medicine test, during which a small amount of radioactive pharmaceutical is injected into a vein, followed by imaging the patient with a gamma camera after a period of time to look for uptake of the radiotracer into the bone. In sports medicine, bone scans have historically been used to help evaluate for stress fractures that do not appear on radiographs. A bone scan will show areas of increased metabolic uptake, but the imaging pattern is nonspecific and does not differentiate between infection, neoplasm, and stress injury. Bone scans are not used as frequently as in the past, as MRI can provide more specific information without the associated radiation exposure from the radiopharmaceutical. Indications for bone scan include evaluation for stress fractures, generalized bone pain to detect tumor, bone metastases in a neoplastic process, or locating a site of infection or inflammatory process [2].

Biochemical Investigations

Serum/Blood

Most pediatric patients with knee pain typically do not require laboratory evaluation. There are a few instances in which to consider obtaining lab work. Individuals who use elicit substances that alter or enhance athletic performance or are used for recreational purposes may be at increased risk for micronutrient deficiencies, iron deficiency anemia, certain liver tumors, and poor bone mineral density. Athletes who also limit caloric intake or particular food groups may also be at risk. These athletes may require additional laboratory work up and vitamin supplementation. If a patient complains of fatigue and a concern for overtraining, one can obtain a CBC, ferritin, thyroid studies, and vitamin D [2] (See Table 4.1 for a list of lab test abbreviations).

Females with menstrual dysfunction may require laboratory evaluation to evaluate for etiology of symptoms; appropriate testing may include LH, FSH, hCG, prolactin, TSH, FT4, estradiol, testosterone (total & free), and DHEA/S. Other testing may include 8 am 17-OH progesterone, progesterone challenge test, and pelvic US [13].

Not all joint pain is musculoskeletal in nature. Juvenile idiopathic arthritis (JIA) is generally defined as joint inflammation with age of onset <16 years old and duration of symptoms >6 weeks. JIA has several subtypes, including oligoarticular (affecting less than 5 joints), polyarticular (affecting 5 or more joints), and systemic.

Table 4.1 Lab test abbreviations

CBC	Complete blood count
LH	Luteinizing hormone
FSH	Follicle-stimulating hormone
hCG	Human chorionic gonadotropin
TSH	Thyroid-stimulating hormone
FT4	Free thyroxine
DHEA/S	Dehydroepiandrosterone sulfate
17-OH progesterone	17 a hydroxyprogesterone
CRP	C-reactive protein
ESR	Erythrocyte sedimentation rate
RF	Rheumatoid factor
CPK	Creatine phosphokinase
ANA	Antinuclear antibody

Polyarticular JIA may be subtyped into rheumatoid factor positive and negative [14]. Symptoms including prolonged morning stiffness that improves with activity, along with persistent joint swelling, warmth, and pain; occasionally painless limp; and fever, rash, and fatigue may indicate a rheumatologic condition. Referral to a rheumatologist is most appropriate, when a rheumatologic condition is suspected. A comprehensive physical examination evaluating for joint effusions, synovial thickening, bony proliferation, and skin findings, among others, will be performed. Initial laboratory evaluation includes CBC, CRP, ESR, RF, CPK, and ANA titers [2], but JIA is a clinical diagnosis and cannot be made based on laboratory studies alone. Because of low specificity, improper timing, and the presence of variability, laboratory values may be normal and falsely disprove the presence of a rheumatologic condition.

Other etiologies of knee pain may include arthritis associated with inflammatory bowel disease and Lyme disease. The presence of blood in the stool, nocturnal stooling, and growth failure can be signs of arthritis associated with inflammatory bowel disease, and referral to Gastroenterology is appropriate in this instance. Lyme disease should be considered with residence in, or travel to, endemic areas and the presence of signs and symptoms consistent with the disease, such as erythema migrans (bulls-eye patterned rash). Serum *Borrelia burgdorferi* enzyme-linked immunosorbent assay (ELISA), followed by western blot, can help make the diagnosis of Lyme disease. It is difficult to culture *B. burgdorferi* in synovial fluid; however, PCR done on synovial fluid may detect its presence. Additionally, synovial fluid usually displays inflammatory markers in this condition, with elevated white blood cell counts [15].

Synovial Fluid Analysis

Children's knees are not generally aspirated for joint fluid to relieve pain. Joint fluid analysis may be indicated, however, to evaluate for infectious or inflammatory processes. Having symptoms of effusion, warmth, erythema, and a possible fever may be indicative of a septic joint. The joint aspirate should be sent for cell count, gram stain, and culture [2]. A concurrent serum laboratory analysis may include CBC, CRP, ESR, RF, ANA titers, and blood cultures.

Chapter Summary

1. Radiographs are routinely obtained as the initial study of choice for a pediatric patient with knee pain and should include multiple views, depending on the indication.
2. Cross-sectional imaging with ultrasound, CT, or MRI is warranted, if a soft tissue injury or occult osseous abnormality is suspected.

3. MRI is useful in the pediatric population because of its superior visualization of soft tissue structures and lack of ionizing radiation exposure.
4. The role of musculoskeletal ultrasound is rapidly expanding, given advances in quality, increased availability, and operator experience. It is particularly useful to evaluate for joint effusion, synovitis, and integrity of superficial tendons and ligaments around the knee.
5. Labwork is not routinely indicated in pediatric patients with knee pain but may be considered to evaluate if there is a concern for non-mechanical etiologies of pain or if there are underlying comorbidities.

References

1. Harris SS, Anderson SJ, editors. Care of the young athlete. 2nd ed; 2009. p. 640.
2. Mortazavi M, Huang R. In: Koutures C, Wong V, editors. General radiology imaging and laboratory testing: What to order and when, in pediatric sports medicine: essentials for office evaluation; 2014. p. 130–7.
3. Strouse PJ, Koujok K. Magnetic resonance imaging of the pediatric knee. Top Magn Reson Imaging. 2002;13(4):277–94.
4. Jain NP, Khan N, Fithian DC. A treatment algorithm for primary patellar dislocations. Sports Health. 2011;3(2):170–4.
5. Leschied JR, Udager KG. Imaging of the pediatric knee. Semin Musculoskelet Radiol. 2017;21(2):137–46.
6. Zbojniewicz AM, Laor T. Focal Periphyseal edema (FOPE) zone on MRI of the adolescent knee: a potentially painful manifestation of physiologic physeal fusion? AJR Am J Roentgenol. 2011;197(4):998–1004.
7. Abdullah SB, Iyer RS, Shet NS, Lesions PO. Semin Musculoskelet Radiol. 2018;22(1):57–65.
8. Kocher MS, et al. Diagnostic performance of clinical examination and selective magnetic resonance imaging in the evaluation of intraarticular knee disorders in children and adolescents. Am J Sports Med. 2001;29(3):292–6.
9. Hemke R, et al. Imaging of the knee in juvenile idiopathic arthritis. Pediatr Radiol. 2018;48(6):818–27.
10. Li M, et al. Diagnostic value of diffusion-weighted MRI for imaging synovitis in pediatric patients with inflammatory conditions of the knee joint. World J Pediatr. 2019.
11. Di Minno MND, et al. Ultrasound for early detection of joint disease in patients with hemophilic Arthropathy. J Clin Med. 2017;6(8).
12. van Vulpen LFD, Holstein K, Martinoli C. Joint disease in haemophilia: pathophysiology, pain and imaging. Haemophilia. 2018;24(Suppl 6):44–9.
13. Joy E, et al. 2014 female athlete triad coalition consensus statement on treatment and return to play of the female athlete triad. Curr Sports Med Rep. 2014;13(4):219–32.
14. Petty R, Laxer R, Lindsley C, Wedderburn L. Textbook of pediatric rheumatology, vol. 7: Elsevier; 2015.
15. Arvikar SL, Steere AC. Diagnosis and treatment of Lyme arthritis. Infect Dis Clin N Am. 2015;29(2):269–80.

Chapter 5
General Management of Pediatric Knee Injuries

Marshall J. Crowther and Calvin J. Duffaut

General management of pediatric knee injuries includes initiating treatment for the relief of symptoms; determining the suitable activity and timetable for an appropriate return to sport and activity; choosing relevant protection, if indicated (examples including bracing, casting, and/or the use of crutches); and addressing any underlying causative factors, if present, to prevent future injuries through rehabilitation and/or physical therapy.

Following the accurate identification of a pediatric knee injury, further evaluation and imaging may determine which injuries can be managed in a primary care setting and which need referral to orthopedic or specialty care. Table 5.1 lists some of the more common exam findings that should alert the practitioner to refer to a higher level of care.

Management of knee injuries is determined first by whether the presenting problem represents an acute injury or involves a more chronic condition. General management considerations for both acute and chronic knee injuries are outlined below.

It is important to remember that, in the skeletally immature pediatric patient, the weakest point of the musculoskeletal system is the physis, or growth plate; thus, injuries to these structures occur more often in youth with open growth plates than do injuries to the ligaments and tendons, which are more commonly seen in the skeletally mature patient. The major physes of the knee joint include the distal femoral and proximal tibial physes, where long bone growth occurs, and the proximal tibial and distal patellar apophyses, where the patellar tendon inserts and originates, respectively.

M. J. Crowther (✉)
Department of Athletics Health & Sports Performance, University of Mississippi Student Health Services, University, MS, USA
e-mail: Crowther@olemiss.edu

C. J. Duffaut
Family Medicine & Orthopaedics, Division of Sports Medicine, UCLA, Santa Monica, CA, USA

© Springer Nature Switzerland AG 2021
N. Coleman (ed.), *Common Pediatric Knee Injuries*,
https://doi.org/10.1007/978-3-030-55870-3_5

Table 5.1 Indications for referral to Sports Medicine/Orthopaedics

Knee effusion (may indicate meniscal, chondral, or ligamentous injury)
Locked knee or inability to flex or extend the knee completely (may indicate meniscal injury or osteochondral lesion)
Ligament instability (especially anterior cruciate ligament (ACL), lateral collateral ligament (LCL), posterior cruciate ligament (PCL) injuries)
Any fracture or osteochondral lesion
Inability to bear weight on the injured knee
Health care provider concern

Management of Acute Injuries

Pediatric acute knee injuries generally occur, due to sudden macro trauma to the knee joint and surrounding structures, usually during contact or high-impact sports. Such a high-intensity, short-duration force can injure the bones (fractures, including epiphyseal and apophyseal injuries), ligaments, and musculotendinous units surrounding the knee joints.

Immediate care of an acute knee injury, like other musculoskeletal injuries, should be treated with a protocol best remembered by the acronym "**RICES**," which includes the following: [1]:

- Rest
- Ice
- Compression
- Elevation
- Stabilization

Another commonly used acronym in this setting is "PRICE," which stands for Protection, Rest, Ice, Compression, and Elevation and accomplishes the same treatment goals as "RICES."

All components of RICES should be used immediately after injury to help alleviate the current symptoms, mitigate further tissue damage from secondary injury, and allow for earlier return of full function and return to play. RICES accomplishes these goals by decreasing the development of swelling, pain, muscle spasm, and neural inhibition [1].

Complete rest involves abstaining from joint motion during the immediate period after the injury, which progresses to "relative rest" as tolerated, meaning limiting joint motion in a way that does not cause further pain and discomfort. The main rationale for the use of rest is not only to decrease the acute pain associated with the injury but also to prevent additional symptoms and delayed recovery, related to "neural inhibition" [1]. Neural inhibition, one of the body's responses to pain, causes a decrease of the surrounding neuromuscular functions (e.g. strength and range of motion). These compensatory changes serve as the body's natural way to "protect" itself from pain and may persist after the initial injury has healed, thus, delaying full recovery and return to a normal activity level.

The use of crutches for knee injuries also can be a component of "rest" in the setting of an acute knee injury, so as to allow for pain-free ambulation and to avoid the neural inhibition that may come with painful walking and limping. Crutches should, therefore, be used until a patient can walk with a normal gait [1].

The use of ice, or cryotherapy, as an acute treatment for injury helps to decrease swelling but also helps to limit secondary injury [1]. Secondary injury may occur to the surrounding uninjured tissue through multiple mechanisms, including inadequate blood flow and tissue metabolic changes. Inadequate blood flow and oxygen supply occurs because of damage to the surrounding blood vessels and hemodynamic changes related to the initial injury. With cooling, the metabolic needs of the surrounding cells and tissues are decreased, making them less susceptible to ischemic injury [1]. With less injured tissue, there is less cellular debris, which lowers tissue oncotic pressure and decreases edema, allowing the repair process to be shorter and resulting in a quicker return to normal activity.

For cryotherapy to be most effective, ice should be applied to the injured tissue as soon after the injury as possible. Ice is best used for 15–20 minutes at least three times a day. Ice can be applied via an ice pack, ice bath, or ice massage. Ice should be avoided prior to physical activity, if the pain involves a nerve, if there is a history of vascular disease, or if there is a history of cold hypersensitivity, such as cold-induced urticaria [1].

Compression of the injured knee aids in controlling and decreasing the edema after the injury. The increased pressure outside of the capillaries helps to decrease filtration pressure. Constant compression applied to an injured knee helps prevent formation of edema, whereas intermittent compression helps remove existing edema by stimulating the lymphatic system. Compression may be provided by elastic knee sleeves, compression stockings, or ace-bandages [1].

Elevation serves to decrease surrounding tissue edema by decreasing capillary hydrostatic pressure. To accomplish this decreased pressure, the injured area should be elevated above the level of the heart.

The final component of RICES is stabilization, which involves supporting the injured leg and knee joint to allow surrounding muscles to relax, reducing neural inhibition and pain. During the neural inhibition process, muscle guarding surrounding the knee joint can occur, causing muscle spasm, which leads to more pain, possibly leading to additional spasm and rigidity of the joint [1]. Early joint stabilization can allow surrounding muscles to relax, avoiding the vicious cycle of pain-spasm-pain. Examples of conventionally used post knee injury stabilization devices include knee immobilizers, hinged knee braces, and patellar stabilizing braces. A knee immobilizer limits knee motion. Patellar stabilization braces can be used in patients with a history of patellar subluxation or dislocation. A temporary hinged knee brace can be helpful in patients that have had a medial or lateral collateral ligament injury, as it will stabilize valgus and varus stressed placed on the knee.

Non-steroid anti-inflammatory drugs (NSAIDs) can be used in the setting of an acute injury to help with reduction of pain and inflammation. It is recommended to limit use of NSAIDs to no longer than 7 days, as longer use may actually delay healing. Patients and parents should be given the appropriate dose and dose interval. The dosing for ibuprofen is 10 mg/kg/dose every 6–8 hours; the typical maximum single dose is 400 mg; and the maximum daily dose regimen is 40 mg/kg/day. Families also need to be aware of the common side effects of NSAIDs, including nausea, bloating, gastritis, gastric and duodenal ulcers, blood-thinning, and renal and hepatic toxicity [2].

After the inflammation has improved and the pain has resolved, the gradual return to play after an acute injury can begin. This is best started with a period of rehabilitation (home exercises or with a physical therapist). Therapy should first work on obtaining full range of motion of the knee. Additional recovery goals include strengthening of the hip abductors, vastus medialis, and core, as well as improving flexibility and biomechanics.

Management of Chronic Injuries

Chronic or overuse injuries are caused by repetitive microtrauma and submaximal stress to the musculoskeletal structures of the knee (and lower extremity) without sufficient rest or recovery time. They are commonly seen in times of rapid increases in training frequency, duration, and/or intensity. In addition, the cartilage of athletes in a rapid phase of growth is more susceptible to the forces of training. Overuse injuries are often related to multiple intrinsic and/or extrinsic factors. Intrinsic factors include growth-related factors, susceptibility of growth cartilage to repetitive stress, the adolescent growth spurt, history of a previous injury, the athlete's previous level of conditioning, anatomical factors, menstrual dysfunction, and psychological and developmental factors. Extrinsic factors can involve training workload (rate, intensity, and progression), training and competition schedules, equipment and footwear, environment, sport technique, and psychological factors (adult and peer influences). Trying to avoid or reduce these risk factors is part of the management of chronic knee injuries [3].

Treatment of intrinsic factors through rehabilitation programs commonly involves the strengthening of the hip, quadriceps, and core musculature to re-establish the normal biomechanics of the knee. Flexibility exercises and an evaluation for any gait abnormalities also should be a component of such a physical therapy program. These types of programs should emphasize developing a foundation of general strength, endurance, and motor skills to improve and maintain optimal sport-specific biomechanics [3].

For extrinsic factors, one must evaluate training volume and intensity, as both are correlated with overuse injuries. Young athletes should avoid year-round training in a single sport. They should also limit participation in tournaments during which several games are played on a single day or extending over consecutive days [3]. A simple rule of thumb is for an athlete to limit formal training hours per week to his/her age in years.

Table 5.2 Knee braces uses

Type of knee brace	When to use
Knee immobilizer or post-operative brace	After acute injury
Patellar stability brace	Patella dislocation/instability
Patellar tendon strap (counterforce brace)	Patellar tendinosis, Osgood-Schlatter disease, Sinding-Larsen-Johansson syndrome
Hinged knee brace	Medial collateral ligament (MCL) or Lateral collateral ligament (LCL) injury

Different types of knee braces and supports can be utilized in patients with chronic knee injuries (Table 5.2). There are a multitude of different types of knee braces available, including both "off-the-shelf," as well as those custom-made for the individual. In general, three categories of knee braces can serve as an overview of how to approach bracing for chronic conditions.

A patella tendon strap, also referred to as a counterforce brace, can be used in patients with knee extensor mechanism conditions, such as Osgood-Schlatter disease, Sinding-Larsen-Johansson syndrome, and patella tendinosis.

For symptoms related to patellar mal-tracking, such as patellar instability and/or chronic patellofemoral pain, a full-length, soft, knee brace that includes a lateral patellar pad or "J" pad may be helpful. In addition to this knee brace, placement of arch supports or custom orthotics into the shoe can be helpful in many of these patients, who have excessive foot pronation, as this can commonly contribute to this type of chronic knee pain [4].

The third type of support to consider is a metal, hinged knee brace. These are commonly utilized for stabilization of the knee in the setting of acute or chronic ligament injuries. A simple "off the shelf" hinged knee brace can be appropriate for medial or lateral collateral ligament injuries. Custom-made braces can also be used for a more specific fit and commonly may be used in the setting of anterior cruciate ligament (ACL) injury after surgical reconstruction. Questions on appropriate bracing can be discussed in conjunction with the patient's physical therapist and/or sports medicine specialist and can be a part of the overall rehabilitation plan for chronic knee injuries.

Another aspect that one must consider in chronic knee injuries is treating over-training and/or burnout. Relative rest, developing realistic perception of competence, and possible consultation with a mental health expert can be a part of this management [3].

Summary

Determination of the appropriate disposition is a critical part of the early management of both acute and chronic knee injuries. Their management may simply involve conservative treatment with rest and RICES protocol or may require more formal bracing and protection. Supplementary treatment may also necessitate referrals to physical therapy and/or sports medicine and orthopedic specialists. Having a general understanding of commonly occurring injuries, the structures involved, and identification of worrisome physical exam findings can significantly aid in this process.

References

1. Knight KL, Draper DO. Therapeutic modalities the art and Science, Chapter 5, immediate Care of Acute Orthopedic Injuries. Philadelphia, PA: Lippincott Williams & Wilkins; 2008. p. 54–75.
2. Zeltzer LK, Krell H. Chapter 71. Pediatric pain management. In: Kliegman RM, Stanton BF, St. Gemell JW, editors. Nelson textbook of pediatrics. 19th ed. Philadelphia, PA: Saunders Elsevier; 2011. p. 360–75.
3. DiFiori JP, Benjamin HJ, Brenner JS, et al. Overuse injuries and burnout in youth sports: a position statement from the American Medical Society for sports medicine. Br J Sports Med. 2014;48:287–8.
4. Coleman N. Sports injuries. Pediatr Rev. 2019;40:278–90.

Chapter 6
Patellar Subluxation and Dislocation

Shelley Street Callender

Introduction

The abnormality of patellar instability, which can result in patellar subluxation/dislocation, involves the anterior compartment of the knee, including the patella and its functional relationship to the femur and quadriceps, which impact the extensor mechanism of the knee. The initial insult is most commonly traumatic but can also be unknown or noncontact in nature [4, 8, 12]. While this injury can occur in athletes in a variety of sports, it is most common in those which involve significant twisting and redirection, i.e., football, basketball, gymnastics, and soccer.

Epidemiology

Patellar subluxation/dislocation is estimated to have an incidence of 11.9 to 43 per 100,000 [7, 8, 12]. The typically affected athlete is between the ages of 15 and 19 years, when this problem begins [4]; however, it can occur in younger age groups. This skeletally immature group often presents with higher rates of recurrence [4, 13]. Patellar subluxation/dislocation in the acute setting is 33% more common in females than males [4]. Both acute and recurrent patellar subluxation/dislocation can result in continued pain and discomfort from cartilage injuries and early arthrosis [8]. Patellar subluxation/dislocation is a cause of hemarthrosis and the second leading cause of knee effusion for the athlete after anterior cruciate ligament (ACL) disruption [10].

S. S. Callender (✉)
Department of Pediatrics, Navicent Health System, Mercer University School of Medicine, Macon, GA, USA
e-mail: Callender.Shelley@navicenthealth.org

© Springer Nature Switzerland AG 2021
N. Coleman (ed.), *Common Pediatric Knee Injuries*,
https://doi.org/10.1007/978-3-030-55870-3_6

Mechanism of Injury

In the acute setting, the athlete has lateral translation of the patella after contact during a contact/collision sport [1]. The same lateral translation can also occur during a noncontact event that involves an aggressive cutting and pivoting maneuver in a contact sport. In either case, the mechanism of injury typically occurs with the knee in slight flexion and the lower leg in a valgus position. One primary stabilizer of the patella is the medial patellofemoral ligament (MPFL), which is often disrupted during acute dislocations [1].

Risk factors in the history and physical examination that predispose the athlete to this problem include, but are not limited to, the following: younger age, trochlear dysplasia, patella alta, and a laterally located tibial tubercle [2]. While there can be a relationship between patellofemoral pain syndrome (PFPS) and patellar subluxation/dislocation (also considered "instability"), they are somewhat different entities. PFPS is insidious in onset and often considered an overuse syndrome, rarely needing surgical intervention. Patellar subluxation, when acute, is typically related to a specific event or injury (contact or noncontact).

On-Field Assessment

The on-field physical examination may be limited in scope by the athlete's discomfort and swelling but must include a neurovascular assessment by checking sensation and proximal and distal pulses [6]. The athlete may have an obvious deformity, with the patella being laterally displaced. In those cases, relocation with the application of gentle pressure along the lateral boarder of the patella and the gradual extension of the knee is often effective. Most often, the patella spontaneously reduces, and the athlete may report a sensation of a movement out and then back into the groove, thereby explaining a double thump or pop sensation.

In-Clinic Assessment

The in-clinic knee examination should start with inspection and include palpation, range of motion, strength testing, and special testing. The athlete may describe discomfort in the front of the knee that is sore, achy, sharp, or stabbing. There is typically no erythema but often an effusion on inspection. Increased patellar motion during patellar tracking on activation of the quadriceps may be observed, and an increase in the Q ankle (quadriceps angle) might be noted. One may find some tenderness to palpation of the patellar facets and/or tenderness surrounding the patella. With active or passive range of motion of the knee, crepitus of the patella is often present, although early after the injury this finding may be absent. One may find patellar looseness (increased patellar motion) or functional laxity of the affected limb. Patellar grind, compression of the patella on the femur with the knee in extension, can be painful, which would be a positive finding. Patellar apprehension, discomfort with passive lateral patellar motion when the knee is in extension or up to 20 degrees of flexion, is also consistent with a history of patellar subluxation/dislocation [4]. Typically, the other ligamentous structures of the knee are intact (i.e., intact valgus and varus stress testing for MCL and LCL integrity, respectively; intact anterior and posterior drawer testing for ACL and PCL integrity, respectively). On strength testing, there is generally quadriceps weakness with resisted knee extension and weakness of the hip abductors [5, 9]. For the skeletally immature athlete, the physis or apophysis should be evaluated, as they, too, when injured, can significantly impact the extensor mechanism; therefore, the exam should include palpation at the inferior patella, tibial tubercle, distal femur, and proximal tibia.

Imaging can be a necessary component of the evaluation of patellar subluxation/dislocation events. Radiographs are important, particularly in those with an acute or initial injury, and should include anterior-posterior, lateral, and merchant (i.e., sunrise) views [2, 12]. There is debate regarding the timing and need for magnetic resonance imaging (MRI). While an MRI is always indicated for evidence of an osteochondral defect on radiographs, some experts would recommend an MRI for all initial dislocations; others would wait to determine the athlete's response to conservative treatment [1, 3, 12, 14].

Management – Rehabilitation

For most with an initial event, the recommended intervention is physical therapy and rehabilitation with or without bracing. For those with repeated subluxation/dislocation or with cartilage damage, surgical interventions should be considered. Effective prevention strategies are lacking in the literature, and further studies surrounding prevention are necessary.

Nonoperative interventions that focus on physical therapy and rehabilitation are the standard treatment for most patients with a first-time patellar subluxation/dislocation [8]. Rehabilitation should focus on ensuring the core is stable and work on the functional action of the patella, as it participates in the extensor mechanism of the knee. Therapy should be progressive, because, at initiation of therapy, the athlete may have limitations in activity, due to discomfort. While some bony structural components cannot be altered, inhibition and activation of muscle structures require repetition in order to change or alter a neuromotor input. Initial intervention should focus on neuromotor input and gradually progress to muscle loading (esp. quadriceps) to improve patellar control and knee extension.

Physician re-evaluation during the initial rehabilitation stage is helpful in order to ensure that the intervention is being successful and to redirect the program, if needed. A follow-up visit offers another opportunity to assess if bracing or taping can be helpful and to determine if there is any improvement in muscle recruitment or neurological input or signaling. If there is no change at all, then consultation with a sports medicine physician or orthopedist may be helpful to assist in reconsidering the diagnosis, re-directing the rehabilitation program, and/or determining the need for advanced imaging.

For a program to be successful, the athlete must actively participate and commit to continuing the exercises between therapy sessions, in addition to incorporating like exercises into their sport preparation activities long term. Often an adolescent athlete will need therapy for a few months and continuation of a home program with incorporation of those exercises into his/her sport training. If the athlete continues to experience high levels of pain, despite adequate physical therapy, a referral to a sports medicine physician or sports surgeon is warranted to determine if consideration for additional evaluation and/or surgical intervention is warranted.

Management – Surgical

Surgical intervention is indicated and more effective in skeletally mature adolescents, who have instability of the patella and have failed appropriate conservative therapy. In the skeletally immature, surgery is often postponed until skeletal maturity has been reached. When there is an unstable osteochondral defect or chondromalacia, surgery includes repair or removal of the defect along with intervention to improve patellar stability, allowing for better outcomes [10, 11, 14]. As such, for the skeletally immature athlete with significant chondromalacia or an osteochondral defect, postponing surgery may not be possible. When surgery is indicated in this skeletally immature group, physeal-sparing procedures should be considered. One of the most common surgical interventions is the medial patellofemoral ligament (MPFL) tightening procedure [2, 10, 11, 14]. Other procedural options include tibial transfers or osteotomies, which can be helpful for patients with significant bony malalignment, and patellofemoral joint space resurfacing techniques, which can be helpful for patients with moderate to severe chondromalacia of the patella.

Outcomes

After an initial event most athletes return to full play in about 3 weeks [6]. Initially, the majority have a partial or complete response to conservative interventions; however, the risk for re-injury is approximately 17% following a first dislocation and 50% or higher subsequently [1]. This re-injury risk seems to be highest in the younger age groups and those with trochlear dysplasia, patella alta, or the presence of a laterally placed tibial tubercle. Up to 96% of those with patellar subluxation/dislocation have trochlear dysplasia [7].

Common Case Presentation

A 15-year-old girl comes in complaining of right knee pain for 1 week. She plays tuba in her marching band. At the end of her last marching band show, she landed awkwardly on her right knee, after stepping in a divot in the grass. She describes feeling a pop sensation and a giving out of her knee. She immediately had pain and discomfort but did not fall to the ground. The patient was unable to continue participation at that time and has not resumed marching band practice since the event. She comes into the office for evaluation because of continued pain and swelling. The pain has improved; the swelling started 1 day after the incident. She has been wrapping the knee with an Ace bandage.

On physical examination, there is a moderate right knee effusion. There is positive patellar apprehension pain and laxity with tenderness along the medial patellofemoral ligament (MPFL). Her passive range of motion is painful and limited to an arc of 30 to 100 degrees. Normal valgus and varus stress testing indicates adequate stability of the medial and lateral collateral ligaments, respectively. She has good endpoints with anterior drawer, posterior drawer, and Lachman's test. McMurray test is negative.

Anterior-posterior, lateral, and merchant (sunrise) radiographs are obtained. The imaging is consistent with patella alta, lateral placement of the patella (Fig. 6.1), and a knee effusion without fracture or dislocation. This imaging is consistent with patella subluxation/dislocation of the right knee. Because this is a first subluxation/dislocation, you decide to order an MRI of the right knee. The MRI results are consistent with lateral dislocation of the right patella without chondromalacia or any chondral defect in the knee.

The patient is placed in the lateral patellar tracking brace and started in physical rehabilitation for neuromuscular training, quadriceps strengthening, and pain

Fig. 6.1 Lateral tracking of patella on merchant (sunrise) X-ray view

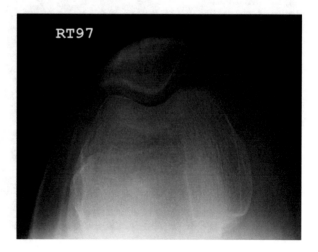

management. In addition, she was started on nonsteroidal anti-inflammatory medications. After 4 weeks of physical therapy, she was able to resume marching band activities.

Uncommon Case Presentation

A 17-year-old boy comes in complaining of right knee pain. He reports a sudden onset of right knee pain after trying to get out of bed. He denies any trauma or a fall. He reports not being able to walk well, since the pain began. He has always been active but stopped playing soccer a few years ago, because of the feeling that his right knee was always going to give out. During his grade school years, when he played soccer, he recalls intermittent swelling in the front of his knee with an associated popping sensation.

On physical examination, there is no knee effusion. He has full active and passive range of motion of the right knee. There is an increase in Q angle, apparent patella alta, and patella laxity with positive patellar apprehension and patellar grind tests. He has intact valgus and varus stress testing, anterior and posterior drawer testing, and a stable endpoint with Lachman's test.

Anterior-posterior, lateral, and merchant (sunrise) radiographs are obtained. The imaging, consistent with patellar subluxation/dislocation, demonstrates the following findings: patella alta, lateral placement of the patella in the femoral trochlear groove, and a possible chondral defect. Because of the radiographic findings, an MRI is obtained. The MRI shows a loose chondral fragment, likely from the patella, trochlear dysplasia, patella alta, and a small effusion (Fig. 6.2).

Fig. 6.2 White area demonstrates a patellar effusion on MRI

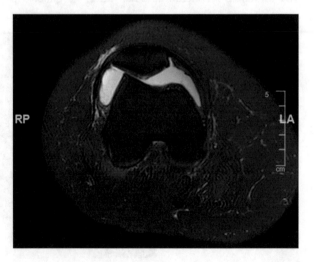

This patient was referred to Orthopedic Surgery for surgical intervention. Before and after surgical correction, the patient is placed in a lateral patellar tracking brace. After surgery, he is started in physical rehabilitation for neuromuscular training, quadriceps strengthening, and pain management. After 8 weeks of physical therapy, he was able to resume regular activities without pain or that almost giving out feeling and is also considering a return to soccer.

Summary

Patellar subluxation/dislocation often has an acute onset with a high incidence of recurrence. Initial injuries without bony defects should start with physical therapy and rehabilitation. These athletes need to incorporate quadriceps strengthening exercises into a routine. Surgical interventions are reserved for those with recurrent dislocations or with bony destruction amendable to repair. The skeletally mature are better candidates for surgical intervention; however, in cases where bony destruction is present in the skeletally immature, surgery, particularly physeal-sparing procedures, should be highly considered. Currently, prevention revolves around maintaining a stable core, ensuring quadriceps strength, and bracing or taping the patella laterally. More studies are needed to establish effective means of prevention (Table 6.1).

Table 6.1 Condition Table

Condition	Patellar dislocation
Description	Instability of patella (subluxation or dislocation)
Epidemiology	Slight female predominance
Mechanism (common)	Traumatic - patella forced laterally
History and exam findings	Athlete felt pain after fall Immediate swelling and instability – not able to return to play Swelling limited flexion on exam Pain with translation of patella
Management	Acute symptoms management Timely rehabilitation Consideration for surgical intervention after multiple occurrences Rehabilitation and quadriceps strengthening are key

References

1. Bessette M, Saluan P. Patellofemoral pain and instability in adolescent athletes. Sports Med Arthrosc Rev. 2016;24(4):144–9.
2. Clark D, Metcalfe A, Wogan C, Mandalia V, Eldridge J. Adolescent patellar instability. Bone Joint J. 2017;99-B(2):159–70.
3. Cline S. Acute injuries of the knee. In: Patel DR, editor. Pediatric practice: sports medicine. China: The McGraw Hill Education; 2009. p. 313–30.
4. DeFroda S, Gil J, Boulos A, Cruz A. Diagnosis and management of traumatic patellar instability in the pediatric patient. Orthopedics. 2017;40(5):e749–57.
5. Gregory AJM. Plica syndrome. [online] UpToDate. 2019. Available at: https://www.uptodate.com/contents/plica-syndrome. Accessed 17 July 2019.
6. Hergenroeder A. Approach to acute knee pain and injury in children and skeletally immature adolescents. [online] UpToDate. 2019. Available at: https://www.uptodate.com/approach-to-acute-knee-pain-and-injury-in-children-and-skeletally-immature-adolescents. Accessed 17 July 2019
7. Keyes S, Price M, Green D, Parikh S. Special considerations for pediatric patellar instability. Am J Orthop. 2018;47(3).
8. Liu JN, Steinhaus ME, Kalbian IL, Post WR, Green DW, Strickland SM, Shubin Stein BE. Patellar instability management: a survey of the international patellofemoral study group. Am J Sports Med. 2017;46(13):3299–306.
9. Patel DR, Lyne D. Overuse injuries of the knee. In: Patel DR, editor. Pediatric practice: sports medicine. China: The McGraw Hill Education; 2009. p. 330–42.
10. Pedowitz J, Edmonds E, Chambers H, Dennis M, Bastrom T, Pennock A. Recurrence of patellar instability in adolescents undergoing surgery for Osteochondral defects without concomitant ligament reconstruction. Am J Sports Med. 2018;47(1):66–70.
11. Redler L, Spang R, Tepolt F, Davis E, Kocher M. Combined reconstruction of the medial patellofemoral ligament (MPFL) and medial quadriceps tendon - femoral ligament (MQTFL) for patellar instability in children and adolescents: surgical technique and outcomes. Orthop J Sports Med. 2017;5(7_suppl6):232.
12. Ries Z, Bollier M. Patellofemoral instability in active adolescents. J Knee Surg. 2015;28(04):265–78.
13. Seitlinger G, Ladenhauf H, Wierer G. What is the chance that a patella dislocation will happen a second time. Curr Opin Pediatr. 2018;30(1):65–70.
14. Smith TO, Donell S, Song F, Hing CB. Surgical versus non-surgical interventions for treating patellar dislocation. Cochrane Database Syst Rev. 2015.

Chapter 7
Patellar Contusion

Clinton J. Ulmer and Nathaniel S. Nye

Anatomy and Normal Function

The patella is a large sesamoid bone within the quadriceps tendon, which continues distally as the patellar tendon. The quadriceps muscle engages the patella into the trochlear groove upon activation, producing extension at the knee. There are very high contact forces between the patellar cartilage and trochlear cartilage during weight bearing and loading. Proper function of the knee extensor mechanism depends upon stability and control proximally in the hip girdle and lumbopelvic core, as well as distally in the ankle and foot core musculature. The patella is important in that it provides somewhat of a fulcrum during knee extension, providing increased mechanical advantage by lifting the contractile force vector away from the hinge point of the knee.

Pathology and Dysfunction

Patellar contusions are very common among the pediatric population. The injury is frequently caused by direct blunt-force trauma during casual play, organized sports, and motor vehicle accidents. Despite the high incidence of patellar contusions, severe complications, such as a patella fracture, are rare [1, 2].

The terms "bone bruise" and "bone contusion" are generally used interchangeably in the literature. They represent a spectrum of radiographically occult bone

C. J. Ulmer
University of Texas Health Science Center at San Antonio, San Antonio, TX, USA

N. S. Nye (✉)
Sports Medicine Clinic, Fort Belvoir Community Hospital, Ft. Belvoir, VA, USA
e-mail: Nathaniel.s.nye.mil@mail.mil

© Springer Nature Switzerland AG 2021
N. Coleman (ed.), *Common Pediatric Knee Injuries*,
https://doi.org/10.1007/978-3-030-55870-3_7

injuries that are best diagnosed with increased signal intensity on T2-weighted magnetic resonance imaging (MRI), which often corresponds with decreased signal on T1-weighted images [3]. Histologic studies demonstrate that relatively minor trauma may cause marrow edema with preserved cancellous bone, while increasing severity of trauma produces trabecular bone microfractures and associated intramedullary hemorrhage [3, 4]. In 1988, Wilson et al. introduced the term *bone marrow edema* to describe this finding [5]. Specific marrow edema patterns are seen with different types of injury and are often described as a footprint left behind from the injury. Direct impact traumatic contusions typically produce uniform edema throughout the patella. The classic bone contusion pattern of lateral patellar dislocation includes marrow edema of the lateral femoral condyle and the inferomedial aspect of the patella [6, 7]. The presentation, diagnosis, and management of patellar subluxation and dislocation are detailed in Chap. 6.

The dysfunction that a young patient will have secondary to contusion or subluxation is primarily due to the soft-tissue injury, with the severity of bone bruising itself showing no consistent association with pain severity or level of function after injury [8]. In the absence of other complications, the dysfunction accompanying a patellar bruise is secondary to pain. The overwhelming majority of patients will return to play at their previous level once recovered from a patellar contusion.

Specific Pointers

While the diagnosis and management of a patellar contusion is generally straightforward, there are a few situations that require specific care. These include patellar subluxation and symptomatic bipartite patella.

The patella is the largest sesamoid bone in the body, forming from one to three ossification centers [9, 10]. Approximately 2% to 6% do not fuse mutually, resulting in a multipartite patella [11]. Of these multipartite patella, 50% are bilateral and are in a male to female ratio of 9:1 [12, 13]. Figure 7.1 illustrates the Saupe

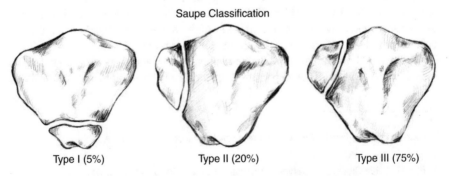

Saupe Classification

Type I (5%)   Type II (20%)   Type III (75%)

Fig. 7.1 The Saupe classification of bipartite patella with respective percentage of presentation in individuals with bipartite patella. Type I – inferior pole (5%), Type II – lateral margin (20%), Type III – superolateral margin (75%)

classification and relative frequency of different types of bipartite patella [14]. Among bipartite patella, approximately 2% become symptomatic [15]. The most common presentation is anterior knee pain in a male athlete under the age of 20, who sustained direct impact to the knee [15–17], though it may become symptomatic with overuse, as well. The pain is typically aggravated by knee extension or direct pressure. Patients will also endorse pain with sudden bending of the knee or crouching [18]. While this injury is painful, it should be noted that traumatic separation of a bipartite patella is exceedingly rare [9].

Differentiating between a bipartite patella and patellar fracture can be difficult in the clinical setting [19]. In the majority of bipartite cases, anterior-posterior plain radiographs will show a separated, well-corticated ossicle, often at the superolateral aspect of the patella [20, 21]. As in most cases, the patient's history can also assist in diagnosis. Overuse and gradual pain development are more likely in a symptomatic bipartite patella. Along with knowledge of the typical location and epidemiology of bipartite patella, skyline views, bone scintigraphy, and MRI can assist in diagnosis [13, 22, 23]. The presence of bone marrow edema is significant for pathology associated with bipartite patella. MRI studies have demonstrated bone marrow edema in connection with painful bipartite patella, while patients with asymptomatic bipartite patella [13, 21] did not have marrow edema.

Clinically (without advanced imaging), it may be difficult to determine whether a contusive blow has caused injury to the superficial soft tissues only or whether the patella itself has been contused. The distinction is often purely academic; advanced imaging is generally not necessary to distinguish between these two injury patterns, as both are treated conservatively, based on symptoms.

Epidemiology

While the true incidence of patellar contusions is difficult to measure, several epidemiological studies offer insight into the frequency, age groups, gender, and common activities that are related to patellar contusions. Gage et al. reported on emergency department (ED) visits, due to knee in injuries in the United States between 1998 and 2008 [24]. They estimated 666,432 knee injuries were evaluated at emergency departments per year, with patients under age 25 representing 46.1% of these injuries. Among the pediatric population (age less than 18), 29.1% of knee injuries seen at an ED were classified as knee contusions. It should be noted that all knee contusions were grouped into a single category; therefore, the exact number of specific patellar contusions is unknown [24]. Females sustained a higher rate of contusions than males (31.8% vs 22.8%) [24].

Moustaki et al. evaluated the common activities that are related to knee injury in a pediatric population. Of 2167 children injured in non-motor vehicle collisions (i.e., all-cause knee injury but excluding motor vehicle collisions), 43.5% were diagnosed with knee contusion (patella vs. other bone involvement not specified). The authors found that minor knee injuries, such as contusions, were more common among female patients, and often were the result of a fall or direct impact, while playing at home or on a playground, particularly in the summer months [25]. Children who participate in sport have a greater risk of knee injury [25, 26].

These two studies highlight the defining epidemiologic characteristics of general knee contusions in the pediatric population. Knee contusions are very common injuries that are more common in females than males and in children than adults [24, 25, 27, 28]. Patellar contusion is often associated with typical children play activities at home and at school. Children who participate in sport have a greater likelihood of injuring their knee [25, 26].

Diagnosis: History and Examination Findings, Testing

The common presenting history with patellar contusions, like most bone contusions, is trauma with direct impact of the patella. As described above, minor falls during play or athletics are common culprits [25]. Although the inciting event may be obvious, a focused history should include previous history of knee injury, history of bipartite patella, and other symptoms that would suggest a ligamentous injury or patellar subluxation/dislocation. Ability to bear weight on the injured limb immediately after the injury should be ascertained, and, if swelling is reported, the location, timing, and extent of swelling are also important. Understanding the patient's baseline functional status and activities is also helpful.

A complete knee exam, including comparison to the contralateral knee, should be performed and documented. In isolated patellar contusion, the most likely findings are erythema, mild prepatellar swelling (generally without intraarticular effusion), and tenderness to palpation over the patella. The patient will usually have full range of motion but may have pain on full flexion of the knee. To our knowledge, there is no existing published literature on the sensitivity and specificity of these findings for patellar contusion.

It is important to distinguish between a patellar fracture and contusion at presentation. Standard radiographs of the knee (antero-posterior, lateral, and sunrise views) are used to investigate a potential fracture [29]. A key clinical question is whether to order plain films. Two well-known clinical decision rules, the Pittsburgh Decision Rule (PDR) and the Ottawa Knee Rule (OKR), have been developed and validated for the selective use of radiographs in evaluation of acute knee trauma [29–31, 32].

The PDR and OKR were developed in 1994 and 1995, respectively, and have slightly different decision-making criteria within their respective diagnostic protocols (See Tables 7.1 and 7.2). Early, individual studies of PDR and OKR showed sensitivities in the 99–100% range, and many groups subsequently began to study and validate these rules in different populations. A systematic review of the OKR in 2004 showed pooled sensitivity and specificity of 98.5% and 48.6%, respectively, in the general adult population [33]. In 2013, Cheung et al. completed a cross-sectional validation study comparing the two decision rules in a U.S. urban teaching

Table 7.1 Ottawa knee rule

Patients with knee trauma should receive knee radiographs if meeting one or more of the following criteria:
Age 55 or older
Tenderness at head of fibula
Isolated tenderness of the patella
Inability to flex knee to 90 degrees
Inability to walk four weight-bearing steps immediately after the injury and in the emergency department

Table 7.2 Pittsburgh decision rule

Patients with knee trauma should receive knee radiographs if mechanism of injury was blunt trauma or a fall, AND meeting at least one of the following criteria:
Age younger than 12 years or older than 50 years
Inability to walk four weight-bearing steps in the emergency department

hospital in patients over the age of 18. Both the PDR and OKR were found to have a sensitivity of 0.86, but specificity of PDR was higher (0.51 versus 0.27) [34]. A separate retrospective study showed that using the PDR would have resulted in 30% fewer knee films being obtained without missing a single fracture, whereas 25% fewer would have been obtained if the OKR was used [35].

Of note, only the OKR has been specifically validated in children. A 2009 systematic review and meta-analysis of the OKR in children (with only 4 applicable studies included, representing 1130 children) found 99% sensitivity and 46% specificity, with reduction of radiograph ordering between 30–40%. The authors concluded that evidence was sufficient to recommend use of OKR in children over age 5, but evidence was insufficient for children under age 5 [36]. The PDR recommends plain films for all knee trauma patients under the age of 12 whose mechanism of injury was blunt trauma or a fall [29–31]. The relative strengths and respective inclusion criteria should be considered during clinical application.

Management

Uncomplicated patellar contusion requires straightforward conservative management. The patient should undergo activity modification as guided by pain. As commonly accepted for many acute injuries, ice, compression, and elevation may also be used. When pain is not controlled sufficiently with the above measures, consider adding acetaminophen or non-steroidal anti-inflammatory medications as needed. Pediatric patients and their families should expect a complete return to normal play within 1–3 weeks as symptoms resolve. There is currently no research to suggest a specific treatment algorithm or return to play timeline. This is most likely due to the benign prognosis of this injury. Treatment may become more complex, when the patellar contusion is complicated, such as with bipartite patella or prepatellar bursitis.

There are 12 named bursae about the knee, of which the prepatellar bursa is most commonly injured with a patellar contusion [37, 38]. As the name suggests, the prepatellar bursa is located between the patella and the overlying subcutaneous tissue. The recommended initial management of superficial bursitis, secondary to trauma, begins with the same conservative treatment approach taken for a patellar contusion [39], except that compression is prioritized as an important component of treatment. Typically, an elastic bandage is utilized for compression, but neoprene knee sleeves, athletic taping, and other methods may be utilized. If there is concern for possible septic bursitis, a diagnostic aspiration should be performed [39, 40]. Aspiration can also be considered for symptomatic relief; however, the literature suggesting this treatment approach was performed in adults [39–41].

As discussed previously, a bipartite patella can become symptomatic, secondary to trauma. A systematic review from 2016 found that the majority of symptomatic bipartite patella were treated conservatively [22]. Conservative treatment typically involves activity modification, anti-inflammatory medications, stretching exercises of the quadriceps, and the use of dynamic patellar bracing [9, 42]. In cases of severe pain, immobilization of the knee with a brace in 30 degrees of flexion for 2–3 weeks may provide improved pain relief [9, 18, 43]. In the majority of literature discussing this issue, a minimum trial of 3 months of conservative management is advised prior to considering surgical intervention [9, 22].

Demonstration Cases

Case 1 (Common Presentation)

Presentation: A 9-year-old female presented to the clinic with her father. She complained of right knee pain after falling, while skateboarding, the day before. While skateboarding, the patient was wearing a helmet but no knee or elbow pads. She was able to ambulate directly after the injury but reports increased pain over the anterior knee since the fall. She denies any previous history of trauma. Her father is worried she might have broken a bone. Physical exam reveals a slightly antalgic gait, but she is able to bear full weight with walking. Her right knee is swollen over the patella with a few light abrasions. She is diffusely tender over the patella but non-tender along the fibular head, tibial plateau, and femoral condyles. There is no palpable intraarticular effusion. She is able to perform a full double-leg squat without difficulty but reports anterior knee pain with full knee flexion. Her knees are stable to varus, valgus, anterior drawer, and posterior drawer stress. Lachman and McMurray tests are normal.

Clinical Course: Noting blunt force trauma in a patient under age 12, x-rays were ordered based on the Pittsburgh Decision Rule. Standard AP, lateral, and sunrise films showed mild soft tissue swelling overlying the patella but no sign of osseous abnormality or fracture. The patient and her father were instructed on conservative management, including activity modification, pain control with ice, compression, elevation, and occasional NSAIDs as needed. The benefit of safety gear, such as elbow and knee pads, was also discussed. They were told to follow-up in 1–2 weeks if the pain persists.

Case 2 (Uncommon Presentation)

Presentation: A 17-year-old male was playing soccer, when he experienced a direct knee-to-knee impact with a player from the opposing team. He fell to the ground, and athletic trainers responded, helping him to the sideline for evaluation. He was unable to bear weight on his left knee immediately after the injury or in the athletic training room 2 hours later. He was exquisitely tender to palpation over the patella, and moderate diffuse edema of the anterior knee was noted. Range of motion was limited, with a 5-degree extension lag, and he could not flex beyond 90 degrees, due to pain. He was able to flex actively and extend the knee without assistance and was able to lift his leg off the table from a supine position, while keeping his knee mostly straight. No obvious knee effusion was noted, and Lachman and McMurray tests were indeterminate (limited due to pain). The team physician instructed him on non-weight-bearing, gave crutches, and sent him for X-rays. The next day, upon follow up with the team physician and athletic trainer, he continued to show moderate swelling and bogginess over the patella. X-rays showed prominent prepatellar soft tissue edema but no sign of fracture or dislocation. Bedside ultrasound confirmed a diagnosis of prepatellar bursitis, and ice/compression/elevation were prescribed.

Clinical course: After 1 week of conservative management, he was able to wean off crutches but the swelling did not improve. Ultrasound-guided prepatellar bursa aspiration was performed and compression/ice were continued. The swelling thereafter recurred, and aspiration was repeated 1 week later. Upon follow up 3 weeks after injury, he reported continued anterior knee pain with little improvement. Range of motion and strength were somewhat improved, but he was still unable to flex past 110 degrees, due to pain and tightness. There were no clinical signs of septic prepatellar bursitis. An MRI was ordered and showed prominent marrow edema throughout the entire patella with no fracture line. There was evidence of mild residual prepatellar bursitis, and all knee ligaments and cartilage were intact. The patient improved slowly over the ensuing 4 weeks, while doing low-impact rehabilitation daily with the athletic training staff. He was cleared for full return to sport 6 weeks after the initial injury.

Pearls and Pitfalls
- Patellar contusion is typically a self-limiting injury with a full return to play after conservative management.
- A thorough history and physical exam should be performed to evaluate potential patellar subluxation and/or ligamentous injury.
- The Ottawa Knee Rule or Pittsburgh Decision Rule may be used to aid in the decision regarding plain films of the knee. The OKR has been validated in children age 5 and older but not in children under age 5. The PDR has not been specifically validated in children of any age.
- Although uncommon, a symptomatic bipartite patella should be considered in the differential and evaluated appropriately.
- Acute non-septic prepatellar bursitis may develop, secondary to trauma, and is initially managed with rest, ice, compression, and elevation. Aspiration of bursal fluid should be considered for persistent or recurrent effusion.

Chapter Summary

Patellar contusions are common among the pediatric population. Contusions are most frequently caused by direct trauma; however, patellar subluxation also produces a characteristic patellar marrow edema pattern. The hyperemia and increased edema in the subchondral bone can often be visualized on T2-weighted MRI. Patellar contusion is occasionally complicated by prepatellar bursitis and patella fracture. Due to abnormal fusion of the secondary ossification centers, a bipartite or tripartite patella can form in the pediatric population. Although this abnormality is typically asymptomatic, a bipartite patella can become painful after direct trauma. Care should also be taken in the clinical setting to distinguish a bipartite patella from an acute fracture. Patients with a symptomatic bipartite patella should undergo conservative management. If symptoms persist after 3 months, surgical intervention should be considered. Although complications can arise, patellar contusions are typically a self-limiting injury that resolve with appropriate conservative care. Patient education, activity modification, and pain management are cornerstones of treatment. The overwhelming majority of patients will return to play at their previous level once recovered from a patellar contusion (Table 7.3).

Table 7.3   Condition table. Chapter review

Condition	Patellar contusion
Description	Edema and/or intraosseous hemorrhage within the patella caused by direct trauma
Epidemiology	Very common. Out of >660,000 knee injuries seen in emergency departments annually in the United States, 29% are knee contusions. A high proportion of knee contusions are patellar contusions.
Mechanism (common)	Direct blunt-force trauma, usually during play at school/home, during sports, or motor vehicle accidents
History and exam findings	Anterior knee pain with acute onset following trauma, often with swelling. Knee range of motion is usually intact but may be limited by pain. Intact extensor mechanism on exam is helpful for ruling out most patellar fractures.
Management	Uncomplicated patellar contusions heal with conservative care (rest, ice, compression, elevation) until symptoms resolve, followed by gradual return to exercise and full activity. When complications are present, such as symptomatic bipartite patella, patella fracture, patella dislocation, or prepatellar bursitis, specific treatment is required as noted above.

Disclosure   The opinions expressed herein are those of the authors, and do not represent official policy of the US Air Force or the Department of Defense.

References

1. Gettys F, Morgan R, Fleischli J. Superior pole sleeve fracture of the Patella: a case report and review of the literature. Am J Sports Med. 2010;38(11):2331–6.
2. Schmal H, Strohm P, Niemeyer P, Reising K, Kuminack K, Sudkam N. Fractures of the patella in children and adolescents. Acta Orthop Belg. 2010;76(5):644–50.
3. Mandalia V, Fogg A, Chari R, Murray J, Beale A, Henson J. Bone bruising of the knee. Clin Radiol. 2005;60(6):627–36.
4. Rangger C, Kathrein A, Freund M, Klestil T, Kreczy A. Bone bruise of the knee: histology and cryosections in 5 cases. Acta Orthop Scand. 1998;69(3):291–4.
5. Wilson A, Murphy W, Hardy D, Totty W. Transient osteoporosis: transient bone marrow edema? Radiology. 1988;167(3):663–7.
6. Sanders T, Medynski M, Feller J, Lawhorn K. Bone contusion patterns of the knee at MR imaging: footprint of the mechanism of injury. Radiographics. 2000;20(Special Issue):S135–51.
7. Zaidi A, Babyn P, Astori I, White L, Doria A, Cole W. MRI of traumatic patellar dislocation in children. Pediatr Radiol. 2006;36(11):1163–70.
8. Gomez J, Molina D, Rettig S, Kan J. Bone bruises in children and adolescents not associated with ligament ruptures. Orthop J Sports Med. 2018;6(7).
9. Gaheer R, Kapoor S, Rysavy M. Contemporary management of symptomatic bipartite patella. Orthopedics. 2009;32(11):843–9.

10. Canizares G, Selesnick F. Bipartite patella fracture. Arthroscopy. 2003;19(2):215–7.
11. Carter S. Traumatic Separation of a bipartite Patella. Injury. 1989;20(4):244.
12. Thomas A, Wilson R, Thompson T. Quadriceps avulsion through a bipartite patella. Orthopedics. 2007;30(6):491–2.
13. Kavanagh E, Zoga A, Omar I, Ford S, Schweitzer M, Eustace S. MRI findings in bipartite patella. Skelet Radiol. 2007;36(3):209–14.
14. Saupe H. Primäre Krochenmark serelung der kniescheibe. Deustsche Z Chir. 1943;258:386–92.
15. Weaver J. Bipartite patella as a cause of disability in the athlete. Am J Sports Med. 1977;5(4):137–43.
16. Halpem A, Hewitt O. Painful medial bipartite patella: A case report. Clin Orthop Relat Res. 1978;(134):180–1.
17. Iossifidis A, Brueton R. Painful bipartite patella following injury. Injury. 1995;26(3):175–6.
18. Okuno H, Sugita T, Kawamata T, Ohnuma M, Yamad N, Yoshizumi Y. Traumatic separation of a type 1 bipartite patella: a report of four knees. Clin Orthop Relat Res. 2004;420:257–60.
19. Echeverria T, Bersani F. Acute fracture simulating a symptomatic bipartite patella. Am J Sports Med. 1980;8(1):48–50.
20. Ma J, Shi F, Huang C, Gu S. Forensic identification of bipartite patella misdiagnosed as patella fracture. J Forensic Sci. 2017;62(4):1089–91.
21. O'Brien J, Murphy C, Halpenny C, McNeill G. WC. T. Magnetic resonance imaging features of asymptomatic bipartite patella. Eur J Radiol. 2011;78(3):425–9.
22. McMahon S, LeRoux J, Smith T, Hing C. The management of the painful bipartite patella: a systematic review. Knee Surg Sports Traumatol Arhtrosc. 2015;24(9):2798–805.
23. Collings C. Scintigraphic findings on examination of the multipartite patella. Clin Nucl Med. 1994;19(10):865–6.
24. Gage B, McIlvain N, Collins C, Fields S, Comstock R. Epidemiology of 6.6 million knee injuries presenting to United States emergency departments from 1999t Through 2008. Acad Emerg Med. 2012;19(4):1553–2712.
25. Moustaki M, Pitsos N, Dalamaga M, Dessypris N, Petridou E. Home and leisure activities and childhood knee injuries. Injury. 2005;36(5):644–50.
26. Majewski M, Susanne H, Klaus S. Epidemiology of athletic knee injuries: a 10-year study. Knee. 2006;13(3):184–8.
27. Simon T, Bublitz CHS. Emergency department visits among pediatric patients for sports-related injury: basic epidemiology and impact of race/ethnicity and insurance status. Pediatr Emerg Care. 2006;22(5):309–15.
28. Louw Q, Manilall J, Grimmer K. Epidemiology of knee injuries among adolescents: a systematic review. Br J Sports Med. 2008;42(1):2–10.
29. Weber J, Jackson R, Peacock W, Swor R, Carley R, Larkin G. Clinical decision rules discriminate between fractures and nonfractures in acute isolated knee trauma. Ann Emerg Med. 1995;26(4):429–33.
30. Stiell I, Greenburg G, Wells G, McKnight R, Cwinn A, Cacciotti T, et al. Derivation of a decision rule for the use of radiography in acute knee injures. Ann Emerg Med. 1995;26(4):405–13.
31. Seaberg D, Jackson R. Clinical decision rule for knee radiographs. Am J Emerg Med. 1994;12(5):541–3.
32. Tandeter H, Shvartzman P. Acute knee injuries: use of decision rules for selective radiograph ordering. Am Fam Physician. 1999;60(9):2599–608.
33. Bachmann LM, Haberzeth S, Steurer J, ter Riet G. The accuracy of the Ottawa knee rule to rule out knee fractures: a systematic review. Ann Intern Med. 2004;140(2):121–4.
34. Cheung T, Tank Y, Breederveld R, Tuinebreijer W, de Lange-de Klerk E, Derksen R. Diagnostic accuracy and reproducibility of the Ottawa knee rule vs the Pittsburgh decision rule. Am J Emerg Med 2013; 31(4): p. 641–645.
35. Konan S, Zang T, Tamimi N, Haddad F. Can the Ottawa and Pittsburgh rules reduce requests for radiography in patients referred to acute knee clinics? Ann R Coll Surg Engl. 2013;95(3):188–91.

36. Vijayasankar D, Boyle AA, Atkinson P. Can the Ottawa knee rule be applied to children? A systematic review and meta-analysis of observational studies. Emerg Med J. 2009;26(4):250–3.
37. Chatra P. Bursae around the knee joints. Indian J Radiol Imaging. 2012;22:27–30.
38. Samin M, Smitaman E, Lawrence D, Moukaddam H. MRI of anterior knee pain. Skeltal Radiol. 2014;43:875–93.
39. Khodaee M. Common superficial bursitis. Am Fam Physician. 2017;95(4):224–31.
40. Sebastian F, Baumbach S, Lobo C, Badyine I, Mutschler W, Kanz K. Prepatellar and olecranon bursitis: literature review and development of a treatment algorithm. Arch Orthop Trauma Surg. 2014;134(3):359–70.
41. McAfee J, Smith D. Olecranon and prepatellar bursitis. Diagnosis and treatment. West J Med. 1988;149(5):607–10.
42. Palumbo P. Dynamic patellar brace: a new orthosis in the management of patellofemoral disorders. Am J Sports Med. 1981;9(1):45–9.
43. Stocker R, van Laer L. Injury of a bipartite patella in a young upcoming sportsman. Arch Orthop Trauma Surg. 2011;131(1):75–8.

Chapter 8
Sinding-Larsen-Johansson Syndrome

Anastasia N. Fischer

Anatomy and Normal Function

The apophysis at the inferior pole of the patella is a growth center that serves as an attachment site for the patellar tendon and is often referred to as a secondary growth center [1]. It opens at approximately age 10 and closes by approximately age 14 in boys and girls [2, 3]. Located at the origin of the patellar tendon, the apophysis serves as a connection point for the patellar tendon to the tibial tubercle, providing continuity for the quadriceps muscle from the hips to the tibia.

Pathology and Dysfunction

Commonly stressed during phases of rapid growth, when the growth cartilage is weak relative to the tendon, this apophysis can become inflamed, secondary to a relative overuse injury, a condition called Sinding-Larsen-Johansson Syndrome (SLJ) [1, 4]. The usual state of inflexibility at this age can contribute to traction at the apophysis and, ultimately, a local inflammatory response. Advanced cases lead to microavulsions at the proximal attachment of the patellar tendon and de novo calcification and ossification at this junction [4]. These injuries can be considered stress fractures of the apophyseal physis, analogous to a nondisplaced Salter-Harris I injury [1].

A. N. Fischer (✉)
Division of Sports Medicine, Nationwide Children's Hospital, Dublin, OH, USA

Department of Pediatrics, The Ohio State University College of Medicine, Columbus, OH, USA
e-mail: Anastasia.Fischer@NationwideChildrens.org

© Springer Nature Switzerland AG 2021
N. Coleman (ed.), *Common Pediatric Knee Injuries*,
https://doi.org/10.1007/978-3-030-55870-3_8

Epidemiology

Commonly seen in both boys and girls from approximately ages 10–14, SLJ can be seen more often in active children who engage in quadriceps-heavy activities (running, jumping, landing) [3, 4], is a commonly reported injury amongst middle-school athletes [5], and may be more likely to occur during practice than during competition [5]. SLJ is also more likely to be diagnosed in adolescent athletes specializing in a single sport than in those participating in multiple sports [6] and may be noted at an earlier age in boys than in girls [7].

Mechanism of Injury

Children may experience SLJ as a consequence of regular physical activity, excessive physical activity, or an acute hit to the inferior pole of the patella [3].

Diagnosis

History

Most children will complain of an insidious onset of pain over the past few weeks or months, worsened by physical activity, particularly jumps and sudden stops [4].

Exam

Localized swelling at the inferior pole of the patella may be present, but the injury should not be associated with a knee effusion. The inferior pole of the patella will be point tender, but tenderness may extend into the proximal patellar tendon. Range of motion may be full or limited in flexion, due to pain with increased traction of the patellar tendon at the site of injury. Strength may be full or compromised, secondary to pain, but the patient must be able to activate the extensor mechanism of their leg, helping to rule out a patellar sleeve fracture. Pain is commonly reproduced with jumping in the exam room.

Testing

The presence of ossicles at the inferior pole of the patella on lateral knee radiograph is not enough to make the diagnosis of SLJ and soft-tissue swelling at this site should be noted (Fig. 8.1) [1]. This swelling may extend into the proximal patellar

Fig. 8.1 Lateral radiograph showing SLJ

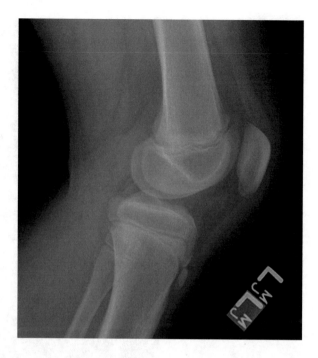

tendon, with calcification/ossification seen in severe cases [4]. Ultrasound evaluation may exhibit cartilage swelling, patellar tendon swelling at its proximal insertion, and patellar fragmentation at the distal pole [2]. Further advanced imaging should not be necessary to make the diagnosis but can be considered if ruling out other pathologies, such as a patellar sleeve fracture.

Management

Relative rest of the knee to encourage a pain-free state is encouraged, as further participation will likely increase pain or prevent resolution. Participation in athletic activities should be encouraged once range of motion is full; strength is equal bilaterally; and the patient can land from jumps and run with minimal pain. A patellar tendon counterforce strap may provide symptomatic relief and can be worn as desired (Fig. 8.2). Stretching of the quadriceps, hamstrings, and calves can also help decrease tension at the apophysis and should be encouraged independently or under supervision with a rehab specialist [3]. Recalcitrant cases should undergo a biomechanics evaluation to ascertain if the knee is twisting or undergoing a valgus moment (tibia deviating away from the midline) that may be preventing full recovery and address neuromuscular deficits [6]. Local injection of corticosteroid into or around the patellar tendon is contraindicated, due to risk of subcutaneous atrophy or tendon injury [4].

Fig. 8.2 Patellar
counterforce straps on an
11-year-old male

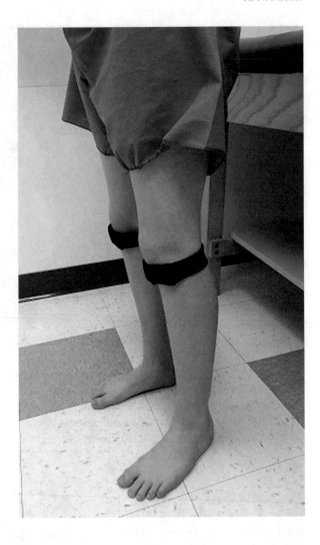

Demonstration Cases

Common Presentation

A 12-year-old boy presents to the office with anterior knee pain that is worsened with physical activity. He can walk with a normal gait and points to the inferior pole of the patella as the site of pain. Exam reveals mild swelling at the inferior pole of the patella, full range of motion with some pain at end range passive flexion and pain reproduced with jumping in the exam room. There is no evidence of internal derangement of the knee (no knee effusion, unstable ligaments, negative meniscal testing). Radiographs reveal an open apophysis at the inferior pole of the patella with surrounding soft tissue swelling. He is prescribed a patellar tendon strap, stretches for knee flexion and extension, and relative rest until his pain improves.

Uncommon Presentation

A 12-year-old boy presents to the office with a report of pain with physical activity, points to the inferior pole of the patella, has radiographs with an open apophysis, but has a normal physical exam of the knee and hip without tenderness at the inferior pole of the patella. This child may have a mild case of SLJ and should be encouraged to warm-up adequately before physical activity and may be given a stretching program and patellar tendon strap. He should be instructed to follow-up if the pain worsens.

Pearls and Pitfalls
- Consider SLJ as a diagnosis when an ambulating, early adolescent patient presents with a history of insidious onset of knee pain at the inferior patella, especially if pain is worsened with physical activity.
- SLJ should be distinguished from a patellar sleeve avulsion fracture, a cartilaginous injury at the inferior pole of the patella associated with an acute injury that removes a child from participation. Common findings of patellar sleeve fractures include a knee effusion, loss of the extensor mechanism of the knee, and a high degree of pain. X-ray may reveal a patella alta deformity and a fragment at the inferior pole of the patella. MRI can help distinguish between the two conditions, if not immediately apparent [8].

Chapter Summary

SLJ is a common cause of insidious onset of knee pain in early adolescent active children. It is an apophysitis affecting the growth center at the inferior pole of the patella with surrounding soft tissue swelling commonly extending into the proximal patellar tendon. Diagnosis is made by tenderness at the site on physical exam and an open apophysis on radiograph with associated swelling. Treatment consists of ensuring pain relief, commonly with relative rest and assisted by a patellar tendon strap; improving flexibility of the surrounding musculature; and ensuring good biomechanical alignment at the knee.

Suggested Websites

https://www.nationwidechildrens.org/specialties/sports-medicine/sports-medicine-articles/why-does-my-knee-hurt-article

Review Table

Sinding-Larsen-Johansson Syndrome	
Description	An apophysitis of the inferior pole of the patella
Epidemiology	Common in children ages 10–14 who are physically active
Mechanism (common)	An overuse injury associated with running and jumping, but occasionally due to blunt trauma
History and exam findings	Insidious onset of pain at the inferior pole of the patella, worse with physical activity, tender to the touch and sometimes with associated swelling
Management	A counterforce patellar tendon strap, stretching of the quadriceps, hamstrings and calves, consider biomechanical analysis to ensure good knee alignment

References

1. Davis KW. Imaging pediatric sports injuries: lower extremity. Radiol Clin N Am. 2010;48(6):1213–35.
2. Draghi F, et al. Overload syndromes of the knee in adolescents: sonographic findings. J Ultrasound. 2008;11(4):151–7.
3. Atanda A Jr, Shah SA, O'Brien K. Osteochondrosis: common causes of pain in growing bones. Am Fam Physician. 2011;83(3):285–91.
4. Browne GJ, Barnett P. Common sports-related musculoskeletal injuries presenting to the emergency department. J Paediatr Child Health. 2016;52(2):231–6.
5. Barber Foss KD, Myer GD, Hewett TE. Epidemiology of basketball, soccer, and volleyball injuries in middle-school female athletes. Phys Sportsmed. 2014;42(2):146–53.
6. Hall R, et al. Sport specialization's association with an increased risk of developing anterior knee pain in adolescent female athletes. J Sport Rehabil. 2015;24(1):31–5.
7. Lau LL, Mahadev A, Hui JH. Common lower limb sport-related overuse injuries in young athletes. Ann Acad Med Singap. 2008;37(4):315–9.
8. Gottsegen CJ, et al. Avulsion fractures of the knee: imaging findings and clinical significance. Radiographics. 2008;28(6):1755–70.

Chapter 9
Patellar Sleeve Fracture

Steven Cuff

Pathology and Dysfunction

A patellar sleeve fracture can be described as an avulsion of a small fragment of bone, and/or periosteum, retinaculum, and cartilage, which typically occurs at the inferior pole of the patella [1, 2]. Articular cartilage is pulled from the deep surface of the patella and periosteum and cartilage from the superficial surface [3].

Specific Pointers

Epidemiology

Patellar fractures, in general, are rare in children, comprising only about 1% of all fractures [3–5]. This is likely the result of the high ratio of cartilage to bone and increased mobility of soft tissues in the pediatric knee [5]. Sleeve fractures, however, account for the majority of such injuries, reported at between 42–72% of all patellar fractures [1, 3, 5]. Patellar sleeve fractures are unique to the pediatric and adolescent population, seen most commonly between 8 and 16 years of age, with a peak incidence of 12.7 years [3, 6]. It is thought that this age group is most susceptible, due to rapid growth with osteochondral transformation at the periphery of the patella, relative patellar instability, and a high intensity of sporting activity [3]. Patellar sleeve fractures predominate in males with a ratio of between 3 and 5:1 [3, 4]. Injuries typically occur in activities involving explosive acceleration, such as jumping, or in high energy sports, like skateboarding [3].

S. Cuff (✉)
Department of Pediatric Sports Medicine, Nationwide Children's Hospital; The Ohio State University College of Medicine, Westerville, OH, USA
e-mail: steven.cuff@nationwidechildrens.org

© Springer Nature Switzerland AG 2021   69
N. Coleman (ed.), *Common Pediatric Knee Injuries*,
https://doi.org/10.1007/978-3-030-55870-3_9

Mechanism of Injury

The most common cause of patellar sleeve fracture is a rapid contraction of the quadriceps muscle, while the knee is in a flexed position [1, 3, 5, 6]. Jumping is typically cited as an inciting mechanism [3, 5, 7], although case reports also describe falls [2, 4, 8] and biking accidents [1, 8].

Diagnosis

Kids with patellar sleeve fractures typically complain of the acute onset of anterior knee pain, swelling, and difficulty straightening their leg [1, 5]. Exam findings include tenderness to palpation over the extensor mechanism, a joint effusion, and a limp. Patients will have difficulty performing a straight leg raise or may be completely unable to do so. A high-riding patella and a palpable gap at the inferior pole of the patella may be present [3, 7]. Plain radiographs may be helpful in making the diagnosis, with a lateral x-ray of the knee being the most likely to show pathology. X-rays may reveal a patella alta, a fracture line through the patella, and/or a small fragment of bone distal to the inferior pole of the patella [5]. MRI can be utilized, if there is a high clinical suspicion of patellar sleeve injury, despite normal x-rays, or to assess the full extent of injury in known sleeve fractures [6]. Ultrasound has also been described as a cost-effective and safe tool for visualizing patellar sleeve fractures [9].

Management

Treatment of patellar sleeve fractures depends upon the amount of displacement of the avulsed bony fragment. If the fracture is nondisplaced or minimally displaced (≤2 mm), then conservative treatment with a cylinder cast with the knee in extension for 4–6 weeks may be considered [1–3]. For displaced fractures, surgical correction with open reduction and internal fixation is the treatment of choice [1, 2].

Demonstration Cases

Common Presentation

A 12-year-old boy presents to the ED after injuring his knee that day during a track meet. He reports the sudden onset of right, anterior knee pain after landing with his knees flexed during the long jump. He is unable to bear weight without significant discomfort and notes that his knee is swollen, and he is having difficulty straightening his knee. On exam, he walks with a limp and has an obvious effusion. His patella appears high-riding, and he is tender to palpation over the patella and patellar tendon. A palpable gap is apparent with palpation at the inferior pole of the patella. X-rays reveal patella alta and a bony fragment displaced 1 cm inferiorly from the base of the patella. MRI confirms the diagnosis of patellar sleeve fracture, and the patient is referred to orthopedics for open reduction and internal fixation of the displaced fracture fragment.

Uncommon Presentation

An 8-year-old girl presents to sports medicine clinic with a 9-month history of right anterior knee pain. She initially injured her knee, when she fell while riding her bike. She was seen in Urgent Care at the time and diagnosed with Sinding-Larsen-Johansson syndrome, when x-rays showed an irregularity at the inferior pole of her patella. Mom reports that she limped after the fall for a few weeks but then symptoms improved; however, the girl has complained of anterior knee pain since the injury with prolonged walking and climbing stairs. The pain is worse with running, jumping, and riding her bike, and she is still unable to straighten her knee fully. On exam she has a somewhat high-riding patella on the right compared to the left side and a firm density palpable inferior to the patella. She lacks ~5 degrees of extension on the right. X-ray reveals abnormal bony formation along the patellar tendon. She is referred to orthopedics for consideration of surgical management of an old patellar sleeve fracture.

Pearls and Pitfalls
- A palpable gap in the patella may be present on exam in significantly displaced fractures; however, this can be difficult to assess in a very swollen knee [2].
- Some patients may still be able to extend their leg actively following a patellar sleeve fracture, due to the presence of a posterior cartilaginous hinge or a cartilaginous sleeve attached to the patella [1].
- Because much of the avulsed fragment is comprised of non-ossified cartilage, x-rays can significantly underestimate the extent of damage or even miss patellar sleeve fractures altogether [5, 8, 10].
- Complications of patellar sleeve fractures include limitation in knee flexion, extensor lag, patella alta, quadriceps atrophy, anterior knee pain, development of ectopic bone within the knee and avascular necrosis [1, 2].

Chapter Summary

Patellar fractures in children are uncommon; however, sleeve fractures comprise the majority of such injuries, are unique to the pediatric and adolescent population, and are more common in boys. They are typically caused by a rapid contraction of the quadriceps muscle, while the knee is in a flexed position, often while jumping or during a fall. These injuries most commonly present with the acute onset of anterior knee pain, swelling, and difficulty straightening the leg and with a limp, tenderness to palpation over the extensor mechanism, an effusion and often an extensor lag on exam. A high-riding patella and a palpable patellar gap may be present, as well. A lateral knee x-ray is helpful in making the diagnosis but can underestimate some injuries, so MRI or ultrasound should be utilized, if there is a high index of suspicion of patellar sleeve fracture. Minimally or nondisplaced fractures can be treated conservatively with casting, while displaced fractures require surgery.

Table for Review

Condition	Patellar sleeve fracture
Description	Avulsion fracture of bone and cartilage from inferior pole of patella
Epidemiology	Most common between 8–16 years old Males > females
Mechanism (common)	Rapid contraction of quadriceps with knee flexed Jumping, falls
History and exam findings	Acute onset of anterior knee pain Swelling/effusion Limp Extensor lag High-riding patella Palpable patellar gap with significant injuries
Management	Nondisplaced/minimally displaced fracture: cylinder cast with knee in extension for 4–6 weeks Displaced fracture: open reduction & internal fixation

References

1. Damrow DS, Van Valin SE. Patellar sleeve fracture with ossification of the patellar tendon. Orthopedics. 2017;40(2):e357–e9.
2. Gao GX, Mahadev A, Lee EH. Sleeve fracture of the patella in children. J Orthop Surg (Hong Kong). 2008;16(1):43–6.
3. Hunt DM, Somashekar N. A review of sleeve fractures of the patella in children. Knee. 2005;12(1):3–7.
4. Gupta RR, Johnson AM, Moroz L, Wells L. Patellar sleeve fractures in children: a case report and review of the literature. Am J Orthop (Belle Mead NJ). 2006;35(7):336–8.

5. Sessions WC, Herring M, Truong WH. Extensor mechanism injury in the pediatric population-a clinical review. J Knee Surg. 2018;31(6):490–7.
6. Dupuis CS, Westra SJ, Makris J, Wallace EC. Injuries and conditions of the extensor mechanism of the pediatric knee. Radiographics. 2009;29(3):877–86.
7. Lindor RA, Homme J. Patellar fracture with sleeve avulsion. N Engl J Med. 2016;375(24):e49.
8. Sullivan S, Maskell K, Knutson T. Patellar sleeve fracture. West J Emerg Med. 2014;15(7):883–4.
9. Ditchfield A, Sampson MA, Taylor GR. Case reports. Ultrasound diagnosis of sleeve fracture of the patella. Clin Radiol. 2000;55(9):721–2.
10. Nath PI, Lattin GE Jr. Patellar sleeve fracture. Pediatr Radiol. 2010;40(Suppl 1):S53.

Chapter 10
Patellofemoral Pain Syndrome

Peter Gerbino

Introduction

Patellofemoral pain syndrome (PFPS) is the most common diagnosis for anterior knee pain in pediatric and adolescent patients [1–4]. It is much more common in adolescent females than males [5]. Unfortunately, there are many causes of anterior knee pain, and without a precise physical examination it is not possible to identify the source or sources of that pain accurately. Too often, the default diagnosis for many of these conditions becomes PFPS.

If that were not bad enough, PFPS has gone by many other names, such as chondromalacia patella, anterior knee pain, idiopathic knee pain, and others. Even worse, many clinicians believe that PFPS has unknown causes and poor treatment options.

Anatomy

The anatomy of the knee is central to understanding the various pathological processes. The patellofemoral mechanism consists of the quadriceps tendon, the patella, the femoral trochlea, the patellar tendon, the tibial tubercle, and the medial and lateral retinaculae (Fig. 10.1). Every one of these structures is innervated with pain fibers with the notable exception of the articular cartilage [6–8]. That means that PFPS pain can theoretically originate in one or more of those structures, but not from the patellar cartilage or femoral trochlea cartilage.

In the optimal situation, the patella would be centered within the trochlea and engage the trochlea at about 30 degrees of flexion [9]. The medial and lateral retinaculae and muscles would be evenly balanced and the quadriceps muscles would

P. Gerbino (✉)
Community Hospital of the Monterey, Peninsula, Monterey, CA, USA

© Springer Nature Switzerland AG 2021
N. Coleman (ed.), *Common Pediatric Knee Injuries*,
https://doi.org/10.1007/978-3-030-55870-3_10

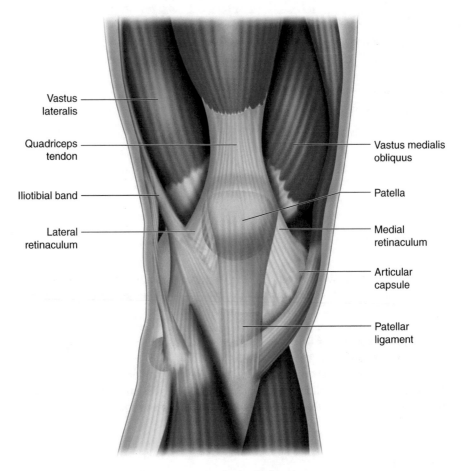

Vastus lateralis

Quadriceps tendon

Iliotibial band

Lateral retinaculum

Vastus medialis obliquus

Patella

Medial retinaculum

Articular capsule

Patellar ligament

Fig. 10.1 Anatomy of the patellofemoral mechanism. All structures are innervated except the articular cartilage

allow full flexion without excessive tension. This is never the case. Patellae tend to track laterally; there can be patella alta or infera; there can be hypermobility; and the quadriceps muscles can be tight. Despite these variations in anatomy and strength and tension, not everyone develops PFPS. As is true throughout the body, variable stress from differing anatomic alignments leads to cartilage and bone toughness in proportion to these stresses. This is an important concept, as many of the treatment protocols involve altering these anatomic variations.

Understanding the functions of the patella is also critical to understanding the possible pathologies. The patella functions as a lever, a pulley, a friction reducer, and a shock absorber. As a lever, it acts to increase the moment arm of the extensor mechanism [9]. It alters the direction of the quadriceps action, a pully function [10]. The articular cartilage functions to provide a smooth gliding surface with the femoral trochlea. Finally, the patella has a shock-absorbing function. It has the thickest articular cartilage [11–13] and subchondral bone [11, 14–16] in the body. It sees forces 6.5 times body weight [17]. It has been shown to compress under physiologic loads [18].

Another concept that is central to understanding PFPS is stress vs. force. Stress is force divided by area. In the patella, stress and pressure are similar. Stress is what leads to stress fractures, increased pressure, and stress-deformation of a structure. Spreading the total force of patellofemoral compression over a broader area decreases focal stress, whereas lateral tracking focuses stress to one part of the patella. This concept is the basis of our understanding of what causes PFPS and how to treat it.

Pathology

The first task is to identify the source or sources of pain. Because there are many potential pain sites and because they are all very near to one another, it is easy to incorrectly identify a particular painful site. If all sites are not examined, all sources of pain cannot be addressed. That situation will frequently lead to oversimplified diagnoses, standardized treatment, and frequent treatment failures.

In a prospective study of 100 consecutive patients with new onset anterior knee pain, we examined the patella, medial and lateral retinaculae, proximal and distal soft tissues, as well as other standard knee structures. We found that loading the patella by pressing it into the trochlea was painful in the majority of patients. This duplicated the pain experienced by climbing stairs, squatting, and jumping. We also found that this patella pain was frequently accompanied by pain in the medial retinaculum and/or by pain in the anterior soft tissues [19]. These findings have been augmented by Luhmann, *et al.* who retrospectively determined that a large number of those with PFPS had pain in the medial patellofemoral ligament portion of the medial retinaculum [20]. These findings confirm what the members of the International Patellofemoral Study Group (IPFSG) have stated, namely that PFPS originates in the patella subchondral bone nerve fibers and can be accompanied by pain in the retinaculae and anterior fat pad [21]. Others have found neoinnervation in the lateral retinaculum of some patients with PFPS accounting for some pain [22].

If we assume that the three most likely components of PFPS are patella subchondral bone pain, medial soft tissue pain, and fat pad pain, we can assess and manage each as needed. For the patella subchondral bone pain fibers to fire, they must be distorted or experience increased intraosseous pressure (stress). The increased pressure theory was first proposed by Lemperg and Arnoldi in 1978 [23]. A second study found that there were elevated intraosseous patella pressures in painful knees [24]. Others have found elevated intraosseous patella pressures associated with patellofemoral pain [25]. Unfortunately, osteotomizing the patella to decrease pressure did not cure PFPS [24]. This means that increased intraosseous pressure may not be a primary cause of PFPS but rather a secondary result of another source of patella stress. It turns out that compressing the patella not only deforms the bone but also increases intraosseous pressure [18, 24, 25]

The theory of patella compression causing the patella component of PFPS conforms to most of the published findings. Ficat determined that lateral compression of the patella was painful [26]. It explains why activities with high patella compression force, such as climbing stairs, squatting, running, and jumping, are painful. It explains why decreasing total force or by redistribution of patellofemoral stresses with braces or taping relieves pain.

If patella compression is the cause of PFPS pain, the next question is why do some patellae become painful and not others, given that most do not have ideal mechanics. It has been speculated that most patellae accommodate to their mechanics and develop thick enough cartilage and subchondral bone that they do not distort enough under pressure to cause pain. This homeostasis can be disrupted by a single excessive force or repetitive sub-injurious loading. That explains why a runner with no history of knee pain can develop PFPS during a marathon. This would mean that PFPS patella pain could arise from a single traumatic overload or multiple sub-threshold compressions or be the result of a patella that can elastically compress to the point where the subchondral bone nerves and pressure sensors are stimulated. It would mean that PFPS is a subchondral patella stress fracture or results from elastic patella subchondral bone deformation. In both cases, the treatment would be to decrease localized stress and total compressive forces and to strengthen the patella subchondral bone.

The "Theatre Sign" or pain in the patellofemoral mechanism after sitting with the knee flexed for an extended period of time is common in PFPS. It has been theorized that this situation can be explained by tension in the soft tissues [20, 22, 27]. Another possible explanation could be that the patella is under continuous compression while sitting increasing deformation and intraosseous pressure to the point where the nerves become stimulated [25]. Extending the knee relieves the pressure and the pain resolves.

These concepts align with the "Patellofemoral pain consensus statement" from The International Patellofemoral Study Group concerning the causes of pain in PFPS [21].

Pathology in the medial soft tissues, when it exists with patella pain, could be from tension in the MPFL [20], medial plica rubbing on the medial femoral condyle and/or medial femoral condyle synovitis.

Pathology in the fat pad comes from enlargement, synovitis, and impingement. These occur typically after prolonged knee inflammation. Fat pad syndrome is described extensively in another chapter.

Epidemiology

PFPS occurs in two main populations, adults with osteoarthritis and adolescents. Thirty percent of adolescents will develop PFPS [28]. Adolescent females will develop PFSS 2–10 times more often than males [28]. If patella compressive overload is the cause of PFPS, anything that causes generalized patella loading or leads to asymmetric patella overload can be implicated. A partial list of possible factors that may be involved is presented in Table 10.1.

Table 10.1 Factors that can lead to generalized or asymmetric patella overload

Increased running mileage
Increased jumping
Running stairs
Poor shock absorption (shoes, surface, muscles)
Anatomic variations
Positive J-sign
Increased Q-angle
Genu valgum
Patella Alta
Patella infera
Lateral patella tilt
Hyperlaxity
Quadriceps weakness
Hip external rotators, abductor weakness
Tight hamstrings
Foot pronation

Sports with a higher incidence of PFPS are those with higher demands on the patellofemoral mechanism and more jumping. These are the running sports, basketball, volleyball, and sports with squatting, such as weightlifting.

Mechanism of Injury

In PFPS, the exact mechanism of injury remains unknown. Despite the lack of clear scientific proof, what is clear is that loading the patella with compressive force is causative. We know what makes the pain worse and we know which interventions decrease pain, so we know that altering patellofemoral compression helps. This can only mean that the mechanism of injury is too much or too focal patellofemoral loading, leading to patella subchondral stress fracture or compression as the source of pain.

Mechanisms of injury for the pain arising in the soft tissues are also poorly understood. A mal-tracking patella could put excess tension on the medial capsular structures. An enlarged fat pad could impinge anteriorly. All soft tissues could become painful from neoinnervation after chronic patellar pain.

Diagnosis

The medical history in PFPS can be variable. Most typically, patients will be adolescent females who state that their knees have been painful for months to years. Pain is noted on ascending and descending stairs, running, jumping, and squatting. Conversely, the pain could have come on acutely after a long run or an increase in training requiring jumping or squatting. Many will report a positive Theatre Sign with patella pain after prolonged sitting.

The physical examination requires a stepwise progression, testing all possible sites of pain and instability. Reserving palpation of the most painful sites for last is always a good strategy. Begin by looking for an effusion or localized edema. Next, assess range of motion, varus and valgus laxity, Lachman and patella mobility. Mobility means how many quadrants the patella can be displaced medially and laterally and whether there is apprehension. If increased mobility is found, test for generalized hyperlaxity. Note whether there is patella alta or infera, lateral tracking, a J-sign, an increased Q-angle, and any crepitus with motion. Test quadriceps and hamstring strength and hip abductor and external rotator strength [29]. Finally, assess sites of tenderness. Check the tibial tubercle, patella tendon, iliotibial band, joint lines, quadriceps tendon, medial and lateral fat pad, medial and lateral retinaculae, and patella. The lateral retinaculum should be checked for tightness, as well as tenderness. The medial retinaculum should be palpated for tenderness in the medial plica, as well as in the MPFL.

The patella exam can be general, assessing for pain by loading the entire patella as one presses it into the trochlea. This is different from some tests where the patella is pressed down and distally as the quadriceps is contracted. That test, sometimes referred to as the patella compression test, the patella grind test or Clarke's Sign is not specific to the patella. It is testing the quadriceps tendon, suprapatellar fat, patella proximal pole, and trochlea. Pressing just the patella into the trochlea limits the test mainly to patella subchondral bone nerves. Performing patella compression with a small bump under the knee eliminates any hypertrophic suprapatellar fat that might impinge and confound the test results (Fig. 10.2).

The patella examination can be further refined. The lateral facet, medial facet, and proximal and distal poles can be individually compressed, isolating each of those sites. Pain elicited with selective compression of the lateral facet isolates the patella damage to that side. This specificity helps determine which interventions will be most effective.

Fig. 10.2 Examination of the patella. Simple compression of the patella into the trochlea isolates the possible sites of tenderness to the patella subchondral bone and trochlea. Flexing the knee 30 degrees ensures that the suprapatellar fat is not within the patellofemoral joint

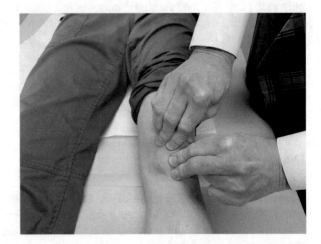

Imaging studies have not been very helpful in PFPS. Radiographs can show lateral patella tilt or pathologies, such as patella osteochondritis dissecans or bipartite patella. MRI can show an enlarged fat pad or plica and, in some cases, show edema in the subchondral bone [30, 31]. Bone scintigraphy has been used to identify subchondral stress fracture. The level of detail needed to see these injuries is high, but patella subchondral injuries in PFPS have been repeatedly documented [32–35].

All elements of the history and physical examination are combined to arrive at a complete diagnosis. A common pattern will be lateral patella facet pain, MPFL and/ or plica pain and lateral fat pad tenderness. Treatment will be tailored to address each of those sites.

Management

If one examines which interventions have been helpful in PFPS, it is possible to understand better the pathological processes in the syndrome. For the pain arising in the patella, all successful interventions involve either reducing the total patellofemoral compression force or altering the distribution of those stresses on the patella. Total force reduction techniques consist of activity modification to limit stairs, running, jumping, squatting, and bent-knee quadriceps strengthening. Increased quadriceps strength has been shown to decrease PFPS pain, so straight-leg isometric quadriceps strengthening is mandatory [36–38]. This exercise also strengthens the vastus medialus obliquus (VMO), which can help realign a patella that tracks laterally.

Altering patellofemoral stresses has been a major intervention to treat PFPS successfully. Patella bracing, McConnell taping, kinesiotaping, and VMO strengthening all alter patella tracking, shifting the pressure points to a different or wider distribution and help treat PFPS [37–39]. This consistent finding lends more credence to the theory that PFPS is a subchondral stress fracture or bone weakness. If there is coexistent fat pad syndrome, the patella brace may put pressure on the lateral fat pad causing pain and so would be contraindicated. Since lateral tracking is the norm, medializing the patella with bracing or taping would also decrease tension in the medial plica and MPFL, decreasing pain from those structures.

Some patients continue to have patella pain, despite these interventions. Anecdotally, it has been found that some of these patients have low vitamin D levels and osteopenia by DEXA [14]. This could mean that their patellae are not stiff enough to withstand normal compressive forces.

In rare circumstances, surgery is required to treat PFPS. In the past, lateral retinacular release was performed for several types of anterior knee pain. It is now understood that this procedure is appropriate for situations with excessive lateral retinacular tightness and/or lateral patella tilt [40]. In situations where patellofemoral pain is the result of recurrent lateral dislocation, lateral retinacular release can be combined with MPFL repair or reconstruction to realign and stabilize the patella [40].

A painful, fibrotic medial plica can be arthroscopically excised. An enlarged fat pad can be partially resected. A painful bipartite patella can be excised or sometimes made less painful by releasing the lateral retinacular attachments to the ossicle [41–43].

Patella alta, patella infera, and severe lateral tracking are more difficult to treat. If non-operative methods are not effective, these conditions can be treated surgically by patella advancement, recession, or anteromedialization of the tibial tubercle and anterior tibial bone [44, 45]. The Fulkerson anteriomedialization of the patella tendon attachment site realigns the patella in the trochlea, shifting focal stresses and elevates the tibial tubercle, decreasing patellofemoral compression force [45]. Measuring the tibial tubercle to trochlear groove (TT-TG) distance has been advanced as a method to determine how much to correct patellar mal-tracking [46]. After any operation, regaining quadriceps, hamstring, and hip strength is critical for optimal success.

Demonstration Cases

Common Presentation

A 14-year-old female presents with a 6-month history of anterior knee pain. There was no trauma. She plays volleyball and notes sharp anterior pain with running, jumping, and climbing and descending stairs. She has the same pain if she sits in a car or at a movie for more than 1 hour.

Physical examination shows decreased quadriceps strength and a laterally tracking patella with a normal Q-angle and no J-sign. There is no effusion and range of motion is −20 to 140 degrees with no pain. The patella translates 2 quadrants medially and laterally, but there is no apprehension. Beighton hyperlaxity exam shows her to be level 4. There is no varus or valgus laxity and Lachman test is negative.

The patellofemoral exam shows lateral tracking with a "bayonet" attachment to the tibial tubercle. There is exquisite pain with loading the lateral facet of the patella. There is milder pain in the MPFL to palpation. The medial plica is non-tender. The lateral fat pad has mild tenderness. Radiographs demonstrate no patella tilt, patella alta, patella infera, bipartite patella, or osteochondral injury.

Diagnosis: PFPS with MPFL and fat pad secondary irritation. Initial treatment is decreased running and jumping, a medializing patellofemoral brace and straight-leg raising exercises until 10 lbs. can be raised easily. If symptoms persist, hamstring and hip strengthening exercises are added. The brace is discontinued when symptoms are resolved.

Uncommon Presentation

An 18-year-old male presents with 2 weeks of anterior knee pain. He has had no past history of knee pain. Symptoms began during a half marathon in the last few miles of the race. Pain is severe and walking is now painful. He cannot run, jump, or climb stairs. He has had no locking or giving way.

On examination there is no effusion. Range of motion is normal but painful in the range of 110–130 degrees of flexion. The only point tenderness is with compression of the patella medial facet. Quadriceps, hamstring, and hip strength are excellent and symmetrical bilaterally. There is no lateral tracking or patella alta. Radiographs are normal.

Diagnosis: PFPS, most likely occult subchondral stress fracture of the medial facet. Treatment is relative rest, so that there is no pain. Bracing or taping is added to unload the medial facet, and steps are taken to ensure adequate calcium and vitamin D in the diet to allow optimal bone healing. Pain should resolve in a few weeks, and patella bone strength should improve over 6–8 weeks.

Pearls and Pitfalls
- The majority of pain in PFPS arises in the patella subchondral bone.
- Suboptimal patellofemoral mechanics do not cause PFPS but can be modified to decrease PFPS pain.
- Secondary sources of pain can be the medial soft tissues and fat pad.
- PFPS results from excessive patella compression forces.
- Failure to address all sources of pain leads to treatment failure.
- Decreasing patellofemoral forces and altering patella stresses leads to pain relief and healing.
- Hip and knee muscle strength, as well as bone strength, must be optimized.
- Surgery is rarely required.
- When surgery is required, changes in tracking and pressure are most beneficial.

Summary

PFPS is extremely common and leads to a large amount of medical care. A consistent pathological lesion has not been identified, but the common sites of pain and methods that reduce that pain present a theory that is reproducible. The most logical conclusion is that patella deformation in compression causes most patellofemoral pain and that medial soft tissues and an enlarged fad pad can add to the pain sources.

Successful treatment involves identifying all the sources of pain and addressing each. Decreasing patella compression forces, altering the stressed areas of the patella subchondral bone, and improving the strength of the patella subchondral bone all contribute to resolving PFPS.

Condition	Patellofemoral pain syndrome
Description	Patella deformation in compression
Epidemiology	30% of adolescents will get PFPS
	Adolescent females are 2–10 times more likely than males to develop PFPS

Condition	Patellofemoral pain syndrome
Mechanism (common)	Excessive patella compression forces
History and exam findings	Chronic anterior knee pain (esp. with climbing stairs, running, jumping, and squatting) Acute anterior knee pain after significant training episode (ex. long run) Composite exam – test all possible sites of pain and instability; common pattern = lateral patella facet pain, MPFL and/or plica pain and lateral fat pad tenderness
Management	Decrease patella compression forces Alter the stressed areas of the patella subchondral bone Improve the strength of the patella subchondral bone

References

1. Dutton RA, Khadavi MJ, Fredericson M. Patellofemoral pain. Phys Med Rehabil Clin N Am. 2016;27(1):31–52.
2. Kodali P, Islam A, Andrish J. Anterior knee pain in the young athlete: diagnosis and treatment. Sports Med Arthrosc Rev. 2011;19(1):27–33.
3. Rothermich MA, Glaviano NR, Li J, Hart JM. Patellofemoral pain. Clin Sports Med. 2015;34(2):313–27.
4. Smith BE, Selfe J, Thacker D, Hendrick P, Bateman M, Moffatt F, et al. Incidence and prevalence of patellofemoral pain: A systematic review and meta-analysis. Screen HR, editor. PLoS One. 2018;13(1):e0190892.
5. Baker MM, Juhn MS. Patellofemoral pain syndrome in the female athlete. Clin Sports Med. 2000;19(2):315–29.
6. Biedert RM, Stauffer E, Friederich NF. Occurrence of free nerve endings in the soft tissue of the knee joint: a histologic investigation. Am J Sports Med. 1992;20(4):430–3.
7. Dye SF, Vaupel GL, Dye CC. Conscious neurosensory mapping of the internal structures of the human knee without Intraarticular anesthesia. Am J Sports Med. 1998;26(6):773–7.
8. Witoński D, Wągrowska-Danielewicz M. Distribution of substance-P nerve fibers in the knee joint in patients with anterior knee pain syndrome. Knee Surg Sports Traumatol Arthrosc. 1999;7(3):177–83.
9. Fujikawa K, Seedhohom B, Wright V. Biomechanics of the patello-femoral joint. Part I: A study of the contact and the congruity of the patello-femoral compartment and movement of the patella. Eng Med. 1983;12:3–11.
10. Grelsamer RP, Colman WW, Mow VC. Anatomy and mechanics of the patellofemoral joint. Sports Med Arthrosc Rev. 1994;2(3):178–88.
11. Eckstein F, Müller-Gerbl M, Putz R. Distribution of subchondral bone density and cartilage thickness in the human patella. J Anat. 1992;180(Pt 3):425–33.
12. Shepherd DET, Seedhom BB. Thickness of human articular cartilage in joints of the lower limb. Ann Rheum Dis. 1999;58(1):27–34.
13. Tecklenburg K, Dejour D, Hoser C, Fink C. Bony and cartilaginous anatomy of the patellofemoral joint. Knee Surg Sports Traumatol Arthrosc. 2006;14(3):235–40.
14. Björkström S, Goldie IF. Hardness of the subchondral bone of the Patella in the Normal state, in chondromalacia, and in Osteoarthrosis. ActaOrthopaedicaScandinavica. 1982;53(3):451–62.
15. Leppälä J, Kannus P, Natri A, Sievänen H, Järvinen M, Vuori I. Bone mineral density in the chronic patellofemoral pain syndrome. Calcif Tissue Int. 1998;62(6):548–53.

16. Putz R, Muller-Gerbl M, Eckstein F, et al. Are there any correlations between superficial cartilagenous alterations and subchondral bone density (CT-OAM) in the femeropatellar joint? Orthop Trans. 1991;15:497.
17. Huberti HH, Hayes WC. Patellofemoral contact pressures. The influence of q-angle and tendofemoral contact. J Bone Joint Surg. 1984;66(5):715–24.
18. Kerr HA, Gerbino PG, Soto R, Zurakowski D, Muller JA. Load-deformation characteristics of the Patella: relationship to intraosseous pressure. Med Sci Sports Exerc. 2007;39(Supplement):S472.
19. Gerbino PG, Griffin ED, d'Hemecourt PA, Kim T, Kocher MS, Zurakowski D, et al. Patellofemoral pain syndrome: evaluation of location and intensity of pain. Clin J Pain. 2006;22(2):154–9.
20. Luhmann SJ, Schoenecker PL, Dobbs MB, Eric Gordon J. Adolescent patellofemoral pain: implicating the medial patellofemoral ligament as the main pain generator. J Child Orthop. 2008;2(4):269–77.
21. Crossley KM, Stefanik JJ, Selfe J, Collins NJ, Davis IS, Powers CM, et al. 2016 patellofemoral pain consensus statement from the 4th international patellofemoral pain research retreat, Manchester. Part 1: terminology, definitions, clinical examination, natural history, patellofemoral osteoarthritis and patient-reported outcome measures. Br J Sports Med. 2016;50(14):839–43.
22. Fulkerson JP, Gossling HR. Anatomy of the knee joint lateral retinaculum. Clin Orthopaed Relat Res. 1980;153:183–8.
23. Lemperg RK, Arnold CC. The significance of intraosseous pressure in Normal and diseased: states with special reference to the intraosseous engorgement-pain syndrome. Clin Orthop Relat Res. 1978;136:143–56.
24. Hejgaard N, Arnoldi CC. Osteotomy of the patella in the patellofemoral pain syndrome: the significance of increased intraosseous pressure during sustained knee flexion. Int Orthop. 1984;8(3):189–94.
25. Graf J, Christophers R, Schneider U, Niethard F. Chondromalacia patellae und intraossärerDruck. ZeitschriftfürOrthopädie und ihreGrenzgebiete. 2008;130(06):495–500.
26. Ficat P, Ficat C, Bailleux A. External hypertension syndrome of the patella. Its significance in the recognition of arthrosis. Rev ChirOrthopReparatriceAppar Mot. 1975;61(1):39–59.
27. Outerbridge RE, Outerbridge HK. The etiology of chondromalacia patellae. Clin Orthop Relat Res. 2001;389:5–8.
28. Gorman McNerney ML, Arendt EA. Anterior knee pain in the active and athletic adolescent. Curr Sports Med Rep. 2013;12(6):404–10.
29. Ireland ML, Willson JD, Ballantyne BT, Davis IM. Hip strength in females with and without patellofemoral pain. J Orthopaed Sports Phys Therapy. 2003;33(11):671–6.
30. Chhabra A, Subhawong TK, Carrino JA. A systematised MRI approach to evaluating the patellofemoral joint. Skelet Radiol. 2011;40(4):375–87.
31. Draper CE, Quon A, Fredericson M, Besier TF, Delp SL, Beaupre GS, et al. Comparison of MRI and 18F-NaF PET/CT in patients with patellofemoral pain. J Magn Reson Imaging. 2012;36(4):928–32.
32. Draper CE, Fredericson M, Gold GE, Besier TF, Delp SL, Beaupre GS, et al. Patients with patellofemoral pain exhibit elevated bone metabolic activity at the patellofemoral joint. J Orthop Res. 2012;30(2):209–13.
33. Hejgaard N, Diemer H. Bone scan in the patellofemoral pain syndrome. Int Orthop. 1987;11(1):29–33.
34. Morrey BF. Diffusely increased bone Scintigraphic uptake in patellofemoral pain syndrome. Yearbook of Orthopedics. 2006;2006:8.
35. Naslund JE. Diffusely increased bone scintigraphic uptake in patellofemoral pain syndrome. Br J Sports Med. 2005;39(3):162–5.
36. Gökçen N. Which predicts quadriceps muscle strength in knee osteoarthritis: biological markers or clinical variables? Archiv Rheumatol. 2017;32(1):32–8.

37. Crossley K, Bennell K, Green S, McConnell J. A systematic review of physical interventions for patellofemoral pain syndrome. Clin J Sport Med. 2001;11(2):103–10.
38. Crossley KM, van Middelkoop M, Callaghan MJ, Collins NJ, Rathleff MS, Barton CJ. 2016 patellofemoral pain consensus statement from the 4th international patellofemoral pain research retreat, Manchester. Part 2: recommended physical interventions (exercise, taping, bracing, foot orthoses and combined interventions). Br J Sports Med. 2016;50(14):844–52.
39. Collins NJ, Barton CJ, van Middelkoop M, Callaghan MJ, Rathleff MS, Vicenzino BT, et al. 2018 consensus statement on exercise therapy and physical interventions (orthoses, taping and manual therapy) to treat patellofemoral pain: recommendations from the 5th international patellofemoral pain research retreat, Gold Coast, Australia, 2017. Br J Sports Med. 2018;52(18):1170–8.
40. da FLPRM, Kawatake EH, Pochini A de C. Lateral patellar retinacular release: changes over the last ten years. RevistaBrasileira de Ortopedia (English Edition). 2017;52(4):442–9.
41. Felli L, Formica M, Lovisolo S, Capello AG, Alessio-Mazzola M. Clinical outcome of arthroscopic lateral Retinacular release for symptomatic bipartite Patella in athletes. Arthrosc J Arthroscop Relat Surg. 2018;34(5):1550–8.
42. Oohashi Y. Regarding "clinical outcome of arthroscopic lateral Retinacular release for symptomatic bipartite Patella in athletes". Arthrosc J Arthrosc Relat Surg. 2018;34(8):2269–70.
43. Vieira TD, Thaunat M, Saithna A, Carnesecchi O, Choudja E, Cavalier M, et al. Surgical technique for arthroscopic resection of painful bipartite patella. Arthrosc Tech. 2017;6(3):e751–5.
44. RM B, Alta TPMP. A comprehensive review of current knowledge. Am J Orthop (Belle Mead NJ). 2017;46(7):290–300.
45. Fulkerson JP. Anteromedialization of the Tibial Tuberosity for Patellofemoral Malalignment. Clin Orthop Relat Res. 1983;177:176–81.
46. Pandit S, Frampton C, Stoddart J, Lynskey T. Magnetic resonance imaging assessment of tibial tuberosity–trochlear groove distance: normal values for males and females. Int Orthop. 2011;35(12):1799–803.

Chapter 11
Osgood Schlatter's Disease

Matthew Sedgley

Anatomy and Normal Function

The extensor mechanism of the quadriceps, quadriceps tendon, patella, and patellar tendon form a kinetic chain that attaches at the tibial tuberosity. The extensor mechanism of the pediatric or adolescent knee is different from that of an adult. While there are still the same bones, open growth plates are present. In general, a growth plate is a metabolically active zone of the bone that allows pediatric patients to contribute to their growth. Primary ossification centers in the leg that typically help with height gain are located at the diaphysis of bones and are developed prenatally. Secondary ossification centers develop postnatally. One such secondary ossification site, called the tibial tuberosity apophysis, is at the attachment of the patellar tendon to the tibia [1].

The tibial tuberosity develops from being completely cartilaginous, usually at age 10 or less, to an apophysis from ages 11 to 14, to complete bone via fusion proximally with the tibial epiphysis from ages 14 to 18. Due to its cartilage nature in youth, the tibial tuberosity is the weakest point along the extensor chain, as opposed to the patellar tendon being weakest in adults.

Pathology and Dysfunction

The pathology of Osgood Schlatter's Disease (OSD) starts with rapid bone growth in the leg at the distal femur and proximal tibia. The elongation of the femur can cause pulling at the apophysis. Repeated use of the quadriceps extensor mechanism

M. Sedgley (✉)
MedStar Union Memorial Hospital, Westminster, MD, USA
e-mail: matthew.d.sedgley@medstar.net

© Springer Nature Switzerland AG 2021
N. Coleman (ed.), *Common Pediatric Knee Injuries*,
https://doi.org/10.1007/978-3-030-55870-3_11

(e.g., running, jumping sports, leg extensions) places further tension at the tibial tuberosity. This repeated stress could initially cause pain and inflammation, resulting in inflammation of the cartilage. This is referred to as osteochondritis. In more severe cases, and with continued repetitive stress upon the apophysis, the tibial tuberosity may fragment. A load of excessive use during growth makes this condition more likely [2].

Epidemiology: Age, Gender, Common Sports

Without large databases, the exact epidemiology of OSD is hard to pinpoint. OSD is, however, a condition of skeletally immature athletes. Both girls and boys experience OSD during growth spurts, girls from age 8 to 13 and boys from age 10 to 15. Common sports with affected athletes include lacrosse, basketball, soccer, figure skating, and gymnastics. Symptoms are reported bilaterally in 20–30% of cases [2]. Given that equal numbers of boys and girls present with OSD to general practice clinics in the UK, there appears to be no role of gender being a true risk factor [1, 3].

Mechanism of Injury: Common/Likely, Uncommon/ Less Likely

The mechanism of OSD is often associated with a running or jumping sport in a skeletally immature knee joint [4]. This is because these sports require adolescent athletes to contract their quadriceps muscles more frequently. This contraction increases the forces along the extensor mechanism. As mentioned above, this pulling, coupled with rapid growth, places stress at the tibial tuberosity. This repetitive injury eventually can cause irritation and micro-trauma [5]. When not addressed with rest, the area can become inflamed and enlarged. In severe cases the apophysis can fragment. Less commonly, one sudden traumatic event (e.g., a sprint, landing on the tibial tubercle, or significant leap) can aggravate the underlying condition. Medical providers must be cautious in these scenarios to exclude other causes of pain caused by the trauma.

Diagnosis: History and Exam Findings, Testing

Diagnosis of OSD is predominantly clinical. There is a history of a sport that involves running or jumping, coupled with anterior lower knee pain. There is no history of instability, loss of range of motion, or swelling. The tibial tubercle is often enlarged in the affected knee on inspection. There is no history of fevers or chills, suggesting osteomyelitis [6]. There is also no night pain or unexplained weight loss to suggest malignancy [7].

Children with OSD are tender to palpation at the tibial tuberosity [8]. There is no tenderness of the patella. Athletes do not report hip pain and have a normal hip examination. There is often a report of overuse in jumping or running sports [5]. Physical examination may reveal pain with single leg hop on the affected side.

Radiographs may be helpful, as they can show widening or fragmentation of the growth plate and exclude other diagnoses. While not required, radiographs are helpful in excluding tumors, both benign and malignant. Failure to respond to a trial of conservative care is the most commonly recommended indication for radiographs [6]. Magnetic resonance imaging (MRI) may be helpful in grading severity but is not often required, unless suspicion exists for other causes of anterior knee pain, such as a stress fracture from overuse. If the condition is recurrent, MRI may be useful in distinguishing acute conditions, like a bone stress injury, from chronic situations, like recurrent OSD.

Newer technologies, like portable musculoskeletal (MSK) ultrasound (US) machines, are being used more often [9]. US can easily be used in the clinic at the time of the visit. It is very cost-efficient and may be used on the contralateral side for comparison. Additionally, there is no radiation. Similar to x-ray and MRI, US may not be necessary for diagnosis of OSD. Due to radiation, computed tomography (CT) and bone scan with SPECT (single photon emission CT) are not recommended unless another diagnosis, like stress fracture, is being considered and MRI is not an option [9, 6].

Management

Patients with OSD often respond to a course of rest for a few weeks. While simple, this is the mainstay of treatment protocols. True rest can be challenging, as these athletes are often used to being active many hours a week in one or more sports. Rest and activity modification reduce the stress and load generated with knee extension activities. This, in turn, gives the apophysis a break from these forces to heal. Icing can be also helpful. Some sources recommend an infrapatellar strap which may be of some help with pain, but there is not evidence in the literature to support this.

Gentle stretching of the thigh muscles and over-the-counter analgesics (e.g., ibuprofen or acetaminophen) generally decrease the pain over a few weeks. Many clinicians also recommend patellar straps for the pain; however, their effectiveness in the literature has not been proven or disproven. Athletes with severe pain may take months to recover, and cases lasting 12 to 24 months have been reported [8]. Rest and reassurance with education is important to share with the patient and parent as part of treatment.

Other less commonly used treatments for OSD include steroid injections and surgical intervention. Steroid injections are discouraged, as the risks outweigh the benefits. Steroid injections increase the potential for infection, bleeding, pain, and reactions to the injectate. In addition, subcutaneous fat atrophy may occur [5]. Allergies to lidocaine or other anesthetics could also be a concern. Steroids, even if helpful for pain relief, have an effect that wears off in a few weeks. If the tibial tuberosity has fragmented and that fragment is causing irritation, despite a trial of rest and activity modification, surgery with arthroscopic removal of the fragment may be helpful; this is rarely required, unless the pain persists beyond 2 years [6, 10, 11].

Case reports have presented ortho-biologicals (e.g., autologous blood products, such as platelet-rich plasma, PRP) as novel treatments for patients with recalcitrant presentations. Such options would carry risks similar to steroid injections, without the risk of reacting to a foreign substance. As these procedures are often cash-only procedures, their general availability is relatively low. Case reports in the literature are confounded, as the patients receiving the PRP had also received patellar tendon straps, taping, and physical therapy [8].

Demonstration Cases

Common Presentation

A 14-year-old male presents to the sports medicine clinic with his mother complaining about right anterior knee pain for 6 weeks. His pain is located at the anterior proximal tibia. The area of pain is enlarged, compared to his left knee. He denies swelling in the joint, trauma, and instability. There is no hip pain or limping. He denies fevers, chills, and night pain. His pain is better with ice and rest. Returning to year-round soccer, basketball, and lacrosse makes the pain worse. On examination there is no effusion, but the tibial tubercle is enlarged on the right leg versus the left. Palpation reveals tenderness at the tibial tuberosity of the right knee only. Range of motion is normal. There is no ligament laxity on physical examination. McMurray's grind test is normal. Gait is normal. No radiographs are performed.

Uncommon Presentation

A 15-year-old tennis player presents with bilateral anterior knee pain. She plays 6 days per week for many hours each session. She has a healthy diet and reports normal menstruation. She was diagnosed with OSD in the past, and periods of rest have kept the pain away. A full recovery had been made last year. She has recently increased her practice time with a new coach and now notes significant swelling at the patellar tendon insertion at the tibial tuberosity. She has tried patellar straps, ice, and rest. She denies numbness, fevers, and chills. Examination is benign without laxity of the ligaments and with normal range of motion and excellent symmetric strength. Kneeling is painful. She has bilaterally enlarged tibial tubercles. X-ray shows fragmentation of the tibial tuberosity, best seen on the lateral view. Due to the recurrent nature of the knee pain bilaterally, an MRI was performed, showing no ligament, tendon, or meniscus injury; however, there was evidence of inflammation seen in the tibial tubercle, best seen on the axial views. No stress fracture or tumors were seen.

> **Pearls and Pitfalls**
> While knee pain is a common presentation in adolescent athletes, not every presentation can be assumed to be from OSD. Even if the patient presents with a history of overuse, OSD should not be the sole consideration. Hip pathology could possibly present with a history of limping; slipped capital femoral epiphysis (SCFE) may present with knee pain. A patient with tears to ligaments, tendons, or cartilage may present with knee pain but also with a significant effusion. Neoplasms of the distal femur and knee joint may present with pain and other symptoms, like night pain. Other conditions of internal knee derangement, like an osteochondral defect (OCD) or meniscus tear, may be the source of pain, when there is a history of knee instability, such as buckling, locking, or giving out.
>
> While OSD may be made worse with a sudden traumatic event, it usually presents over time. On physical examination the location of knee pain is anterior, and there is tenderness at the tibial tuberosity [4]. It should be emphasized that rest of the knee helps, and hip examination is normal. Lack of improvement with rest and time should prompt reconsideration of the etiology of the adolescent patient's knee pain.
>
> Imaging, such as x-ray, is often unnecessary but can often be reassuring, with the exception of revealing a widened apophysis at the tibial tuberosity. Physical examination of a patient with OSD should demonstrate normal findings in the hip and the knee, with the exception of tenderness at the tibial tuberosity [4].

Chapter Summary

OSD is a known cause of knee pain in the skeletally immature athlete. Typically resulting from overuse, OSD is located at the tibial tuberosity. Diagnosis is often clinical; excluding other potential diagnoses is key. Imaging, if warranted, may help exclude other suspected causes of knee pain or grade the severity of OSD. Treatment mainly involves the use of rest, ice, and gentle stretching. The duration of OSD pain, while often only a few weeks, can last many months. Outside of the potential for painful ossicles developing, the pain of OSD typically does not return, when the growth plate fuses.

Suggested Helpful Websites, Videos, Etc., for Readers to Obtain Additional Information

https://www.aafp.org/afp/2006/0315/p1014.html
   https://www.uwhealth.org/sports-medicine/clinic/osgood-schlatter-disease/10109
   https://www.ncbi.nlm.nih.gov/books/NBK441995/
   https://www.ncbi.nlm.nih.gov/pmc/articles/PMC5457541/
   https://www.ncbi.nlm.nih.gov/pmc/articles/PMC5738486/
   http://www.aappublications.org/content/14/8/2.5

Chart/Table for Review

Condition	Osgood Schlatter's disease
Description	Inflammation at the tibial tuberosity in adolescent athletes that occurs with high levels of athletic activity prior to the growth plate closing.
Epidemiology	Girls from age 8 to 13 and boys from age 10 to 15.
Mechanism (common)	Running and jumping sports causing micro-trauma at the apophysis
History and exam findings	History is of inferior knee pain at the tibial tuberosity without other findings suggestive of internal derangement; Exam is normal except for enlargement and/or tenderness at the tibial tuberosity.
Management	Success is often seen with rest, icing, and gentle stretching of quadriceps. Rarely, surgery for fragment removal is needed but can be helpful.

References

1. Michaleff ZA, Campbell P, Protheroe J, Rajani A, Dunn KM. Consultation patterns of children and adolescents with knee pain in UK general practice: analysis of medical records. BMC Musculoskeletal Disord. 2017;18(1):239. https://doi.org/10.1186/s12891-017-1586-1.
2. Smith JM, Varacallo M. Osgood Schlatter Disease. StatPearls [Internet]. Treasure Island (FL): StatPearls Publishing; 2019, May 5 latest update.
3. Circi E, et al. Treatment of Osgood-Schlatter disease: review of the literature. Musculoskelet Surg. 2017;101:195–200. https://doi.org/10.1007/s12306-017-0479-7.
4. University of Wisconsin Hospitals and Clinics Authority. Osgood-Schlatter disease. Obtained from https://www.uwhealth.org/sports-medicine/clinic/osgood-schlatter-disease/10109. Date of access 1 Sept 2019.
5. Cassas KJ, Cassettari-Wayhs A. Childhood and adolescent sports-related overuse injuries. Am Fam Physician. 2006;73(6):1014–22.
6. Binazzi R, et al. Surgical treatment of unresolved Osgood–Schlatter lesion. Clin OrthopRelat Res. 1993;(289):202–204.
7. Bloom OJ, Mackler L, Barbee J. Clinical inquiries. What is the best treatment for Osgood-Schlatter disease? J Fam Pract. 2004;53:153–6.

8. Danneberg DJ. Successful treatment of Osgood-Schlatter disease with autologous-conditioned plasma in two patients. Joints. 2017;5(3):191–4. https://doi.org/10.1055/s-0037-1605384. eCollection 2017 Sep.
9. Bianchi S, Martinoli C. Pediatric ultrasound, pp 946–8, 957. In: Martinoli C, Vale M, editors. Ultrasound of the musculoskeletal system. New York: Springer; 2007.
10. Nierenberg G, et al. Surgical treatment of residual Osgood–Schlatter disease in young adults: role of the mobile osseous fragment. Orthopedics. 2011;34(3):176.
11. DeBarardino TM, Branstetter JG, Owens BG. Arthroscopic treatment of unresolved Osgood-Schlatter lesions. Arthroscopy. 2007;23(10):1127.e1–3. https://doi.org/10.1016/j. arthr.2006.12.004.

Chapter 12
Anterior Cruciate Ligament Injury

Shelley Street Callender

Introduction

The anterior cruciate ligament (ACL) is one of the four main ligamentous structures of the knee. It stabilizes the knee from rotational forces and attaches the femur and the tibia. The anatomical location of the ACL is from the anterolateral femoral condyle to the medial tibial condyle. Knowledge about the ACL has grown over the last two decades, as the general population becomes more familiar with its structure, function, potential injures, and rehabilitation. Much of this added awareness is due to the increased frequency of ACL tears and the high-profile athletes who have successfully returned to play after such injuries.

Epidemiology

ACL injury has become one of the most common ligamentous injuries of the knee. While the skeletally mature athlete can have a mid-substance ACL tear, the young athlete most often tears the ACL at the origin on the femur. Adolescent females are 1.6 times more likely to have ACL tears per athletic exposure than their male counterparts [2]. A variety of anatomical, biomechanical, and hormonal reasons with varying levels of evidence have been postulated for this difference, including a higher body mass index, patella alta, increased quadriceps angle (Q-angle), ligament laxity, genu valgum, dynamic valgus landing, and unbalanced quadriceps strength [1, 2, 5].

S. S. Callender (✉)
Department of Pediatrics, Navicent Health System, Mercer University School of Medicine,
Macon, GA, USA
e-mail: Callender.Shelley@navicenthealth.org

© Springer Nature Switzerland AG 2021
N. Coleman (ed.), *Common Pediatric Knee Injuries*,
https://doi.org/10.1007/978-3-030-55870-3_12

Mechanism of Injury

Most ACL injuries occur during a non-contact landing injury in a contact sport or during a forced rotation of the knee while making a sudden turn, resulting in rapid deceleration and external rotation of the knee [1]. The less frequent contact-related ACL injury, due to direct trauma in contact-collision sports, is seen primarily in male-dominated sports (i.e., American Football). The athlete will often describe feeling and/or hearing a "pop" with immediate discomfort and instability of the knee. He/she often is unable to continue participation. In addition to the sudden pain and instability, affected athletes will develop rapid knee swelling, due to an effusion, in this case a hemarthrosis, during the first few hours after injury.

On-Field Assessment

The on-field physical examination may be limited in scope by the athlete's discomfort and swelling but must include a neurovascular assessment. For the neurovascularly intact athlete, who has findings consistent with an ACL tear, acute treatment consists of instating knee immobilization, maintaining a non-weight-bearing status, and starting cryotherapy. Absence, or decreased intensity, of lower extremity pulses on the affected side can indicate compromise of neurovascular integrity, which may suggest a total knee dislocation (i.e., disruption of three or more ligaments in the knee at one time). As the mechanism of an ACL injury can resemble that of a knee dislocation, checking the neurovascular integrity of the limb is critical, as a knee dislocation is a surgical emergency that warrants immediate orthopedic evaluation and intervention to preserve the integrity of the lower leg.

In-Clinic Assessment

The initial knee effusion and limited range of motion noted on field often remain present at the follow-up evaluation in the clinic. The degree of motion limitation is due, in part, to the severity of the knee effusion and can also suggest the length of time since the injury (ex. chronic injury usually has no effusion). There can be tenderness to palpation of the tibial plateau. Quadriceps strength is compromised, and the anterior drawer and Lachman's maneuvers should lack a solid endpoint. For both tests, the knee is in flexion, and the tibia is quickly pulled forward. In the anterior drawer test, the patient lies supine on the table with the hip flexed, the knee at 90 degrees, and the foot planted on the exam table. The examiner sits lightly on the patients foot and places both hands around the proximal tibia to reach the pulling position. In Lachman's test, the patient lies supine on the table with the hip flexed and knee at 20–30 degrees. The examiner stabilizes the femur in one hand and places the other hand around the proximal tibia to reach the pulling position. Once again, the tibia is quickly pulled anteriorly in the same plane as the joint. A sudden jerking to a stop (i.e., solid endpoint) reflects an intact ACL, as the ACL prevents continued anterior motion of the tibia past the femur. The other ligamentous structures should be intact, unless concomitant damage has occurred. Meniscal pathology is present with an ACL injury about 20%–50% of the time; thus, McMurray maneuver, a circumduction-based meniscus test, can be equivocal with ACL tears, as there can be pain with this motion even in the absence of a true meniscus tear.

Diagnosis is highly suggested by the mechanism of injury described above and by a physical examination consistent with an insufficient ACL. In youth, this injury can be associated with a tibial or fibular fracture, due to the immature bone development and presence of centers of ossification; therefore, knee radiographs, initially AP and lateral views, are recommended. The definitive diagnosis of an ACL tear is determined by obtaining magnetic resonance imaging (MRI) of the knee. The child or adolescent with a suspected or confirmed ACL tear should be referred to a sports medicine physician or a pediatric/sports orthopedic surgeon.

Management – Surgical

In children and adolescents, damage to the ACL can be partial or complete, but often both require surgical intervention. One group with an exception to this requirement is the skeletally immature athlete or those less than 14 years of age with a partial ACL tear, as they are often treated non-operatively [7].

There has been controversy surrounding ACL reconstruction methods and timing following a complete ACL tear. For the skeletally mature athlete, immediate progression to ACL reconstruction remains the recommended course of intervention. Previously, for the skeletally immature, the clinician would initiate conservative therapy until skeletal maturity occurred, after which ACL reconstruction would be completed. Because of the poor outcomes associated with that management plan, repair is now typically performed on a timeline similar to that for the skeletally mature, so as to limit additional damage and long-term problems [6, 9–11]. What we currently know is that those that wait even 6–12 weeks have greater meniscus and chondral damage, placing them at higher risk of early arthritis [2, 3]. Currently, most patients undergo ACL reconstruction within a few weeks of injury. The more challenging question for the skeletally immature athlete with an ACL tear, and his/her surgeon, is the type of physeal-sparing surgical intervention or approach. There are also options for the source and type of graft used to complete the repair. As the concern for centers of growth no longer exists, the surgical approach for the skeletally mature youth athlete is similar to that for an adult. Someone familiar with the challenges of surgical management should be involved in the conversation with the family to facilitate the best decision for the athlete.

The predominance of females with ACL injury in sport does not correlate with the retrospective information gathered regarding those that undergo ACL reconstruction surgery [4]. In fact, in an epidemiology study from New York State, the number of males that had ACL reconstruction was equal to the number of females [4]. This may be due to increased numbers of males who experience trauma in collision sports or to a health care disparity between genders, regarding intervention. In this same study, Dowdell et al. found that those who had public health insurance were less likely to receive ACL reconstruction than those who had private insurance [4].

Management – Rehabilitation

As sustaining an ACL tear on one side increases the risk for tearing the contralateral side and experiencing a second tear on the repaired side, rehabilitation and prevention are important to limit or avoid, respectively, the profound long-term sequelae of having an ACL tear and undergoing reconstruction. Hewett et al. studied preventive measures and found that a functional rehabilitation program, with improvement of the dynamic valgus positioning (see image) and hamstring strength, can result in preventing ACL disturbance. In the group with a prior ACL reconstruction, incorporation of a prevention program is paramount. ACL prevention programs incorporate strength training, jump training, and core muscle strengthening. The athletic programs that incorporate these exercises into their regular warm up and conditioning program successfully promote an environment of injury prevention [8].

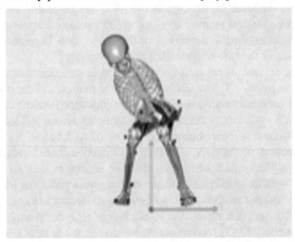

Outcomes

Although more children and adolescents return to play than adults after an ACL tear, many do not return to their prior level of sport. There is also a higher risk of revision due to graft failure and of subsequent ipsilateral and contralateral ACL injuries in pediatric patients compared to their adult counterparts [2]. This is the reason to stress the importance of primary prevention. As noted previously, it is common to have an associated meniscus injury with an ACL tear [3]. Any delay of treatment of these injuries increases the athlete's risk of having more extensive meniscus pathology and/or chondral pathology of the medial femoral condyle and medial tibial plateau [2, 3], which raises the likelihood of early arthritis.

Demonstration Cases

Common Case Presentation

A 16-year-old basketball player is going up for rebound and comes down awkwardly. She reports feeling a pop and immediate giving out of her left knee. She has immediate swelling, pain, and discomfort. She is helped off the court by her basketball coach and certified athletic trainer. Her knee is immobilized, and ice (cryotherapy) is applied.

She comes into the office wearing a knee immobilizer and using crutches for ambulation the following day. Her pain is improved with acetaminophen, nonsteroidal anti-inflammatory medications, and cryotherapy. There is a moderate knee effusion on physical examination. She is unable to flex and extend the knee fully. There is a loose endpoint on anterior drawer and Lachman tests with an intact posterior drawer, suggesting an ACL disruption. She has an equivocal McMurray. Strength testing in all directions of the hip and knee are decreased on the affected side. The remainder of the hip and knee exams are normal.

Complete radiographs are obtained and show no evidence of fracture or dislocation, but there is a large knee effusion. She is encouraged to continue cryotherapy and the assistance with her ambulation. An MRI is obtained, as you suspect an anterior cruciate ligament tear. The MRI demonstrates an ACL tear and a small medial meniscus tear.

The patient is referred to orthopedics for surgical intervention. She is encouraged to begin working on flexion and extension of the knee and to continue cryotherapy for pain control. She has a successful ACL and meniscus repair, completes physical therapy, and returns to sport 9 months later.

Uncommon Case Presentation

An 18-year-old girl is playing intercollegiate basketball. She jumps for a block, lands awkwardly on her right knee, and falls down. She is slow to get up and run to the other end of the court, and she continues to play the remainder of the game without event.

The following day she comes into your office complaining about significant knee swelling. She denies feeling a pop or giving out sensation in her right knee. She reports pain and discomfort that she attributes to the swelling. The pain has been responsive to the nonsteroidal anti-inflammatory medication she took overnight.

On physical examination, there is a moderate knee effusion. She has limited flexion but full extension. She has normal valgus and varus stress tests, suggesting normal medial and lateral collateral ligaments. The anterior drawer test is loose but does have an endpoint; Lachman test is positive; posterior drawer is intact. McMurray test causes her significant pain and discomfort. Strength testing is full and intact without significant abnormality. The remainder of the hip and knee exams are normal.

Complete radiographs are obtained and show no evidence of fracture or dislocation, but there is a large knee effusion. An MRI of the knee is obtained and shows complete rupture of the ACL.

The patient is referred to orthopedics for surgical intervention. She is encouraged to begin working on flexion and extension of the knee and to continue cryotherapy for pain control. She has a successful ACL and meniscus repair, completes physical therapy, and returns to sport 9 months later.

Summary

ACL injuries are increasing in frequency [3]. Primary prevention of the first ACL tear is optimal, as those who have had an ACL tear are at a much higher risk of a repeat injury. For those with a prior ACL tear, secondary prevention and rehabilitation activities should be pursued. While some risk factors (ex. gender) cannot be changed, lower extremity neuromuscular function and balance can be improved to decrease the risk of a tear. Clinicians involved in the care of young athletes should educate athletes, parents, and coaches about the value of incorporating ACL prevention activities into their sport preparation. Most skeletally immature and mature patients with a complete ACL tear should have it reconstructed in a timely manner [3, 7]. For the skeletally immature athlete, there should be consideration for a physeal- or growth plate-sparing procedure.

Condition	Anterior cruciate ligament injury
Description	Tear (complete or partial) of the ACL
Epidemiology	Slight female predominance (1.6:1)
Mechanism (common)	Plant and twist injury with knee in valgus
History and exam findings	Athlete felt/heard a pop, when pivoting
	Immediate swelling and instability – not able to return to play
	Effusion and limited motion on exam
	Absent endpoint with Lachman's and drawer tests
Management	Acute symptoms management
	Timely reconstruction followed by rehabilitation
	Physeal-sparing reconstruction for skeletally immature
	Primary prevention is key

References

1. Boden B, Sheehan F, Torg J, Hewett T. Noncontact anterior cruciate ligament injuries: mechanisms and risk factors. American Academy of Orthopaedic Surgeon. 2010;18(9):520–7.
2. DeFrancesco C, Storey E, Shea K, Kocher M, Ganley T. Challenges in the management of anterior cruciate ligament ruptures in skeletally immature patients. J Am Acad Orthop Surg. 2018;26(3):e50–61.
3. Dekker T, Rush J, Schmitz M. What's new in pediatric and adolescent anterior cruciate ligament injuries? J Pediatr Orthop. 2018;38(3):185–92.
4. Dodwell E, LaMont L, Green D, Pan T, Marx R, Lyman S. 20 years of pediatric anterior cruciate ligament reconstruction in New York state. Am J Sports Med. 2014;42(3):675–80.
5. Hewett T, Myer G, Ford K, Heidt R, Colosimo A, McLean S, van den Bogert A, Paterno M, Succop P. Biomechanical measures of neuromuscular control and valgus loading of the knee predict anterior cruciate ligament injury risk in female athletes: a prospective study. Am J Sports Med. 2005;33(4):492–501.
6. Hewett T, Torg J, Boden B. Video analysis of trunk and knee motion during non-contact anterior cruciate ligament injury in female athletes: lateral trunk and knee abduction motion are combined components of the injury mechanism. Br J Sports Med. 2009;43(6):417–22.
7. Joseph S, Huleatt J, Vogel-Abernathie L, Pace J. Treatment of ACL tears in the skeletally immature patient. Sports Med Arthrosc Rev. 2018;26(4):153–6.
8. Kocher M, Micheli L, Zurakowski D, Luke A. Partial tears of the anterior cruciate ligament in children and adolescents. Am J Sports Med. 2002;30(5):697–703.
9. Patel DR, Lyne D. Overuse injuries of the knee. In: Patel DR, editor. Pediatric practice: sports medicine. China: The McGraw Hill Education; 2009. p. 330–42.
10. Ramski D, Kanj W, Franklin C, Baldwin K, Ganley T. Anterior cruciate ligament tears in children and adolescents. Am J Sports Med. 2013;42(11):2769–76.
11. Tepolt F, Feldman L, Kocher M. Trends in pediatric ACL reconstruction from the PHIS database. J Pediatr Orthop. 2018;38(9):e490–4.

Chapter 13
Patellar Tendon Injury

Kiyoshi Yamazaki

Anatomy and Normal Function

The structure that connects the inferior patella (kneecap) to the proximal end of the tibia (shin) is the patellar tendon. In reality, this structure is a ligament rather than a tendon, composed of fibers connecting two bones together, rather than originating from a muscle body; however, as the superior patella is directly connected to the quadriceps muscle body by the quadriceps tendon, the patellar tendon indirectly serves as a teammate in extending the knee joint [1]. Structurally, the patellar tendon fibers extend over the anterior aspect of the patellar bone joining the descending fibers of the quadriceps tendon. The posterior aspect of the patellar tendon rests on and slides over the infrapatellar fat pad and infrapatellar bursa [1]. In pediatric patients, it is important to remember that the distal patellar tendon fibers attach to the tibial tubercle, which is the precise location of repetitive traction on the growth plate irritated in Osgood-Schlatter's disease.

Pathology and Dysfunction

Known in layman's terms as "jumper's knee," repetitive eccentric overuse of the patellar tendon may result in irritation and/or inflammatory changes described as patellar tendinopathy. Early on in the injury process, this might be labeled tendinitis, but we have recently come to understand the histopathology of this type of overuse tissue injury as a more mucoid degeneration process than simple inflammation [1, 2, 4]. This means that repetitive overuse that exceeds healing rest

K. Yamazaki (✉)
Non-Operative Sports Medicine Physician, HealthFit Clinic, Centura Castle Rock Adventist Hospital, Castle Rock, CO, USA

© Springer Nature Switzerland AG 2021
N. Coleman (ed.), *Common Pediatric Knee Injuries*,
https://doi.org/10.1007/978-3-030-55870-3_13

time can lead to collagen breakdown in the involved tendon [1–3]. The currently accepted term for this condition is patellar tendinosis or patellar tendinopathy. Predisposing conditions, like Osgood-Schlatter, Sindig-Larsen-Johanssen, or patellofemoral (pain) syndrome, can be found in pediatric patients complaining of patellar tendinopathy symptoms, either as concurrent diagnoses or as the initial etiology of their complaint [1, 4].

Specific Pointers

Epidemiology

Because they still have open growth plates, skeletally immature adolescents and children are less likely to sustain patellar tendon injuries than adults. These patients still can acquire this pathology, however, with year-round sports participation and early specialization (i.e., overuse). Pediatric patellar tendinopathy is most commonly seen in jumping sports, like volleyball, basketball, and ice skating, especially in preteens and teens who engage in repetitive submaximal stresses to the tendon [1–4]. The specific site of injury to the extensor mechanism occurs at the attachment at the inferior pole of the patella more often than at the tibial tuberosity. Nearly 20% of jumping athletes complain of this problem at some point in their sports participation, with a slightly greater incidence in males than females, due to increased loading of the patellar tendon in male athletes [4, 5, 6]. Although the subject of ongoing research, the gender difference in risk can range from almost equivalent to twice as likely in male v female athletes [5, 6]. In addition, decreased quadriceps and hamstring flexibility serves as a risk factor in developing this injury. In contrast to patellar tendinopathy, the presence of tears and complete rupture of the patellar tendon should prompt providers to consider secondary causes of tissue weakness, such as performance-enhancing drugs, bone/kidney disease, quinolone use, or trauma [1–4].

Mechanism of Injury

Patellar tendon injury most often occurs as a result of repetitive forceful contraction of the extensor mechanism of the knee. The eccentric contraction process of controlled lengthening of the tissues under an excessive load is what results in the microtears within the tissue matrix that develop into patellar tendinopathy. As such, the landing phase of a jump contributes more to the injury pathway than the take-off phase [1–4].

Diagnosis

The history and physical examination of the pediatric patient will provide the main diagnostic evidence for patellar tendon injury/dysfunction. These patients and their family members will usually present with insidious onset of anterior knee pain and tenderness at the proximal patellar tendon. The stage of injury is defined by the extent of life interference caused by the infrapatellar pain. Early Stage I patellar tendon injury will be characterized by discomfort after activity/sport, while a Stage II injury will cause pain at the beginning and end of activity/sport; advanced Stage III injury pain occurs both at rest and during activity/sport. Complete patellar tendon rupture, classified as a Stage IV injury, will not be discussed in detail in this chapter [1–4].

On examination, the patient will report point tenderness at the proximal patellar tendon, worse with the knee in extension rather than flexion. A positive Basset Sign describes this phenomenon of tenderness to palpation of the relaxed patellar tendon and lack of tenderness to palpation of the taut tendon. Activation, as well as over-stretching, of the extensor mechanism will also elicit discomfort. It is uncommon to find knee joint effusion, ligament instability, or direct bony tenderness in the pediatric patient with isolated patellar tendinopathy [1–4].

X-ray imaging should typically be normal, aside from occasional proximal calcifications found in more chronic cases or bony changes consistent with concurrent Sinding-Larsen-Johansson or Osgood-Schlatter's traction apophysitis. Though not usually necessary for the diagnosis of patellar tendinopathy, ultrasound (US) and magnetic resonance imaging (MRI) can display unique findings with this condition. US will reveal focal hypoechoic regions with enlargement of the tendon and occasional neovascularization in more chronic cases. An MRI may show increased signal within the deep region of the tendon distal to the patellar attachment [1–4].

Management

The mainstay of patellar tendinopathy management is non-operative, consisting of ice, relative rest, NSAIDS, counterforce strapping, and physical therapy. This approach has resulted in pain-free return to activity within 6 months for 90% of patients with isolated patellar tendinopathy [1–4, 7]. The early phases of rehabilitation should focus on pain reduction, quadriceps flexibility, and isometric strengthening; only after symptoms have resolved should rehabilitation progress to eccentric exercises. While some clinicians advocate for steroid injection in intractable cases, steroid usage is not recommended, due to the risk of patellar tendon rupture and the evolving understanding of steroid's potentially collagen-disruptive effects on tendon tissue [1–4, 8]. In more severe or recalcitrant cases, needle tenotomy, orthobiologics, or operative tenotomy may be considered. Needle tenotomy, which involves fenestration (creating multiple windows or holes) of the stalled degenerative tendon fibers, combined with an orthobiologic injection, like platelet-rich plasma (PRP), can be utilized as a non-operative means of restoring the diseased tendon. The goal with this technique is to prime the damaged tissue target and then introduce concentrated autologous bioactive factors to restart the healing cascade. Surgical tenotomy, the traditional operative version of this procedure (involving resection, debridement, and reattachment of the damaged tendon), can be performed if the needle tenotomy and orthobiologic approach fail. Finally, regardless of the treatment course chosen, once the patient's patellar tendon has healed from injury (exhibiting full passive and active range of motion without pain), it is essential to initiate a preventative exercise protocol to help avoid reinjury and allow for a successful return to sport and activity.

Demonstration Cases

Common Presentation

An 11-year-old male volleyball athlete presents to the sports medicine clinic with about 1 month of left anterior knee pain. He states that the pain came on insidiously during the season and denies ever feeling a pop or definitive moment of injury. The pain is worse when he ascends or descends stairs, as well as when he jumps or runs. Although his pain is relieved temporarily by ice, rest, and oral NSAIDs, it returns whenever he tries to run quickly or play volleyball. Recently, he has been complaining of this anterior knee pain even at rest. Physical examination reveals point tenderness at the proximal patellar tendon, especially when his knee is kept in extension. There is no joint effusion found, and both ligament and meniscus testing were negative. On-site x-ray images do not show any acute fracture or dislocation; the growth plates are open. A counterforce brace was selected and applied to facilitate relative rest while the athlete remained active, and a detailed sports medicine rehab program was initiated with physical therapy. This athlete was able to return to play volleyball immediately, while in the brace, and progressed appropriately to full sports clearance in about 8 weeks.

Uncommon Presentation

A 14-year-old left-handed female cheerleader is accompanied by her mother, as she presents to the sports medicine clinic with a complaint of 8 months of anterior right knee pain. The patient states that she first noticed a dull ache inferior to her kneecaps, when both of her knees began to ache off and on, especially when she would kneel or squat down deeply. The family was told these were symptoms of growing pains that, though irritating, would eventually subside once the patient finished growing. After joining competitive cheerleading 6 months ago, the patient noted increased intensity and frequency of her knee pain, right worse than left. While the discomfort was still anterior, it seemed to move upward toward the inferior pole of her kneecaps. The pain worsened with tumbling and aerial activities. As she continued to participate in competitive cheerleading, despite her pain, she noticed knee discomfort with simple walking to class or getting on and off a chair. Currently, she avoids any squatting and opts to bend at the waist to pick something up from the floor. Her only relief comes from rest and avoidance of running, squatting, and cheerleading stunts. Physical examination reveals point tenderness from the inferior pole of the patella down to the mid-body of the patellar tendon, especially when her knee is kept in extension. There is also mild tenderness at the tibial tubercle and, what appears to be, a bony prominence there. There is no joint effusion, and both ligament and meniscus testing are negative. On-site x-ray images do not show any acute fracture or dislocation; the growth plates are open; some micro-fragmentation at the tibial tuberosity is noted. A counterforce brace was selected and applied to facilitate relative rest while the athlete remained active, and a detailed sports medicine rehab program was initiated with physical therapy. This athlete was able to return to play volleyball immediately, while in the brace, and progressed appropriately to full sports participation in about 10 weeks. There was expected residual tenderness and mild ache at her tibial tubercles, which spontaneously resolved with the closure of her growth plates around her seventeenth birthday.

Pearls and Pitfalls
- Not all anterior knee pain in pediatric patients is Osgood-Schlatter's disease; a thorough history and hands-on examination is essential in making the complete diagnosis and successful management plan.
- Even for patients with patellar tendinopathy and a baseline of Osgood-Schlatter's disease, utilization of counterforce bracing and physical therapy techniques can dramatically relieve patient discomfort and allow return to sports, while the athlete is still actively growing.
- Bone and joint injuries, such as tibial avulsion or growth plate fractures, can masquerade as patellar tendon injuries; an effusion, direct bony or joint line tenderness, and pain with weight-bearing should be absent in pure patellar tendinopathy. The presence of these findings should raise the suspicion for other diagnoses and prompt further workup.
- The presence of a complete tear or rupture of the patellar tendon in the pediatric patient without a known traumatic injury should signal consideration of secondary causes of tissue weakness such as performance-enhancing drugs, bone or kidney disease, or quinolone use.

Chapter Summary

Patellar tendon injury is a fairly common etiology of pediatric anterior knee pain. While most always a non-surgical injury, this ailment can cause months of morbidity and loss of sports playing time in athletes. For this reason, proper diagnosis relies on detailed history-taking and a non-presumptive physical examination of the knee, which will result in a management plan for successful healing and rapid return to sport for the pediatric athlete. Early recognition of this diagnosis can help clinicians avoid unnecessary pain, delay in return to sports participation, and progression to stalled healing, tendinosis, or tear. Once the patient's patellar tendon has healed from injury, it is essential to initiate a preventative rehab protocol to help avoid reinjury in the future.

Condition Summary Table

Condition	Patellar tendon injury/patellar tendinopathy
Description	Repetitive overuse injury of knee extensor tendon that can lead to severe pain and dysfunction
Epidemiology	Boys slightly more than girls, jumping athletes
Mechanism	Repetitive forceful eccentric contraction
History and Exam	Insidious patella tendon pain and tenderness, especially in extension, without effusion/instability
Management	PRICE (Protect, Rest, Ice, Compression, Elevation) for acute symptoms, counterforce strap, PT; avoid steroid injection due to rupture risk. For intractable cases, needle/surgical tenotomy, orthobiologics may be considered

References

1. Brockmeier SF, Klimkiewicz JJ. Overuse Injuries. In: Johnson MD, Mair MD, editors. Clinical sports medicine. Inc.: Mosby; 2006. p. 625–6.
2. Ferretti A. Epidemiology of Jumper's knee. Sports Med. 1986;3(4):289–95.
3. Fischer, SJ, et al. Overuse Injuries In Children. orthoinfo.aaos.org [Internet]. Rosemont, IL. The American Academy of Orthopaedic Surgeons. 2012. Available from: https://orthoinfo.aaos.org/en/diseases—conditions/overuse-injuries-in-children/. Accessed 15 May 2019.
4. Wheeless, III, CR. Patellar Tendonitis (Jumper's Knee). wheelessonline.com [Internet]. Durham, NC. Accessed 12 April 2019.
5. Karahan M, Errol B. Muscle and tendon injuries in children and adolescents. Orthopedic Trauma Journal. 2004;38(1):37–46.
6. Jansen I. The influence of sex and skill level one patellar tendon loading during landing: University of Wollongong Research Online [Internet]; 2013. Available from http://or.uow.edu.au/theses/4257. Accessed 12 March 2019

7. Rudavsky A, Cook J. Physiotherapy Management of Patellar Tendinopathy (Jumper's knee). J Physiother. 2014;60(3):122–9.
8. Wei MD. A et al. the effect of corticosteroid on collagen expression in injured rotator cuff tendon. J Bone Joint Surg (Am Vol). 2006;88(6):1331–8.

Chapter 14
Quadriceps Tendon Injury

Kelly Davis and Katherine Rizzone

Anatomy and Function

The quadriceps muscle group is made up of four muscles: the vastus lateralis, vastus medialis, vastus intermedius, and the rectus femoris. All three vastus muscles originate on the femur. The vastus lateralis originates at the greater trochanter of the femur. The vastus intermedius is the deepest muscular layer and originates on the anterior surface of the upper two-thirds of the femur. The vastus medialis originates at the intertrochanteric line of the femur. The rectus femoris is superficial to the other three muscles and originates from the pelvis. The rectus femoris has two origination points: one on the upper rim of the acetabulum and a second on the anterior inferior iliac spine. All four muscles then converge together to form the quadriceps tendon that inserts onto the patella. The tendon then continues distally as the patellar tendon and inserts onto the tibial tubercle.

These four muscles act together to accomplish the quadriceps' primary function of knee extension. They also act as stabilizers of the knee, assist in hip flexion (rectus femoris), and assist in internal and external rotation of the knee (vastus medialis and lateralis, respectively). The quadriceps muscle is the only muscle that acts to extend the knee joint.

Another important role of the quadriceps muscle is as an antagonist to the hamstrings. Over-activation of the quadriceps may lead to imbalanced forces on the anterior cruciate ligament (ACL), potentially increasing the risk of injury. The balance of activation of the quadriceps with the hamstrings is an important part of ACL injury prevention.

K. Davis (✉)
Children's Hospital of Orange County, Orange, CA, USA
e-mail: kdavis@posocortho.com

K. Rizzone
Orthopaedics and Pediatrics, University of Rochester, Rochester, NY, USA
e-mail: katherine_rizzone@urmc.rochester.edu

© Springer Nature Switzerland AG 2021
N. Coleman (ed.), *Common Pediatric Knee Injuries*,
https://doi.org/10.1007/978-3-030-55870-3_14

In addition to the four primary muscles, there is a fifth muscle called the articularsi genus. This is a small flat muscle deep to the vastus intermedius that is responsible for tightening the synovial membrane during knee extension to prevent impingement of the synovial tissue between the femur and the patella [1].

The lateral circumflex femoral artery (LCFA) is the primary blood supply to the quadriceps muscle.

The muscle is innervated by the femoral nerve branches L2–L4.

Pathology and Dysfunction, Evaluation and Management

Quadriceps Tendinitis

Quadriceps tendinitis is inflammation of the quadriceps tendon from overloading of the knee's eccentric extensor mechanism. This leads to microscopic tears in the tendon, resulting in pain with activity. Risk factors include participating in running and jumping sports, such as basketball, volleyball, track, long jump, and high jump [2]. It is most commonly seen in adult male athletes.

On exam, the patient will have tenderness to palpation in the area of the quadriceps tendon, swelling, and pain with resisted knee extension. X-rays and ultrasound imaging can be performed to rule out other pathology. Magnetic resonance imaging (MRI) should be obtained, if there is concern for a tendon rupture.

Treatment for quadriceps tendinitis includes rest from the aggravating activity, ice, anti-inflammatory medication, and physical therapy. Physical therapy typically focuses on quadriceps muscle flexibility and eccentric strengthening to help alleviate the pain.

Quadriceps Tendon Tear

Quadriceps tendon tears are an uncommon injury (1.37/100,000) [3]. Males are four-to-eight times more likely to experience this injury than females [3, 4]. Tears are very rare in the pediatric population and mainly occur in men 40 years of age and older. Risk factors for a quadriceps rupture include a history of a chronic comorbidity, such as diabetes, renal failure, gout, rheumatoid arthritis, lupus, obesity, or hyperparathyroidism. Anabolic steroids, corticosteroid injections, and fluoroquinolone usage can also be associated with tendon ruptures [5].

Rupture of the tendon can occur, due to direct trauma or excessive eccentric loading of the quadriceps muscle. In athletes, tears are associated with a sudden forceful contraction of the quadriceps muscle during knee extension. This occurs when the foot is planted and the knee is slightly flexed. The tendon rupture usually occurs distally, one to two centimeters superior to the tendon insertion onto the superior patella. This area of the quadriceps tendon is a zone that is relatively hypovascular making it more vulnerable to rupture [6].

On exam, there is often pain and swelling at the superior aspect of the patella. In complete ruptures, the patient will be unable to perform knee extension and there can be a palpable defect just superior to the patella. In partial tears, the patient will have pain over the quadriceps tendon and will have difficulty extending the leg against resistance.

If a tear is suspected, plain films of the femur and knee should be performed to rule out a patellar or femur fracture. A complete tear of the tendon should be suspected on x-rays, if the patella appears inferior on the lateral view. If concerned, a contralateral lateral film can be taken for comparison. X-rays will not accurately visualize the soft tissue of the tendon. An ultrasound and/or an MRI should be performed to evaluate the integrity of the tendon. In complete quadriceps tendon ruptures or partial injuries resulting in loss of knee extension, prompt surgical evaluation and tendon repair is the most appropriate management. A partial tear with an intact extensor mechanism can be treated with knee immobilization in extension for 6 weeks followed by progressive knee range of motion and strengthening [7].

Quadriceps Muscle Strains

Quadriceps strains are a common acute injury in athletes. Strain injuries are more frequently seen in athletes participating in sprinting and jumping sports, such as soccer, rugby, and football [8]. A strain injury is due to an overstretching or sudden forceful eccentric contraction of the muscle with the knee flexed and the hip extended. The partial tearing of the fibers usually occurs at the ends of the muscle at the musculotendinous junction [9]. The rectus femoris is the most frequently injured quadriceps muscle. It is the only quadriceps muscle that crosses two joints, the hip joint and the knee joint, thus placing it at greatest risk for injury [9].

On exam, patients will have pain over the anterior thigh in the injured area and pain with resisted hip and knee motion testing. Grading of the strain can help provide guidance on eventual return to play. Grade I strains are due to minor tearing of the muscle and present with mild to moderate pain, full strength, and no palpable muscle defect. Grade II strains indicate more severe muscle fiber tearing and present with significant pain, decreased strength, and an occasional palpable defect. Grade III strains are a result of a complete tear of the muscle and present with severe pain, total loss of strength, and a palpable defect in the muscle [8]. Hematoma collection and bruising can be late findings after a strain occurs.

X-ray imaging should be considered to rule out any underlying fracture of the femur. X-ray images are often normal in the acute injury. Musculoskeletal ultrasound or MRI imaging can be performed to evaluate further the size of any developing hematoma and to evaluate for complete versus partial quadriceps muscle or tendon tears.

Treatment for quadriceps strains is focused on symptomatic treatment of the pain with compression, ice, anti-inflammatories, and rest from sports. Cryotherapy for quadriceps strains has been shown to decrease the pain associated with the injury [10]. After the initial period of rest (3–5 days), physical therapy should be initiated to introduce stretching, range of motion, and, eventually, strengthening. Once the athlete is pain-free, demonstrates full range of motion of the hip and knee, and has near full strength, when compared to the non-injured leg, gradual return to play can be initiated. Operative treatment may be considered for some cases of complete muscle tears that involve the musculotendinous junction or if there is persistent pain after conservative treatment.

Quadriceps Contusions

Quadriceps contusions are a common injury in athletes participating in contact sports, such as football, soccer, karate, judo, and rugby [11]. Contusions are a result of a direct blunt force trauma to the muscle. The muscle belly of the quadriceps rectus femoris is the most common location, in which to sustain a contusion [12].

On exam, patients will have pain and swelling over the area with decreased motion at the knee. Occasionally, a palpable mass can be felt if there is a large hematoma collection in the thigh.

X-ray imaging should be considered to rule out any underlying fracture of the femur. Musculoskeletal ultrasound or MRI imaging can be done to evaluate further the size of the hematoma and identify any concomitant quadriceps muscle or tendon tears that may also be present.

Treatment after a contusion injury consists of quadriceps muscle immobilization with the knee flexed to 120° for 24 hours. Anti-inflammatory medication can be taken to help decrease pain and inflammation in the area. After the initial period of immobilization, physical therapy and early motion should be started. Therapy should focus on passive and active stretching, as well as knee range of motion. As pain and motion improve, therapy can advance to quadriceps strengthening and eventual return to sport-specific activity, once strength and range of motion is equal to the contralateral side.

Complications can occur following quadriceps contusions. Due to the large amount of potential space in the quadriceps muscle area, extensive bleeding can generate a large hematoma [13]. This can lead to the development of compartment syndrome in the thigh, which is a surgical emergency that needs to be recognized and addressed rapidly. Myositis ossificans can also develop in the area of the contusion as it heals, approximately 3 weeks after the initial injury. There is more information on both of these conditions in the sections that follow.

Myositis Ossificans

Myositis ossificans, also known as heterotopic ossification, is a post-traumatic proliferation of bone and cartilage within a muscle following the formation of an intramuscular hematoma. This process occurred in 9–20% of muscle strains or contusions in studies of post-traumatic quadriceps hematomas [14, 15]. The formation of heterotopic bone after injury is more common in males than females. It most commonly occurs in adolescents and young adult athletes and is rare in athletes under the age of 10 years old. The quadriceps femoris and adductor muscles of the thigh are two of the most common sites for the formation of heterotopic bone [11].

Heterotopic ossification occurs as a result of liquefaction and formation of nonspecific sheets of cells that form at the center of the damaged muscle after the initial muscle injury. Local tissue exposure to inflammatory markers further recruits inflammatory cells and macrophages into the necrotic tissue of the muscle, which cause release of osteogenic bone mediators. These mediators encourage the formation of heterotopic bone in the damaged muscle. The new bony formation is laid down in an outside-to-inside pattern, which helps to distinguish it from an osteosarcoma, which typically begins centrally and then progresses outward. In the center of the myositis ossificans lesion is a mass of immature fibroblasts [16].

On exam, signs typically include a palpable firm mass, pain, tenderness, erythema, soft tissue swelling, and stiffness with progressive loss of range of motion. X-rays, an MRI, and/or ultrasound are the imaging modalities of choice to make the diagnosis. X-ray images (see Figs. 14.1 and 14.2) will show a peripheral ring of mature trabecular calcification with no calcification visible in the center of the lesion.

Myositis ossificans treatment includes rest, ice, anti-inflammatory medication, compression, and physical therapy. Anti-inflammatory treatment with indomethacin is considered the standard, but the use of ibuprofen, naproxen, or diclofenac are also effective treatment options [17–19]. Two additional therapies that are available for cases that are resistant to conservative treatments include bisphosphonates and extracorporeal shock wave therapy. Bisphosphonates have a similar structure to inorganic pyrophosphatates. These molecules play an important role in calcium–phosphate metabolism. Bisphosphonate suppresses bone turnover, slowing down the mineralization process by binding to hydroxyapatite, which decreases the transformation of amorphous calcium phosphate into hydroxyapatite crystals [20]. Bisphosphonates should not be used in the treatment of myositis ossificans in premenopausal women. Extracorporeal shock wave therapy has been utilized with the theory that the sound waves will disrupt the heterotopic bone formation [21, 22]. Neither of these additional therapies have been widely studied, and they have only been studied in conjunction with traditional therapies. More information is needed before using these therapies in place of standard management.

Fig. 14.1 Myositis
ossificans bony formation
after a quadriceps
contusion injury on lateral
knee x-ray

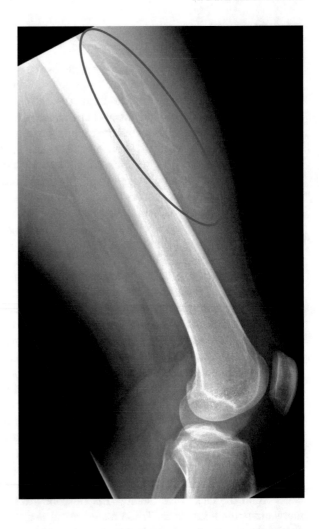

If the symptoms caused by myositis ossificans do not resolve with appropriate conservative therapy, surgical resection should be considered. Patients with persistent pain should be referred to an oncologic orthopedist for evaluation and eligibility as a surgical candidate. If the bony lesion is still metabolically active on a bone scan, resection may need to be postponed given the high rate of recurrence of the lesion after resection [23].

Fig. 14.2 Myositis ossificans bony formation after a quadriceps contusion injury on AP view knee x-ray

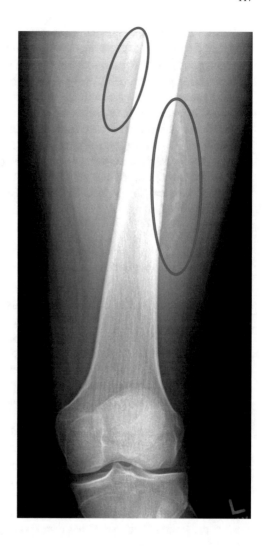

Saphenous Nerve Entrapment

The saphenous nerve is a sensory branch of the femoral nerve that provides sensation to the medial leg. It is the largest and longest branch of the femoral nerve. Its course runs deep to the sartorius muscle traveling laterally to medially as it descends distally in the thigh. It exits through Hunter's canal at the medial knee and then travels distally into the calf [24]. The exit site at the medial knee can be a site for entrapment of the nerve.

Saphenous nerve entrapment is a rare and often challenging diagnosis to make. On exam, it presents as vague medial knee pain with occasional radiation down the medial aspect of the leg into the foot [25]. It is often misdiagnosed as other more common etiologies of medial knee pain, such as a medial meniscus tear, medial collateral ligament sprain, or patellofemoral pain. Compression of the nerve can also be caused by kneeling for a prolonged period. This is called surfer's neuropathy.

Treatment is most often non-operative. Ice, anti-inflammatories, and heat can help relieve the pain. The use of knee pads or refraining from kneeling is beneficial in the case of surfer's neuropathy. For more refractory cases of nerve pain, injection with an analgesic medication and steroids can be effective in treatment and pain relief [22]. Surgical decompression can be performed, if pain is not improved with conservative treatments.

Compartment Syndrome

The thigh is composed of three compartments: the anterior compartment, medial compartment, and posterior compartment. The compartments of the thigh are much larger than those found in the forearm and lower leg. Due to the larger sizes of the compartments, a significantly higher amount of increased pressure is needed to create an environment conducive to compartment syndrome. The anterior compartment of the thigh is most often affected, potentially due to femur fractures, external compression, direct blunt trauma, quadriceps contusions, and atraumatic prolonged muscle use [26].

Athletes who participate in ball sports, such as soccer, basketball, and handball, have been shown to be at increased risk for trauma to the thigh and a resulting compartment syndrome [27–29]. Athletes participating in bodybuilding and spinning have also been shown to be at risk due to excessive use of the quadriceps muscles in these sports [30, 31].

Pain in the anterior thigh out of proportion to the mechanism of injury is often the first presenting symptom. Other symptoms include pain with passive stretching, weakness, and hyperesthesia [32, 33].

Treatment for compartment syndrome is rapid identification with surgical intervention and fasciotomy to relieve compartment pressures. Although compartment syndrome in the thigh is an uncommon injury, it is a surgical emergency, requiring a high index of suspicion for diagnosis and rapid treatment. Delays in treatment can result in significant muscular ischemia with possible loss of the limb or even death.

Rhabdomyolysis

Rhabdomyolysis is an uncommon but potentially life-threatening event that can be caused by excessive extreme exercise. After strenuous exercise, there is breakdown of the skeletal muscle, resulting in the release of creatine kinase (CK), aldolase, lactate dehydrogenase, and myoglobin into the bloodstream. The breakdown products are then filtered out of the blood and excreted from the body by the kidneys. The more strenuous and the longer the duration of activity, the more muscle breakdown is sustained. In high concentrations, this can lead to renal tubular obstruction and acute renal failure [34].

Young male athletes are at highest risk of developing rhabdomyolysis after activity. Other risk factors for developing rhabdomyolysis include use of creatine supplements, alcohol use, concurrent viral infection, sickle cell trait, extreme exercise, competition settings, and hot humid weather [35, 36].

Muscle soreness and dark tea-colored urine are common complaints. Other symptoms include muscle stiffness, nausea, headaches, increasing fatigue, cramps, disorientation, and confusion [31, 33]. A urine analysis should be performed to evaluate for myoglobinuria, and blood levels of creatine kinase, lactate dehydrogenase, and liver enzymes should be checked, if there is suspicion of rhabdomyolysis. In acute rhabdomyolysis, CK levels will be in the thousands. A high index of suspicion is needed with rapid onset of treatment to prevent serious renal injury and/or death.

Treatment for rhabdomyolysis includes aggressive fluid rehydration and supportive care, while monitoring for electrolyte imbalances, renal failure, compartment syndrome, and hemodynamic instability. In severe cases, dialysis may be needed until the patient's kidney function has recovered [31].

Once fully recovered, a slow gradual return to previous activity is needed to monitor carefully for the reoccurrence of symptoms. The return protocol monitors urine and CK levels at rest, at initiation of light activity, and then ultimately as the athlete gradually returns to full sport. Maintaining hydration and adequate rest with activity are also key components of successful return to sport and prevention of future recurrence [33].

Specific Pointers

Epidemiology: Pathology is more common in young male athletes participating in contact sports, kicking sports, and sports that require a lot of jumping. There is a higher incidence of injury among football, rugby, mixed martial arts, judo, karate, and soccer athletes. A second peak of injury is evident in men older than 40 years old, especially those with additional risk factors, such as renal disease, steroid use, and diabetes.

Mechanism of injury: Common causes of quadriceps injury are overuse and direct trauma to the muscle in athletes. Less common causes of injury can include anabolic steroids, fluoroquinolones, or corticosteroid injections. Chronic comorbidities, such as diabetes, renal failure, gout, rheumatoid arthritis, lupus, obesity, or hyperparathyroidism, can also be rare causes of tendon rupture.

Diagnosis: History and physical exam. On exam, evaluate for an extension lag or inability to extend the knee, a palpable defect of the quadriceps tendon, and swelling. Additional testing includes plain film x-rays, ultrasound, and/or MRI.

Management: Anti-inflammatory medications and physical therapy are the primary management for quadriceps tendinitis, contusions, and myositis ossificans. Prolonged immobilization should be avoided in these cases. Quadriceps tendon tears should be treated with immobilization and referral to surgery. Maintain a high index of suspicion for serious complications including compartment syndrome and rhabdomyolysis. Prompt intervention is required for treatment and can be life or limb saving.

Demonstration Cases

Common Presentation

A 17-year-old male athlete active in rugby presents after being kneed in his right anterior thigh by an opposing player during a game earlier that day. He notes pain in the anterior mid-thigh. He is only able to weight-bear minimally on the right with a limp. Ice was applied at the time of injury on the field.

On exam, there is mild swelling of the thigh with loss of full knee extension due to pain. He has tenderness to palpation of the anterior compartment of the thigh. No bruising. Normal sensation. Mild 4/5 weakness with quadriceps knee extension testing, with otherwise normal strength of the hamstring, calf, and foot.

His history and physical exam are consistent with the diagnosis of a quadriceps muscle contusion. X-rays of the thigh may be performed to rule out an underlying fracture. Treatment consists of immobilization for a 24-hour period with the knee in 120 degrees of flexion, followed by mobilization with physical therapy, ice, and anti-inflammatories. Evaluation for compartment syndrome, large hematoma, and myositis ossificans should be performed throughout the healing process. Return to play is determined by the resolution of his pain, normal range of motion of the knee, and normal strength with testing of the quadriceps muscle.

Uncommon Presentation

A 21-year-old male amateur bodybuilder presents with inability to extend the right knee after missing a step when walking downstairs 2 days ago. He reports feeling a painful pop in his knee, followed by inability to bear weight and swelling. Pain is located over the anterior proximal knee. When prompted, he does report a history of intermittent anabolic steroid use over the past several years, when training for bodybuilding competitions.

On exam, there is notable swelling over the anterior knee. When seated, he is unable to extend the knee. There is a palpable defect in the area of the quadriceps tendon. X-rays performed demonstrate an inferiorly displaced patella with edema without fracture.

History and physical exam are concerning for a complete tear of the quadriceps tendon. An MRI is performed and confirms the diagnosis. The knee is immobilized in extension and prompt surgical referral for evaluation and surgical repair is the next appropriate step in management.

Pearls and Pitfalls
- Although uncommon, it is important not to miss a quadriceps tendon tear.
- Do not forget to ask about anabolic steroid use, even in high school athletes.
- Do not immobilize a quadriceps strain/muscle belly tear for too long. Prolonged immobilization can lead to development of myositis ossificans. Early physical therapy and motion is key.
- Maintain a high index of suspicion for serious complications after quadriceps muscle injuries: myositis ossificans, compartment syndrome, or rhabdomyolysis.

Chapter Summary

The quadriceps muscle group consists of four muscles (vastus lateralis, vastus medialis, vastus intermedius, and rectus femoris) that converge together to form the patellar tendon. They act in conjunction to produce knee extension. Quadriceps injuries are sustained more frequently in contact and collision athletes. Severe injury to this muscle group is rare in the pediatric population. Quadriceps tendinitis and contusion injuries are much more common than serious injury to the muscle (compartment syndrome, myositis ossificans, or rhabdomyolysis) and account for about 90% of quadriceps injuries [9]. Although rare, serious complications after a quadriceps injury can occur. Close follow-up and monitoring are required with rapid intervention as needed.

Helpful Resources

Websites: orthobullets.com, orthoinfo.aaos.org

Table for Review

Condition	Quadriceps tendinitis	Quadriceps tendon tear	Quadriceps muscle strains	Quadriceps contusions	Myositis ossificans	Saphenous nerve entrapment	Compartment syndrome	Rhabdomyolysis
Description	Inflammation of the tendon	Complete rupture of the tendon	Overstretching of the muscle fibers leading to partial or complete tearing	Bruising of the muscle due to direct blunt force to the muscle	Post-traumatic proliferation of bone and cartilage in muscle	Entrapment of the saphenous nerve at the medial knee	Increased pressure due to bleeding or external compression	Skeletal muscle breakdown after strenuous activity resulting in elevated CK levels (>1000)
Epidemiology	Athletes in running and jumping sports Males > Females	Men > age 40-years-old Anabolic steroid use	Jumping and sprinting – soccer, rugby, football	Contact athletes – football, rugby, martial arts	Adolescents and young adults. Rare before age 10. Males > Females	Rare and often misdiagnosed	Soccer, basketball, and handball athletes	Young male athletes
Mechanism	Repetitive overloading of the knee's extensor mechanism leading to microscopic tears	Direct trauma or excessive eccentric loading of the muscle	Overstretching or sudden forceful eccentric contraction of the quadriceps muscle	Direct trauma to the muscle	Inflammation leading to bony formation in muscular hematomas after injury	Prolonged compression of the saphenous nerve with kneeling	Increased pressure accumulation in the anterior compartment of the thigh often due to bleeding after injury	Strenuous prolonged exercise, often in hot humid conditions
History and exam findings	Pain with activity, tenderness of the tendon on palpation, and pain with resisted knee extension	Swelling, pain, and inability to extend the knee	Pain on exam with decreased strength with knee extension and possible palpable muscular defect	Contact sport athlete with direct trauma to the muscle. Pain and swelling over the area with decreased motion at the knee. Occasionally a palpable mass can be felt if there is a large hematoma collection in the thigh	Muscle contusion with continued pain and firm palpable mass, swelling, loss of motion. Ossification on x-rays	Medial knee pain with radiation down the leg into the foot	Pain on exam out of proportion to history, swelling, pain with passive stretching, weakness, hyperesthesia	Muscle soreness, cramps, dark urine, headaches, nausea, confusion
Management	Rest, ice, anti-inflammatories, physical therapy	X-ray, ultrasound and/or MRI imaging Surgical repair	Rest, ice, compression, cryotherapy (i.e., exposure to extreme cold, ex. – 100 °C), anti-inflammatories with prompt start of physical therapy	Immobilization with knee in 120 degrees flexion for 24 hours followed by physical therapy, ice, anti-inflammatories	Rest, ice, indomethacin, compression, physical therapy. +/− bisphosphonates or extracorporeal shock wave therapy	Ice, anti-inflammatories, heat, avoid kneeling, knee pads	Rapid identification with surgical interventions and fasciotomy	Supportive care with aggressive fluid resuscitation and monitoring of renal function and hemodynamic status

References

1. Quiring DP, Warfel JH. The extremities. 2nd ed. Philadelphia: Lea & Febiger; 1963.
2. Garner RM, Gausden BE, Berkes TM, Nguyen GJ, Lorich GD. Extensor mechanism injuries of the knee: demographic characteristics and comorbidities from a review of 726 patient records. J Bone Joint Surg Am. 2015;97(19):1592–6.
3. Clayton RAE, Court-Brown CM. The epidemiology of musculoskeletal tendinous and ligamentous injuries. Injury. 2008;39:1338–44.
4. Ilan DI, Tejwani N, Keschner M, Leibman M. Quadriceps tendon rupture. J Am Acad Orthop Surg. 2003;11(3):192–200.
5. Pope JD, Plexousakis MP. Quadriceps tendon rupture. Treasure Island: StatPearls Publishing; 2018.
6. Yepes H, Tang M, Morris SF, Stanish WD. Relationship between hypovascular zones and patterns of rupture of the quadriceps tendon. J Bone Joint Surg Am. 2008;90:2135–41.
7. Nori S. Quadriceps tendon rupture. J Family Med Prim Care. 2018;7(1):257–60.
8. Kary JM. Diagnosis and management of quadriceps strains and contusions. Curr Rev Musculoskelet Med. 2010;3:26–31.
9. Järvinen TAH, Järvinen TLN, Kääriäinen M, Kalimo H, Järvinen M. Muscle injuries: biology and treatment. Am J Sports Med. 2005;33(5):745–64, 20p.
10. Bleakley C, McDonough S, MacAuley D. The use of ice in the treatment of acute soft-tissue injury: a systematic review of randomized controlled trials. Am J Sports Med. 2004;32:251–61.
11. Beiner JM, Jokl P. Muscle contusion injuries: current treatment options. J Am Acad Orthop Surg. 2001;9(4):227–37.
12. Ryan JB, Wheeler JH, Hopkinson WJ, Arciero RA, Kolakowski KR. Quadriceps contusions: west point update. Am J Sports Med. 1991;19:299–304.
13. Jackson DW, Feagin JA. Quadriceps contusions in young athletes: relation of severity of injury to treatment and prognosis. J Bone Joint Surg Am. 1973;55:95–105.
14. Beiner JM, Jokl PJ. Muscle contusion injuries: current treatment options. Am Acad Orthop Surg. 2001;9(4):227–37.
15. Jackson DW, Feagin JA. Quadriceps contusion in young athletes. J Bone Joint Surg Am. 1973;55:95–105.
16. Walczak BE, Johnson CN, Howe BM. Myositis ossificans. J Am Acad Orthop Surg. 2015;23(10):612–22, ISSN: 1940-5480.
17. Macfarlane RJ, Ng BH, Gamie Z, Masry MA, Velonis S, Schizas C, et al. Pharmacological treatment of heterotopic ossification following hip and acetabular surgery. Expert Opin Pharmacother. 2008;9(5):767–86.
18. Baird EO, Kang QK. Prophylaxis of heterotopic ossification – an updated review. J Orthop Surg Res. 2009;4:12. Published online 2009 Apr 20.
19. Barthel T, Baumann B, Noth U, Eulert J. Prophylaxis of heterotopic ossification after total hip arthroplasty (a prospective randomized study comparing indomethacin and meloxicam). Acta Orthop Scand. 2002;73:611–4.
20. Mani-Babu S, Wolman R, Keen R. Quadriceps traumatic myositis ossificans in a football player: management with intravenous pamidronate. Clin J Sport Med. 2014;24(5):e56–8.
21. Torrance DA, Degraauw C. Treatment of post-traumatic myositis ossificans of the anterior thigh with extracorporeal shock wave therapy. J Can Chiropr Assoc. 2011;55(4):240–6.
22. Buselli P, Coco V, Notarnicola A, Messina S, Saggini R, Tafuri S, et al. Shock waves in the treatment of post-traumatic myositis ossificans. Ultrasound Med Biol. 2010;6(3):397–409.

23. Thorndike A. Myositis ossificans traumatica. J Bone Joint Surg. 1940;22:315–23.
24. Kalenak A. Saphenous nerve entrapment. Oper Tech Sports Med. 1996;4(1):40–5.
25. Mozes M, Ouaknine G, Nathan H. Saphenous nerve entrapment simulating vascular disorder. Surgery. 1975;77:299–303.
26. Tarlow SD, Achterman CA, Hayhurst J, et al. Acute compartment syndrome in the thigh complicating fracture of the femur. A report of three cases. J Bone Joint Surg Am. 1986;68:1439–43.
27. Robinson D, On E, Halperin N. Anterior compartment syndrome of the thigh in athletes-indications for conservative treatment. J Trauma. 1992;32:183–6.
28. Diaz JA, Fischer DA, Rettig AC, et al. Severe quadriceps muscle contusions in athletes: a report of three cases. Am J Sports Med. 2003;31:289–93.
29. Riede U, Schmid MR, Romero J. Conservative treatment of an acute compartment syndrome of the thigh. Arch Orthop Trauma Surg. 2007;127:269–75.
30. Bidwell JP, Gibbons CE, Godsiff S. Acute compartment syndrome of the thigh after weight training. Br J Sports Med. 1996;30:264–5.
31. Bertoldo U, Nicodemo A, Pallavicini J, et al. Acute bilateral compartment syndrome of the thigh induced by spinning training. Injury. 2003;34:791–2.
32. Uzel A-P, Bulla A, Henri S. Compartment syndrome of the thigh after blunt trauma: a complication not to be ignored. Musculoskelet Surg. 2013;97:81–3.
33. Burns BJ, Sproule BJ, Smyth H. Acute compartment syndrome of the anterior thigh following quadriceps strain in a footballer. Br J Sports Med. 2004;38:218–20.
34. Khan FY. Rhabdomyolyis: a review of the literature. Neth J Med. 2009;67(9):272–83.
35. Knochel JP. Catastrophis medical events with exhaustive exercise: "White collar rhabdomyolysis". Kidney Int. 1990;38:709–19.
36. Kim J, Lee J, Kim S, Ryu HY, Cha KS, et al. Exercise-induced rhabdomyolysis mechanisms and prevention: A literature review. J Sport Health Sci. 2016;5:324–33.

Chapter 15
Infrapatellar (Hoffa's) Fat Pad Conditions

Valerie E. Cothran and Svetlana Dani

Anatomy and Normal Function

The infrapatellar fat pad (IPFP), also known as Hoffa's fat pad, is the largest of three fat pads in the anterior knee (Fig. 15.1). The pediatric IPFP, much like the adult IPFP, is an intracapsular but extrasynovial structure, bordered anteriorly by the patellar tendon, superiorly by the inferior pole of the patella, inferiorly by the proximal tibia and the deep infrapatellar bursa, and posteriorly by the joint synovium. It is attached to the anterior horns of both the medial and lateral menisci. The IPFP is the largest soft tissue structure in the knee joint.

Function

The exact role of the IPFP is not completely understood. It is a soft mobile structure and changes position as the knee moves through range of motion. It becomes lateralized and moves posteriorly in flexion. During extension, it moves anteriorly, away from the anterior tibia. It is easily deformable, which allows the expansion of the synovial compartment and facilitates the distribution of the joint fluid. It is made of adipocytes and connective tissue. Additionally, it is a potent generator of stem cells, which allows the IPFP cells to differentiate into osteoblasts and chondrocytes but also predisposes it to scarring [12]. The IPFP has been shown to play both a

V. E. Cothran (✉)
Primary Care Sports Medicine, University of Maryland, Department of Family and Community Medicine, College Park, MD, USA
e-mail: vcothran@som.umaryland.edu

S. Dani
University of Maryland, College Park, MD, USA

© Springer Nature Switzerland AG 2021
N. Coleman (ed.), *Common Pediatric Knee Injuries*,
https://doi.org/10.1007/978-3-030-55870-3_15

Fig. 15.1 A midsagittal
view of the knee joint. (1)
IPFP, (2) posterior fat pad,
(3) anterior suprapatellar
fat pad, (4) posterior
suprapatellar fat pad. The
IPFP is located inferior to
the patella and posterior to
the patellar tendon. It is
covered by the joint
capsule (white arrow) and
is anterior to the synovium
(black arrow); thus, it is an
intracapsular but
extrasynovial structure

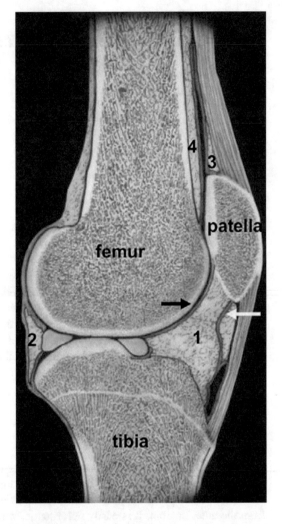

biomechanical role in patella stabilization, as well as an inflammatory role in the
knee joint by secreting pro-inflammatory or anti-inflammatory cytokines, which
may play a role in degenerative osteoarthritis later on in life.

Innervation

The IPFP is heavily innervated, which makes it very sensitive to pain. The predominant nerve supply to the IPFP is the posterior tibial nerve, which provides the majority of fibers to the popliteal plexus. Fibers course from the popliteal plexus
innervating the posterior capsule and the cruciate ligaments and then course anteriorly up to the IPFP [1].

Blood Supply

The IPFP blood supply comes from the upper and lower geniculate arteries. Its vascularization is an anastomosis made of two vertical arteries and two or three horizontal arteries connecting the vertical arteries. These anastomoses allow for rich vascularity at the periphery but poor blood supply in the center (Fig. 15.2) [1, 8].

Pathology and Dysfunction

Pathologic conditions affecting the IPFP are typically caused by inflammation and fibrosis associated with trauma. Trauma may be from a direct blow, acute hyperextension, chronic irritation, or postsurgical scarring (due to trauma from portals placed during arthroscopic surgery).

Epidemiology

IPFP injuries occur more commonly in young women. Athletes that participate in sports that require forceful terminal extension of the knee, such as dance, gymnastics, swimming, martial arts, and jumping field events (high jump, long jump, and triple jump), are also at a higher risk [2]. In both athletes and nonathletes, individuals with ligamentous laxity are at increased risk, likely due to hypermobility, causing repetitive hyperextension of the knee.

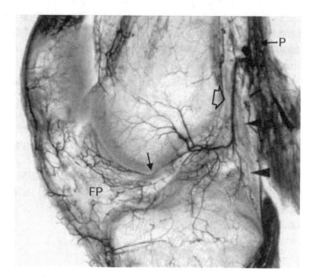

Fig. 15.2 Vascularization of the infrapatellar fat pad (IPFP). Spalteholz preparation of a 2 cm thick sagittal section of the right knee from a 33-year-old male showing the anastamotical connection between the IPFP and the anterior cruciate ligament (small arrow); middle genicular artery (open arrow), posterior capsule (arrowheads) [12]. FP = fat pad; P = popliteal artery

Mechanism of Injury

The most common disorder of the IPFP is Hoffa's disease or IPFP impingement, an intrinsic injury to Hoffa's fat pad stemming from impingement of the IPFP between the femur and the tibia during extension [9]. This causes inflammation of the fat pad, which leads to hypertrophy and then to a cycle of bleeding, acute inflammation, and, ultimately, chronic inflammation with necrosis, fibrosis, and even ossification of the IPFP [3, 10].

Diagnosis (History/Exam Findings/Testing)

Patients often report anterior knee pain, especially when climbing and descending stairs. Physical examination of the athlete with IPFP impingement should begin the same as for other knee injuries. On inspection, there may be no visible gross signs. Often there is localized swelling adjacent to the patellar tendon. Some patients may have a small joint effusion. There may be diffuse tenderness over the patellar tendon. The IPFP can be palpated by placing a finger on either side of the proximal patellar tendon. Passive and active knee extension and flexion should be assessed and compared to the contralateral side. Young athletes may have pain with terminal extension and may exhibit decreased range of motion as compared to the unaffected side. Strength testing of the affected knee should be compared to the contralateral side. There may be pain with resisted knee extension.

As with other components of the knee, there is a special test to evaluate for IPFP impingement, Hoffa's Test. To start Hoffa's test, the patient is made to lie supine on the examination table with the knee in flexion (30°–60°). The examiner puts pressure on the anterior fat pat by placing a finger on either side of the proximal patellar tendon. The patient is instructed to straighten the knee. The test may also be performed with passive extension of the knee by the examiner. The test is positive when the pain is reproduced with extension of the knee.

Imaging can be obtained but is often unnecessary for IPFP impingement, unless other injuries are also suspected, based on the patient's history and exam. Plain radiographs are often normal. In some cases, a small joint effusion or soft tissue swelling may be seen. Ultrasound (US) is a cost-effective, point-of-care imaging modality that may be used to evaluate the IPFP. It may demonstrate enlargement and/or decreased echogenicity within the IPFP. Color Doppler US may demonstrate the increased vascularity associated with inflammation. Dynamic US may demonstrate impingement of the fat pad during terminal extension. Magnetic resonance imaging (MRI) allows a detailed assessment of the normal anatomy of the IPFP and other internal knee structures [6].

Management

Conservative treatment is first-line therapy: relative rest, anti-inflammatory medications, local cryotherapy, and physical therapy (strengthening of the quadriceps). Evaluation of biomechanics with corrective physical therapy is important for rehabilitation and for prevention of future issues [3]. Avoidance of terminal extension should be reinforced. Superficially, taping the knee can reduce the amount of tilt of the patella. Injections of corticosteroids into the IPFP have been effective in treating pain. This should be done with caution to avoid fat atrophy. If the above measures fail, arthroscopic resection is the treatment of choice [4].

Inflammatory and Neoplastic Conditions

Inflammatory and neoplastic diseases can arise in the fat pad, as well. Although the majority are benign lesions, malignant tumors have been observed. These patients present with pain and swelling of the anterior knee. A palpable lump is seen sometimes. There is usually no history of trauma. The most common pediatric IPFP benign tumor is a hemangioma. These lesions are responsive to conservative treatment and will usually become asymptomatic with time. If symptoms of pain and the feeling of fullness persist, resection of the hemangioma is recommended [5, 7].

The pediatric malignant tumors of the IPFP observed in literature are synovial sarcomas, which seem to be unique to the pediatric population. Differences in the presentation of benign and malignant tumors have not been observed. MRI is the diagnostic study of choice for the evaluation of IPFP tumors. An x-ray may be helpful in identifying calcifications, which can be seen in synovial sarcomas. US may be helpful, as well. A combination of a soft tissue mass with calcifications or ossifications should raise the suspicion of a synovial sarcoma in pediatric patients. A biopsy is required to confirm the diagnosis. Open arthrotomy and excision ensures complete removal, which is not always possible with arthroscopy [5, 7].

Ganglion cysts arising from the IPFP have been described in the pediatric population, as well. They present with prolonged painless swelling at the anterior aspect of the knee. MRI is the diagnostic tool of choice for evaluation, if the cyst causes pain and discomfort, arthroscopic resection is the definitive cure.

IPFP Herniation

In children with a painless knee mass at the anterolateral aspect of the infrapatellar region, herniation of the IPFP through a defect in the lateral retinaculum should be suspected. This is seen mostly in the pediatric population and is likely due to congenital weakness of the lateral retinaculum. These children present with a painless mass and are not tender to palpation. There is never any history of preceding trauma or overlying skin changes. The mass is not visible or palpable during full-knee extension. A dynamic US is the best modality for evaluation and will show a focal defect in the anterolateral aspect of the lateral retinaculum with Hoffa's fat pad herniating through the defect during knee flexion and reducing with knee extension. If US is not available, an MRI may offer the answer. Consider obtaining views in knee flexion. When diagnosed, this condition can be managed conservatively; however, there are case reports of painful IPFP herniations. In those cases surgical repair of the lateral retinaculum defect is possible and helpful [11, 13].

Chapter Summary

Although we lack completely understanding about the function of the IPFP, it can present with significant pain and disability. The first-line therapy for IPFP impingement is conservative treatment, although steroid injections and surgery have been effective, when conservative measures fail. We must keep inflammatory and neoplastic conditions in the differential, especially if the patient presents with a knee mass. IPFP herniation may be seen in the pediatric population, as well.

Chart/Table

Condition	Infrapatellar fat pad impingement
Description	Impingement of the IPFP during terminal extension of the knee.
Epidemiology	Seen more commonly in young women and in individuals with ligamentous laxity.
Mechanism (common)	Overuse – Chronic terminal extension.
History and exam findings	Anterior knee pain. Point tenderness over the IPFP (adjacent to the proximal patellar tendon). Increased with terminal extension of the knee.
Management	Relative rest. Activity modification (avoid terminal extension). Physical therapy. Surgical excision is reserved for recalcitrant cases.

References

1. Benninger B (2016) Knee. In: Gray's anatomy, 40th ed. Standring S (Ed). London: Elsevier. 2016, p 1395.
2. Bernhardt DT. Overuse injuries of the knee. In: Harris SS, Anderson SJ, editors. Care of the young athlete. 2nd ed. Elk Grove Village, Illinois: American Academy of Orthopedic Surgeons, American Academy of Pediatrics; 2010. p. 421.

3. Dragoo JL, Johnson C. McConnell evaluation and treatment of disorders of the infrapatellar fat pad. J Sports Med. 2012;42:51.
4. Hannon J, Bardenett S, Singleton S, Garrison JC. Evaluation, treatment, and rehabilitation implications of the infrapatellar fat pad. Sports Health. 2016;8(2):167–71.
5. Helpert C, Davies AM, Evans N, Grimer RJ. Differential diagnosis of tumours and tumour-like lesions of the infrapatellar (Hoffa's) fat pad: pictorial review with an emphasis on MR imaging. Eur Radiol. 2004;14(12):2337–46.
6. Jacobson JA, Lenchik L, Ruhoy MK, Schweitzer ME, Resnick D. MR imaging of the infrapatellar fat pad of Hoffa. Radiographics. 1997;17(3):675–91.
7. Albergo JI, Gaston CLL, Davies M, Abudu AT, Carter SR, Jeys LM, Tillman RM, Grimer RJ. Hoffa's fat pad tumours: what do we know about them? Int Orthop. 2013;37:2225–9.
8. Kohn D, Deiler S, Rudert M. Arterial blood supply of the infrapatellar fat pad. Anatomy and clinical consequences. Arch Orthop Trauma Surg. 1995;114:72–5.
9. Larbi A, Cyteval C, Hamoui M, Dallaudiere B, Zarqane H, Viala P, et al. Hoffa's disease: a report on 5 cases. Diagn Interv Imaging. 2014;95:1079–84.
10. Mace J, Bhatti W, Anand S. Infrapatellar fat pad syndrome: a review of anatomy, function, treatment and dynamics. Acta Orthop Belg. 2016;82:94–101.
11. Rocha R, Ramos R, Campos J et al. Focal herniation of Hoffa's fat pad through a retinaculum defect. 2011.Obtained 11/26/2019 at http://www.eurorad.org/case.php?id=9401.
12. Wickham MQ, Erickson GR, Gimble JM, Vail TP, Guilak F. Multipotent stromal cells derived from the infrapatellar fat pad of the knee. Clin Orthop Relat Res. 2003;412:196–212.
13. Menzies-Wilson R, Twyman R. A case report: painful Hoffa's fat pad herniation. Current Orthopaedic Practice. 2018;29(5):510–1.

Chapter 16
Posterior Cruciate Ligament Injury

Stephanie Lamb, Steven Koch, and Nathaniel S. Nye

Anatomy and Normal Function

The posterior cruciate ligament (PCL) is the largest ligament in the knee and is nearly twice as strong as the ACL. The PCL is an intra-articular ligament and is surrounded by a synovial sheath [1–3]. The PCL lies between two meniscofemoral ligaments: the ligament of Humphrey is anterior to the PCL, while the ligament of Wrisberg lies posterior to the PCL [1]. It originates along the anterolateral aspect of the medial femoral condyle, within the intercondylar notch, and inserts on the posterior aspect of the tibial plateau just distal to the joint line [2, 4]. Its blood supply comes from the middle genicular artery, and it is innervated by branches of the tibial nerve [1, 2].

The primary function of the PCL is to resist excessive posterior translation of the tibia relative to the femur; however, the PCL plays an important role in rotational stability, as well [2, 3]. The PCL is comprised of two bundles, the larger anterolateral bundle (ALB) and the smaller posteromedial bundle (PMB). Historically, these two bundles were believed to function independently in a reciprocal nature, with the ALB acting in knee flexion and the PMB acting during knee extension; however, recent research suggests that they actually function synergistically and play a crucial role in stabilizing the knee during all angles of knee flexion [2, 3].

S. Lamb · S. Koch
Sports Medicine Clinic, 559th Medical Group, JBSA-Lackland, TX, USA

N. S. Nye (✉)
Sports Medicine Clinic, Fort Belvoir Community Hospital, Ft. Belvoir, VA, USA
e-mail: Nathaniel.s.nye.mil@mail.mil

© Springer Nature Switzerland AG 2021
N. Coleman (ed.), *Common Pediatric Knee Injuries*,
https://doi.org/10.1007/978-3-030-55870-3_16

Specific Pointers

In acute cases, pain and guarding may make initial examination both difficult and unreliable. Re-examination within 1 week of injury and additional diagnostic imaging should be considered for proper diagnosis.

PCL avulsion fractures are easily missed on radiographs but are best seen on lateral views. Stress views (posterior tibial stress or kneeling views) are helpful to rule out instability.

MRI is highly sensitive and specific in acute cases but may give false negatives in cases of chronic PCL deficiency.

Pathology and Dysfunction

Reports of PCL injuries in children are rare; thus, the natural history of PCL deficiency in the pediatric population is unknown. PCL injuries in children with open physes most commonly involve an avulsion fracture at either the femoral or tibial insertion site. Mid-substance tears are rarely seen until after the physes have closed [4–8]. Femoral-sided avulsion fractures are more commonly reported than tibial-sided avulsion fractures in the pediatric population [5, 9].

As knowledge of the anatomy and biomechanics of the PCL grows, so has understanding of the importance of the PCL. PCL deficiency leads to abnormal loading and kinematics with functional activities. These abnormal biomechanics, along with chronic instability, are linked to increased risks of articular cartilage degeneration, osteoarthritis, meniscal injury, and subsequent total knee replacement [2, 10, 11].

Epidemiology

Due to the infrequency of PCL injuries in children, the epidemiology is not yet certain. PCL injuries are more common in boys [6, 12, 13]. PCL injuries are more commonly seen in sports, especially ballistic or pivoting sports that carry risk of falling on a flexed knee or a direct blow to the anterior tibia, such as football, basketball, skiing, soccer, track, and gymnastics [14]. Other common activities for PCL injuries in children include falling off bicycles, knee hyperextension on trampolines, and falling off playground equipment, such as monkey bars [9, 14].

Mechanism of Injury

Traffic accidents and sport/play activities are the most common causes of PCL injuries in children. Typical mechanisms include a posteriorly directed force applied to the anterior aspect of the tibia, while the knee is in a flexed position ("dashboard injury") and falling onto the knee with the foot in a plantarflexed position. Non-contact mechanisms are less common and include knee hyperflexion and hyperextension [3, 5, 6].

Diagnosis

History

Children typically present with pain, swelling, limited range of motion, and difficulty bearing weight after acute injury occurs [1, 3, 7, 9]. Symptoms are typically mild and vague. Unlike with ACL injury, no "pop" or "tear" is usually reported [1].

From a functional standpoint, some children are able to compensate for their PCL deficiency rather well, and symptoms may not present right away. Children with delayed symptoms generally report having repeated episodes of effusion, pain in the anterior knee, and difficulty performing regular activities, due to calf fatigue and pain. They may also report difficulty with squatting and sitting cross-legged on the ground [7].

Exam Findings

Acute PCL injuries typically present with a knee effusion, tenderness in the popliteal space, and limited range of motion at the knee. There may be a contusion, laceration, and/or abrasion on the anterior aspect of the tibia, providing clues to the specific mechanism of injury. The posterior drawer test, posterior sag sign, quadriceps active test, Clancy sign, and dial tests are all used to assess the integrity of the PCL. The posterior sag sign is the most sensitive test for PCL integrity, while quadriceps active test is the most specific test. The posterior sag test is performed with the patient in a supine position with both the hips and knees flexed to 90 degrees while the provider supports the lower legs. Posterior sagging of the tibia signifies a positive test. The quadriceps active test uses the same patient and provider positioning required for the posterior drawer test (see Fig. 16.1). In a PCL-deficient knee, the tibia will be dynamically reduced, when the patient performs an isometric quadriceps contraction. A positive Clancy sign is the loss of normal medial and lateral tibial plateau prominences beneath the femoral condyles with palpation when the knee is flexed to 90 degrees and neutrally rotated. The dial test is used to assess for combined lesions to the posterior lateral corner (PLC) of the knee by assessing external rotation asymmetry. Increased external rotation of 10 degrees or more is considered abnormal. With the patient in either a supine or prone position, the provider should apply an external rotation force to both feet with the knees at 30 degrees of flexion and then again at 90 degrees of flexion. Increased external rotation at 30 degrees only is consistent with isolated PLC injury, while increased external rotation at 30 and 90 degrees is consistent with PLC and PCL injury. Laxity may be

Fig. 16.1 The quadriceps active test is performed in the same starting position as the posterior drawer test, with the knee flexed to 90⁰ and the foot flat on the exam table. The examiner then stabilizes the ankle and asks the patient to flex their quadriceps, watching for auto reduction of the knee

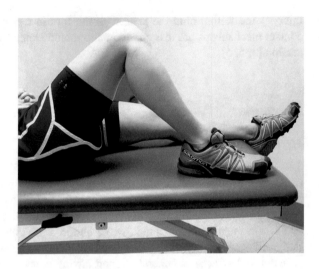

easily missed in acute stages, due to reflexive muscle spasm and painful mobilization. Clinical examination should include careful comparison to the contralateral knee [1, 3, 5, 7, 8, 11].

Tests, such as the posterior drawer test, allow PCL tears to be graded based on the position of the medial tibial plateau relative to the medial femoral condyle, while the knee is in 90° of flexion. In this position, the medial tibial plateau is roughly 10 mm anterior to the medial femoral condyle. With grade I injuries, 0–5 mm of laxity is seen with posterior drawer, and the tibia is still anterior to the femoral condyles, but the distance is slightly diminished. Grade II injuries are characterized by 5–10 mm of laxity, and the tibia is even with the femoral condyles. Grade III injuries (complete PCL rupture) typically demonstrate greater than 10 mm of laxity, and the tibia can be pushed posteriorly beyond the medial femoral condyle [3, 4, 15].

Testing

Imaging tools, such as radiographs and MRI, should be included as part of the clinical evaluation. Plain radiography is recommended as first-line imaging, due to low cost, high availability, and high specificity for associated injuries, such as fracture, but has a low sensitivity for PCL tears. Standard weight-bearing radiographs should be used to assess joint space and congruity and to detect bony abnormalities. Lateral views are important for identifying an avulsion fracture. Fragments displaced more than 10 mm on radiographs are easily visualized, but fragments displaced less than 10 mm are easily overlooked [5]. Posterior stress radiographs provide an objective measurement of posterior knee laxity and may be helpful for diagnosis, if instability is noted during physical exam. Alternatively, kneeling stress radiographs may be

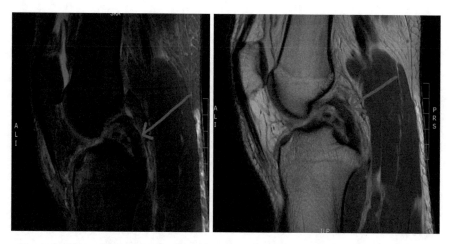

Fig. 16.2 Femoral sided avulsion of PCL without fracture seen on MRI, sagittal PDFS image. Note buckling of the PCL

used to measure the magnitude of posterior tibial displacement on the femur and allow for comparison between injured and uninjured sides [1, 3, 5].

MRI is highly accurate in diagnosing acute PCL tears and is useful for ruling out derangement of other internal knee structures (see Fig. 16.2); however, in chronic cases, MRI is less sensitive (may give false negatives), because the natural process of tissue healing after a PCL tear may mimic the MRI appearance of a native, uninjured PCL [1, 3].

Management

Due to the rarity of PCL injuries in pediatric populations, management is generally comparable to accepted protocols for adult populations [4, 7, 8]. Some isolated midsubstance tears and many non-displaced or minimally displaced avulsion fractures are often given a trial of nonoperative management, reserving surgical intervention for cases with persistent symptoms of pain or instability. Surgical reduction and internal fixation should be considered for avulsion fractures with greater than 5–7 mm displacement [5, 11]. Given that chronic PCL deficiency in adults is associated with instability and degenerative changes, it stands to reason that optimization of treatment is even more crucial in pediatric populations to preserve knee function.

A three-phase rehabilitation protocol has been utilized for both nonoperative and postoperative treatment [5]. Phase one consists of immobilization and limited weight bearing for 6 weeks, while focusing on quadriceps strengthening and hamstring stretching. To optimize ligament healing in the initial phase of rehabilitation, posterior tibial translation should be avoided. This is most commonly done by using a hinged knee cage brace with progressive range of motion; however, a dynamic anterior drawer brace or a cylindrical cast with posterior support to preserve the appropriate tibiofemoral alignment may also be used [3, 5, 15, 16]. Full weight bearing is resumed during the second phase, while continuing to focus on knee and hip strength and range of motion. The third phase focuses on returning to sport-specific activities and begins approximately 12 weeks following injury [5, 17].

Demonstration Cases

Common Presentation

PATIENT 1: 14-year-old male complaining of left posterior-medial knee pain x 11 days.

Mechanism of injury was falling while playing soccer. Special tests included a (+) posterior drawer, (+) tibial sag, and (+) quadriceps-active test. Standard radiographs of the knee were normal. Given the exam findings, an MRI was obtained and demonstrated a complete avulsion of the tibial attachment of the PCL with the ligament substance intact. The patient was treated by open reduction with internal fixation, using bioabsorbable anchors. Postoperatively, the patient completed a rehabilitation program and recovered fully, returning to play at 6 months after surgery [11].

PATIENT 2: 12-year-old female complaining of right knee pain x 7 days.

Mechanism of injury was blunt force trauma while in a flexed-knee position. Special tests included a (+) posterior drawer, (+) posterior tibial sag, and a (+) quadriceps-active test. X-rays demonstrated avulsion fracture at the tibial insertion of the PCL. MRI revealed intact PCL mid-substance with avulsion fracture of the tibial insertion, with fragment displaced 10 mm, but no other internal derangement of the knee was noted. The patient was treated via open reduction with internal fixation using a 4.00 mm cannulated screw and washer. The patient recovered without complication, with return to limited sporting activity at 9 months and to full sporting activity at 12 months.

DISCUSSION: PCL avulsion fracture in pediatrics may or may not be apparent on plain radiographs. When x-rays are negative but clinical suspicion for PCL injury remains, an MRI should be obtained.

PRECAUTIONS: Surgical fixation may disturb the physes; therefore, care should be taken with surgical planning.

Uncommon Presentation

PATIENT: 9-year-old male with left knee injury 3 hours ago.

Mechanism of injury was a fall from a climbing frame. The patient became suspended upside-down by a screw caught on his left trouser leg. Physical exam demonstrated a (+) posterior drawer. After non-stress radiographs demonstrated posterior displacement of the tibial plateau, an MRI demonstrated a femoral-sided avulsion fracture of the PCL. The fracture was reduced operatively with transosseous non-absorbable femoral sutures. Traumatic vascular damage required repair with saphenous vein bypass graft. At 1-year post-op, follow-up examination demonstrated intact peripheral perfusion and sensation. There were no degenerative changes [18].

Pearls and Pitfalls
- Because pediatric PCL injuries are uncommon, relatively little data exist on the epidemiology, natural history, and optimal management of these injuries.
- Long-term PCL deficiency in adult populations may be associated with increased degenerative joint disease, and this can likely be extrapolated to children.
- Pediatric PCL injuries are typically divided into ligament avulsion from the tibial attachment, avulsion from the femoral attachment, or mid-substance tear.
- Pain and guarding in acute injury may make the initial exam difficult and unreliable.
- Children may not complain of symptoms right away; those with delayed presentation may complain of calf pain and fatigue, difficulty sitting cross-legged, and difficulty with squatting.
- MRI is excellent for diagnosis of acute PCL injuries but less sensitive for chronic PCL deficiency. Stress radiographs are preferred for evaluation of suspected chronic PCL injuries.
- Easily visualized fragments on radiographs are typically displaced more than 10 mm, but fragments displaced less than 10 mm are easily overlooked. This is important because surgical fixation is often recommended for fragments displaced more than 5–7 mm.
- Surgery must be performed with care to avoid disturbing open physes, which may cause growth disturbances.

Chapter Summary

Pediatric PCL injuries are rare, and diagnosis and management can be challenging. A detailed initial exam with repeated follow up evaluations are important for proper diagnosis. The initial diagnosis is frequently missed, due to a seemingly normal physical exam and radiographs, and delayed treatment can lead to secondary changes in the knee. Management is adapted from treatment algorithms used in

Table 16.1 Chapter summary

Condition	PCL Tear
Description	Mid-substance tear, avulsion fracture from femoral attachment, avulsion fracture from tibial attachment
Epidemiology	More common in boys; more common in football, basketball, skiing, soccer, track, and gymnastics
Mechanism	Direct blow to anterior tibia; falling on knee with foot in plantarflexed position
History and exam findings	Effusion and tenderness in popliteal space, limited range of motion, positive posterior drawer test, posterior sag test, quadriceps active test; radiographs may show avulsion fracture and are useful for obtaining objective measurements of laxity; MRI useful in acute injuries but less reliable in chronic cases
Management	Isolated mid-substance tears and non-displaced or minimally displaced avulsion fractures treated nonoperatively; surgical intervention for displaced avulsion fractures and cases in which conservative treatment has failed

adult populations. A trial of nonoperative treatment is usually recommended for mid-substance tears or minimally displaced avulsion fractures, while surgical treatment is recommended for displaced avulsion fractures or conservative treatment failure. Optimization of treatment is crucial in pediatric populations to preserve knee function and prevent long-term degenerative joint disease (Table 16.1).

Disclosure The opinions expressed herein are those of the authors, and do not represent official policy of the US Air Force or the Department of Defense. The authors have no conflicts of interest or financial relationships related to this work.

References

1. Dempsey IJ, Gwathmey FW, Miller MD. Posterior cruciate ligament repair and reconstruction. In: Operative techniques: knee surgery. 2nd edition. Elsevier; 2018. P. 194-206. https://doi.org/10.1016/B978-0-323-46292-1.00022-8.
2. Logterman SL, Wydra FB, Frank RM. Posterior cruciate ligament: anatomy and biomechanics. Curr Rev Musculoskelet Med. 2018;11(3):510–4. https://doi.org/10.1007/s12178-018-9492-1.
3. Pache S, Aman ZS, Kennedy M, Nakama YN, Moatshe G, Ziegler C, et al. Posterior cruciate ligament- current concepts review. Arch Bone Jt Surg. 2018;6(1):8–18.
4. Mencio GA, Swiontkowski MF. Green's skeletal trauma in children: fifth edition; 2014. p. 1–658.
5. Katsman A, Strauss EJ, Campbell KA, Alaia MJ. Posterior cruciate ligament avulsion fractures. Curr Rev Musculoskelet Med. 2018;11(3):503–9. https://doi.org/10.1007/2Fs12178-018-9491-2.
6. Wegmann H, Janout S, Novak M, Kraus T, Castellani C, Singer G, et al. Surgical treatment of posterior cruciate ligament lesions does not cause growth disturbances in pediatric patients. Knee Surg Sports TraumatolArthrosc. 2018; https://doi.org/10.1007/s00167-018-5308-5.
7. Hurni Y, De Rosa V, Gonzalez JG, Mendoza-Sagaon M, Hamitaga F, Pellanda G. Pediatric posterior cruciate ligament avulsion fracture of the tibial insertion: case report and review of the literature. Surg J (NY). 2017;3(3):e134–8. https://doi.org/10.1055/s-0037-1605364.

8. Al-Ahaideb A. Posterior cruciate ligament avulsion fracture in children: a case report with long-term follow-up and comprehensive literature review. Eur J OrthopSurgTraumatol. 2013;23(Suppl 2):S257–60. https://doi.org/10.1007/s00590-012-1146-1.
9. Jang KM, Lee SH. Delayed surgical treatment for tibial avulsion fracture of the posterior cruciate ligament in children. Knee Surg Sports TraumatolArthrosc. 2016;24(3):754–9. https://doi.org/10.1007/s00167-015-3929-5.
10. Wang SH, Chien WC, Chung CH, Wang YC, Lin LC, Pan RY. Long-term results of posterior cruciate ligament tear with or without reconstruction: a nationwide, population-based cohort study. PLoS One. 2018;13(10):e0205118. Published 2018 Oct 3. https://doi.org/10.1371/journal.pone.0205118.
11. Pandya NK, Janik L, Chan G, Wells L. Case reports: pediatric PCL insufficiency from tibial insertion osteochondral avulsions. ClinOrthopRelat Res. 2008;466(11):2878–83. https://doi.org/10.1007/s11999-008-0373-6.
12. Shah N, Mukhopadhyay R, Vakta R, Bhatt J. Pre-pubescent posterior cruciate ligament (pcl) reconstruction using maternal allograft. Knee Surg Sports TraumatolArthrosc. 2016;24(3):768–72. https://doi.org/10.1007/s00167-016-3991-7.
13. Sørensen OG, Faunø P, Christiansen SE, Lind M. Posterior cruciate ligament reconstruction in skeletal immature children. Knee Surg Sports TraumatolArthrosc. 2017;25(12):3901–5. https://doi.org/10.1007/s00167-016-4416-3.
14. Kocher MS, Shore B, Nasreddine AY, Heyworth BE. Treatment of posterior cruciate ligament injuries in pediatric and adolescent patients. J PediatrOrthop. 2012;32(6):553–60. https://doi.org/10.1097/BPO.0b013e318263a154.
15. Scott CEH, Murray AW. Paediatric intrasubstance posterior cruciate ligament rupture. BMJ Case Rep Published 2011 Nov. Available from: 10.1136/bcr.09.2011.4803.
16. Wang D, Graziano J, Williams RJ, Jones KJ. Nonoperative treatment of PCL injuries: goals of rehabilitation and the natural history of conservative care. Curr Rev Musculoskelet Med. 2018;11:290–7. https://doi.org/10.1007/s12178-018-9487-y.
17. Senese M, Greenberg E, Lawrence JT, Ganley T. Rehabilitation following isolated posterior cruciate ligament reconstruction: a literature review of published protocols. Int J Sports PhysTher. 2018;13(4):737–51. https://doi.org/10.26603/ijspt20180737.
18. Hesse E, Bastian L, Zeichen J, Pertschy S, Bosch U, Krettek C. Femoral avulsion fracture of the posterior cruciate ligament in association with a rupture of the popliteal artery in a 9 year old boy: a case report. Knee Surg Sports TraumatolArthrosc. 2006;14(4):335–9. https://doi.org/10.1007/s00167-005-0677-y.

Chapter 17
Popliteus Injury

Valerie E. Cothran

Anatomy and Normal Function

The popliteus is the deepest muscle of the knee joint. It is a thin flat triangular muscle that forms part of the floor of the popliteal fossa [2].

Origin and Insertion

It is said to have a reverse origin and insertion, as its proximal attachment is its tendinous portion, whereas its muscle belly sits distally [3, 4]. The tendinous origin lies on the anterior part of the popliteal groove on the lateral surface of the lateral femoral condyle anteroinferior to the proximal attachment of the LCL.

Attachment

There is a direct attachment to the lateral meniscus, produced by the popliteomeniscal fascicles (variable) [4]. The muscular attachment to the tibia lies just proximal to the soleal line (popliteal line) but below the tibial condyles (Fig. 17.1). The popliteus also has a constant and strong attachment to the fibula through the popliteofibular ligament (Fig. 17.2).

V. E. Cothran (✉)
Primary Care Sports Medicine, University of Maryland, Department of Family and Community Medicine, Baltimore, MD, USA
e-mail: vcothran@som.umaryland.edu

© Springer Nature Switzerland AG 2021
N. Coleman (ed.), *Common Pediatric Knee Injuries*,
https://doi.org/10.1007/978-3-030-55870-3_17

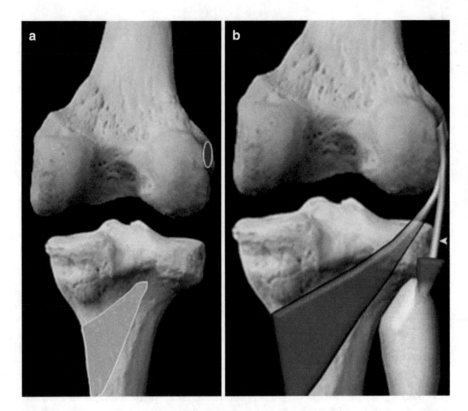

Fig. 17.1 Attachments and course of the popliteus. (**a**) Drawing of the knee (posterior view) shows the muscular belly (blue) and tendinous attachment (red) of the popliteus. (**b**) Posterior drawing of the knee shows the course of the popliteus musculotendinous unit in relation to the LCL (arrowhead) and biceps femoris (partially resected). Yellow = fibula [2]

Course

The popliteus muscle takes a unique path as its tendon courses through the popliteal hiatus to become intracapsular (though extra-articular and extrasynovial); it then passes under the arcuate ligament and becomes extracapsular before finally joining its muscle belly.

Function

The popliteus muscle and tendon provide both static and dynamic functions at the knee. It provides static stability, primarily resists external rotation, and has been termed the fifth ligament of the knee [5]. It also provides some stability to posterior tibial translation, as well as to varus stress. In the non-weight-bearing state, when

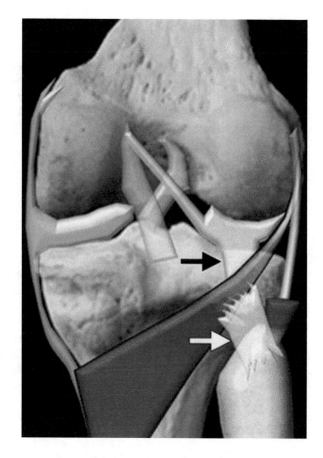

Fig. 17.2 Attachments of the popliteus to neighboring structures of the posterolateral knee. The popliteus has a constant and strong attachment to the fibula through the popliteofibular ligament (white arrow). The attachment of the popliteus to the posterior horn of the lateral meniscus (black arrow) is more variable [2]

the knee is in terminal extension, it "unlocks the knee" by internally rotating the tibia. In the weight-bearing state, the popliteus acts on the femur to externally rotate it on the leg [2]. When the knee flexes, it retracts the posterior meniscus via the popliteomeniscal fascicles (variable). This helps to prevent meniscal injury.

Innervation

The popliteus is innervated by the tibial nerve (L4, L5, S1).

Blood Supply

The popliteus receives its blood supply from the medial inferior genicular branch of the popliteal artery and the muscular branch of the posterior tibial artery.

Pathology and Dysfunction

Pathologic conditions affecting the popliteus muscle range from a muscle strain or tendinopathy to complete tendon rupture. The severity of the injury may be graded or classified using historical muscle injury classification systems. Chronic dysfunction may lead to subtle attenuation or thickening of the tendon, which has been shown to cause repetitive lateral pain and popping (snapping popliteal tendon).

Specific Pointers

Epidemiology

Popliteus muscle strain and popliteal tendinopathy occur more commonly in athletes that run on hills or banked surfaces [6, 7]. They are also more commonly seen in athletes with increased pronation of the ankle and excessive internal rotation of the tibia [8]. In nonathletes, popliteal injury can be seen in hiking and backpacking [9].

Popliteal tendon ruptures are rare in isolation. In an imaging study of 24 popliteal tendon injuries, only 8.3% were isolated [5, 10]. Popliteal tendon ruptures occur more often after trauma in combination with other posterolateral corner knee injuries.

Mechanism of Injury

Popliteus Muscle Strain/Popliteal Tendinopathy

Mild-to-moderate popliteus muscle injuries typically occur as a result of chronic overuse of the muscle tendon unit with downhill running. The popliteus functions to stabilize the knee by preventing anterior femoral translation and tibial external rotation while running [9].

Popliteal Tendon Rupture

A more severe popliteus muscle injury, a popliteal tendon rupture, often occurs after direct anteromedial force and is usually associated with other posterolateral corner knee injuries. When a popliteal tendon rupture occurs in isolation, the mechanism of injury has been less well defined. It may be due to direct or indirect trauma. There have been many case reports that identify several proposed mechanisms including the following: direct blow to the anteromedial knee, sudden forcible external rotation of the tibia in a partially flexed knee [11], sudden forced varus in an externally rotated leg, and forced hyperextension with the tibia in internal rotation. Popliteal tendon ruptures may also be seen in road traffic accidents or falls, during which the knee is hyperextended.

Diagnosis (History/Exam Findings/Testing)

Popliteus Muscle Strain/Popliteal Tendinopathy

Patients often report the insidious onset of posterior or posterolateral knee pain, usually during weight bearing, when the knee is between 15 and 30 degrees of flexion, or during the early swing phase of gait [12, 13]. Athletes may also report a recent increase in activity, especially downhill running or running on banked surfaces [6, 12].

Historically, athletes will describe symptoms beginning at 2–3 miles of running. It is often severe enough to prevent continued running [9]. Injuries isolated to the muscle belly present as posterior pain, whereas injuries isolated to the tendon present with more posterolateral pain. With continued use, symptoms occur even earlier during activity and, in chronic cases, will occur at the commencement of running.

Physical Examination of a Popliteus Muscle Strain/Popliteal Tendinopathy

There are often no visible gross signs of popliteal injury on examination. Occasionally, there may be localized swelling at the area of the popliteal tendon. Palpation of the popliteal tendon may elicit pain. The popliteal tendon should be palpated at its origin, inferior and anterior to the LCL. This is best done with the patient's leg in the Fig. 4 position.

Passive and active knee extension and flexion should be assessed and compared to the contralateral side. Passive and active internal and external rotation of the tibia should also be assessed at 90° of knee flexion. There may be pain with full passive external rotation, as well as with active internal rotation. Strength testing of the affected knee should be compared to the contralateral side. There may be subtle weakness with internal rotation of the leg.

Special tests to evaluate for a popliteus muscle strain or popliteal tendon injury include Garrick's Test and the Shoe Removal Maneuver. Additional tests should be performed to rule out other concomitant injuries. Lachman's Test (assesses ACL stability), Posterior Drawer (assesses PCL stability), Valgus Stress Test (assesses MCL stability); Varus Stress Test (assesses LCL stability); Dial Test, Posterior Lateral Drawer, and ER Recurvatum (Posterolateral Corner): all are negative in isolated popliteal tendon ruptures. Although McMurray's Test should be negative in isolated popliteal tendon ruptures, due to the relationship of the popliteal tendon with the posterior horn of the lateral meniscus, there may be posterior joint line pain with this maneuver.

Garrick's Test

The patient may be seated, supine or prone with the knee at 90°. The examiner grasps the heel and foot and brings the tibia into internal rotation. The examiner then instructs the patient to hold that position, while an external rotation force is applied to the foot and heel (the patient is holding internal rotation against resistance). A positive test is pain or tenderness over the proximal aspect of the popliteal tendon with this maneuver.

Shoe Removal Maneuver

The patient is instructed to remove contralateral shoe by internally rotating affected leg to reach the contralateral heel (as you would do to remove the shoe while standing). A positive test is posterior or posterolateral pain during the maneuver.

Symptoms are best reproduced by allowing the athlete to exercise just prior to the physical exam. Having the patient run downhill just prior to evaluation may assist in localizing pathology [12].

Imaging

Imaging is not necessary to confirm the clinical suspicion of a popliteus injury. It may be used for confirmation and to rule out any concomitant injuries.

Plain radiographs are often normal. In chronic cases, there may be calcifications visualized within the tendon. Musculoskeletal ultrasound (US) has recently emerged as an alternative to advanced imaging. Advantages of US include the increasing availability of bedside US equipment, the relatively low cost of the procedure, the capacity for dynamic evaluation, and the use of nonionizing radiation [14]. Due to its relatively superficial origin, US is an excellent point-of-care imaging modality for viewing popliteal tendon injuries (Fig. 17.3). US may show focal tendon enlargement, hyperechoic or hypoechoic signal within the tendon, or fluid within the tendon sheath.

The popliteus is visualized clearly on MRI. There may be increased signal within the muscle or tendon. Focal tendon enlargement may also be identified.

Popliteal Tendon Rupture

With a popliteal tendon rupture, patients often report the acute onset of sharp posterolateral pain, often with a perceived pop after trauma (direct or indirect). Many patients report the inability to return to activity because of severe pain with ambulation. Some will report perceived instability with ambulation.

Fig. 17.3 Ultrasound image of the lateral knee shows a normal popliteal tendon at its origin

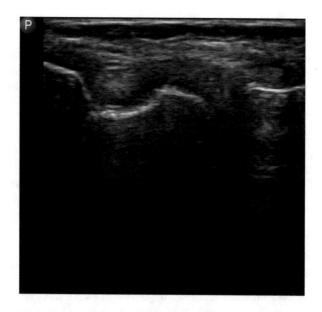

Physical Examination of a Popliteal Tendon Rupture

There may be localized swelling at the area of the popliteal tendon. Due to the intracapsular path of the popliteal tendon, there may also be an effusion. Palpation should proceed along the popliteal tendon from its origin inferior and anterior to the LCL. Significant swelling or inability to palpate popliteal tendon may indicate a complete avulsion. A neurologic exam should be done to rule out concomitant injuries to the common peroneal nerve. Decreased sensation over the proximal anterolateral lower leg (common peroneal nerve), distal anterolateral lower leg (superficial peroneal nerve: SPN), dorsum of the foot (SPN), or first webspace (deep peroneal nerve: DPN) is suggestive of injury to the associated nerve. Additionally, weakness in ankle dorsiflexion (DPN), great toe extension (DPN), or ankle eversion (SPN) should be assessed. Passive and active knee extension and flexion should be assessed and compared to the contralateral side. Patients may exhibit decreased ROM or pain with both terminal flexion and extension. Passive and active internal and external rotation of the tibia should also be assessed at 90° of knee flexion. There may be pain with full passive external rotation, as well as with active internal rotation. Strength testing of the affected knee should be compared to the contralateral side. There may be weakness with internal rotation of the tibia with the knee flexed to 90°.

Special tests to evaluate for a popliteal tendon rupture include Garrick's Test and the Shoe Removal Maneuver. Additional tests should be performed to rule out other concomitant injuries, as noted above.

Imaging

Plain radiographs may demonstrate displaced ossified fragments avulsed from the lateral femoral condyle. US may be used to identify partial and complete tendon ruptures. Popliteal tendon ruptures are easily identified on MRI.

Management

Popliteus muscle strain and popliteal tendinopathy are treated as other muscle strains and tendinopathies throughout the lower extremity. Treatment plans typically include relative rest, anti-inflammatory medication, training modification (may start with running on level surfaces or in the opposite direction on the track), flexibility training, and evaluation of lower extremity biomechanics with corrective physical therapy [9].

Treatment of popliteal tendon ruptures has not been well established, as there is no consensus on the management of isolated popliteal tendon injuries. Support in the literature exists for success with both operative and nonoperative treatments (14). Operative treatment should be considered, if there is any instability on exam. Operative treatment should also be considered, when the popliteal tendon rupture is associated with an osteochondral avulsion that could be reattached. Partial popliteal tendon tears have also been successfully treated with surgical repair. Nonoperative treatment, consisting of ice, rest, and range of motion exercises, has also been successful (14). Physical therapy should start with non-weight-bearing stability exercises and advance to weight-bearing stability exercises as tolerated.

Demonstration Cases

Common Presentation

A competitive distance runner presents with the sudden onset of posterolateral knee pain. The symptoms occurred suddenly midway through a training run; there was no inciting event. The patient denies an indirect or direct trauma. The patient did not hear or feel a pop; "it just started to hurt mid run." The physical exam revealed a small effusion, sharp localized pain in the posterolateral knee at the lateral femoral condyle in the area of the origin of the popliteal tendon. MRI of the knee confirmed an isolated popliteal tendon rupture.

MRI – coronal, sagittal, and axillary images of an isolated rupture of the popliteal tendon.

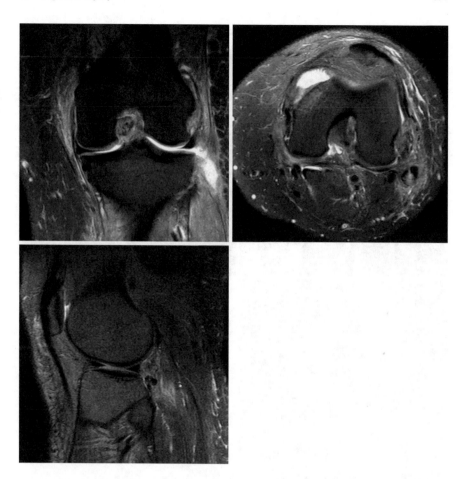

The athlete was treated conservatively with rest, symptom control with oral anti-inflammatory analgesics as needed, and physical therapy. She returned to nonrestricted running after 6 weeks of physical therapy and graded activity progression.

Uncommon Presentation

A professional soccer player presents with the immediate onset of posterior lateral knee pain and swelling after a direct trauma. The athlete was chasing down a ball, made a quick cut in the opposite direction, and was struck on the medial side of his knee by an opposing player (i.e., he sustained a varus force on a fixed and externally rotated knee). The physical exam revealed a small effusion and localized swelling in the area of the origin of the popliteal tendon. The athlete was tender to palpation in the posterolateral knee. This pain was increased with full active extension. MRI of the knee confirmed an isolated popliteal tendon rupture.

MRI –Coronal and axial view of an acute isolated rupture of the popliteal tendon.

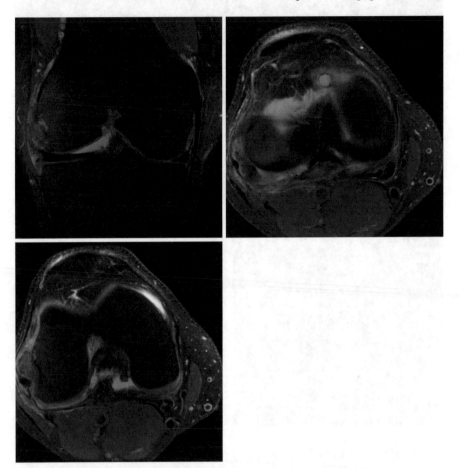

The athlete was given the option of operative debridement versus physical therapy. He elected for operative debridement but was lost to follow-up.

Pearls and Pitfalls
- Popliteus muscle strain or popliteal tendinopathy should be considered in runners with posterior or posterolateral knee pain.
- Posterolateral pain associated with an acute effusion in a stable knee should lead to suspicion of an isolated popliteal tendon injury.
- Isolated popliteal tendon ruptures are rare; thus, concomitant injuries must be ruled out, specifically injuries to the posterolateral corner, PCL, posterior horn of the lateral meniscus, common peroneal nerve, and/or tibial nerve.

Chapter Summary

Popliteal tendinopathy has been reported as the cause of lateral and posterolateral knee pain.

Overuse injuries to the popliteus muscle develop gradually and are more common in runners. These injuries tend to be a result of biomechanical issues (overpronation). Popliteal tendinopathy is commonly seen in athletes who run on hills or banked surfaces or after downhill running, walking, or hiking [1, 6].

Rupture of the popliteal tendon may occur after a significant force to the knee. This injury is more commonly seen in combination with an injury to other structures in the posterolateral corner of the knee. When a popliteal tendon rupture occurs in isolation, the mechanism of injury has been less well defined. It is commonly seen in road traffic accidents or falls, during which the knee is hyperextended. It might also be injured through impacts that force the knee into a varus position.

Suggested Helpful Websites

https://www.sportsinjurybulletin.com/popliteus-assessment-and-rehabilitation

Chart/Table

Condition	Popliteus muscle strain / popliteal tendinopathy
Description	Overuse or tearing of the muscle fibers or muscle tendon unit of the popliteus muscle
Epidemiology	Seen more commonly in distance runners
Mechanism (common)	Downhill running or running on banked surfaces
History and exam findings	Posterior or posterolateral knee pain Point tenderness at the tendon origin (lateral femoral condyle) Increased with resisted internal rotation of the tibia (with the knee at 90° of flexion
Management	Relative rest Activity modification (running on flat surfaces or in the opposite direction on the track) Flexibility training Gait and biomechanical evaluation followed by corrective PT

Condition	Popliteal tendon rupture
Description	Complete tear of the popliteal tendon from its proximal attachment to the femur.
Epidemiology	Rarely seen in isolation.
Mechanism (common)	Acute direct/indirect trauma to the anteromedial knee. Sudden forcible external rotation of the tibia in a partially flexed knee. Sudden forced varus in an externally rotated lower leg. Forced hyperextension with the tibia in internal rotation.
History and exam findings	Posterior or posterolateral knee pain after trauma. Knee effusion may be present. Point tenderness at the tendon origin (lateral femoral condyle). Increased pain with resisted internal rotation of the tibia (with the knee at 90° of flexion).
Management	Currently, there is no consensus on the best treatment for isolated popliteal tendon rupture. Both operative and nonoperative treatments have been proposed. Operative treatment is best performed in the first 3 weeks. Operative treatment should be considered if there is any instability on exam. Operative treatment may also be considered when the popliteal tendon rupture was associated with a bony avulsion. Nonoperative treatment consists of rest and PT. PT should begin with range of motion and advance to non-weight-bearing stability exercises followed by weight-bearing stability exercises as tolerated.

References

1. Mayfield GW. Popliteus tendon tenosynovitis. Am J Sports Med. 1977;5(1):31–6. https://doi.org/10.1177/036354657700500106.
2. Jadhav SP, More SR, Riascos RF, Lemos DF, Swischuk LE. Comprehensive review of the anatomy, function, and imaging of the popliteus and associated pathologic conditions. Radiographics. 2014;34(2):496–513.
3. Blake SM, Treble NJ. Popliteus tendon tenosynovitis. Br J Sports Med. 2005;39(12):e42. https://doi.org/10.1136/bjsm.2005.019349.
4. Chuncharunee A, Chanthong P, Lucksanasombool P. The patterns of proximal attachments of the popliteus muscle: form and function. Med Hypotheses. 2012;78(2):221–4.
5. LaPrade RF, Wozniczka JK, Stellmaker MP, Wijdicks CA. Analysis of the static function of the popliteus tendon and evaluation of an anatomic reconstruction: the "fifth ligament" of the knee. Am J Sports Med. 2010;38(3):543–9. https://doi.org/10.1177/0363546509349493.
6. Safran M, Zachazewski JE, Stone DA. Instructions for sports medicine patients. 2nd ed. Philadelphia: Elsevier/Saunsers; 2012. p. 822–6.
7. Rzonca EC, Baylis WJ. Common sports injuries to the foot and leg. Clin Podiatr Med Surg. 1988;5:591–612.
8. DeLee J, Drez D. De lee & Drez'sorthopaedic sports medicine. Philadelphia: Saunders; 2003.
9. Brown TR, Quinn SF, Wensel JP, et al. Diagnosis of popliteus injuries with MR imaging. Skelet Radiol. 1995;24:511–4.

10. Guha AR, Gorgees KA, Walker DI. Popliteus tendon rupture: a case report and review of the literature. Br J Sports Med. 2003;37(4):358–60.
11. Boden B. Knee and thigh overuse tendonopathy. In: Maffulli N, Renstrom P, Leadbetter WB, editors. Tendon injuries basic science and clinical medicine; 2005. p. 158–64. Retrieved from https://link.springer.com/content/pdf/10.1007/b137778.pdf.
12. English S, Perret D. Posterior knee pain. Curr Rev Musculoskelet Med. 2010;3(1–4):3–10. Published 2010 Jun 12. https://doi.org/10.1007/s12178-010-9057-4.
13. Wang Q, Huang QH, Yeow JTW, Pickering MR, Saarakkala S. Quantitative analysis of musculo-skeletal ultrasound: techniques and clinical applications. Biomed Res Int. 2017;2017:9694316. https://doi.org/10.1155/2017/9694316.
14. Sileo MJ, Schwartz MC. Isolated rupture of the popliteus muscle with painful ossification in a skeletally immature athlete-a case report. Bull NYU HospJt Dis. 2009;67:387–90.

Chapter 18
Hamstring Injury

Jonathan Napolitano and Atul Gupta

Introduction

Hamstring strains and tears are among the most common injuries seen in sports. Involvement of the distal hamstring is a rare yet important consideration in the evaluation of a pediatric patient with posterior knee pain. Understanding the contributions of the hamstring to knee function lays a foundation for how injuries to these muscles cause dysfunction and pain at the knee. This chapter's aim is to provide an overview of the hamstring complex, pathology associated with its distal components, and spectrum of treatments available to improve function and pain outcomes.

Anatomy and Function

The hamstrings are a group of three biarticular muscles, crossing both the hip and knee joints posteriorly. During the gait cycle, the hamstring muscles antagonize the quadriceps and are responsible for both hip extension and knee flexion with concentric contraction. At higher speeds, this group of muscles plays a role in deceleration of both hip flexion and knee extension with eccentric contraction. Additionally, the hamstrings serve to stabilize both the hip and knee joints throughout the gait cycle. The distal hamstring tendons act in conjunction with the anterior cruciate ligament (ACL) to prevent anterior tibial translation; therefore, hamstring strengthening has

J. Napolitano (✉)
Sports Medicine, Nationwide Children's Hospital, Westerville, OH, USA
e-mail: Jonathan.Napolitano@nationwidechildrens.org

A. Gupta
Department of Physical Medicine and Rehabilitation, Virginia Mason Medical Center, Seattle, WA, USA
e-mail: Atul.gupta@vmmc.org

© Springer Nature Switzerland AG 2021
N. Coleman (ed.), *Common Pediatric Knee Injuries*,
https://doi.org/10.1007/978-3-030-55870-3_18

become an important component of ACL prevention programs [1]. Each of these muscles has a large distal tendon that originates deep within the muscle belly and runs close to the entire length of the muscles [2]. The central tendon is attached to the muscle fibers in a symmetric pennate arrangement, like a feather. These long tendons allow for a "spring" effect of contraction and lengthening that accentuates performance but also leads to injury susceptibility [3]. From medial to lateral, this muscle group includes the semimembranosus, the semitendinosus, and the biceps femoris (Fig. 18.1).

The semimembranosus originates from the superolateral portion of the ischial tuberosity of the pelvis. The proximal tendon of the semimembranosus is the longest proximally of the three hamstring muscles and courses both medial and anterior to the other muscles of the posterior thigh [4]. The muscle belly of the semimembranosus is the largest of the three, generating the greatest force but also the slowest velocity [5]. The distal tendon of the semimembranosus inserts on the posterior aspect of the medial tibial condyle. The distal tendon of the semimembranosus crosses that of the medial gastrocnemius at the posteromedial knee. This intersection has been identified as the most common location for the "stalk" of a

Fig. 18.1 Hamstring anatomy

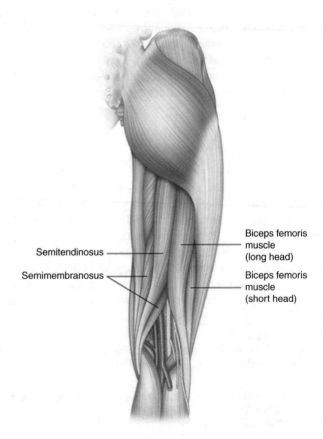

Semitendinosus

Semimembranosus

Biceps femoris muscle (long head)

Biceps femoris muscle (short head)

popliteal cyst. There is a chapter on popliteal cyst, which can provide more information on that condition.

The semitendinosus and long head of the biceps femoris originates from the inferomedial portion of the ischial tuberosity dividing from a conjoint tendon to become two separate muscles. The semitendinosus is named for its long distal tendinous component formed at the midpoint of the posterior thigh, and the longest distal tendon of the three hamstrings [1]. The distal tendon courses medially over the medial femoral condyle, to the anterior medial tibia condyle, where it joins the tendons of the gracilis and sartorius to form the pes anserine. There is a chapter on pes anserine pain, which can provide more information on that condition.

From the conjoint tendon the long head of the biceps femoris courses laterally down the thigh deep to the Iliotibial band. The short head of the biceps originates from the lateral supracondylar ridge of the femur, thus acting only at the knee joint and not at the hip. The origin of the short head of the biceps is commonly used as the level to differentiate a proximal from distal hamstring injury [6]. The distal tendons of the long and short heads of the biceps femoris form a complex network of attachments to the fibular head, the iliotibial band, the lateral collateral ligament, the posterior lateral tibial condyle, and the posterolateral joint capsule at the level of the posterior horn of the lateral meniscus [7]. This complex is key to providing rotatory stability to the posterolateral corner of the knee. There is a chapter on posterolateral corner injury, which can provide more information on that condition.

The semimembranosus, semitendinosus, and long head of the biceps femoris are innervated by the tibial component of the sciatic nerve, primarily the L5 nerve root but with additional input from S1 and S2. The medial hamstring reflex can be used to evaluate the L5 nerve root. The short head of the biceps femoris is innervated by the common fibular branch of the sciatic nerve and can be tested in electromyography as the last muscle innervated before the common fibular nerve crosses the fibular head, a common site of entrapment or injury.

Pathology and Dysfunction

The powerful and complex hamstring muscle group is highly vulnerable to injury. Hamstring injuries account for up to 29% of all injuries in athletes [8]. In the pediatric, skeletally immature athlete, the weakest link in the kinetic chain is the ischial apophysis, which begins to ossify between the ages of 15 and 17. This apophysis does not fuse to the ischium until the ages of 19 to 25 [9]. Injuries to the hamstrings themselves are more common proximally than distally. The most common location of muscle injury is the proximal myotendinous junction [6, 10, 11]. These proximal injuries are out of the scope of this book on knee injuries, and the remainder of this chapter will focus on middle-to-distal hamstring injuries.

Hamstring injuries are typically the result of an eccentric muscle contraction or elongation against contraction and not caused by contact. Hamstring injuries range from a mild strain to a complete rupture. In the mildest injuries, only the myofibrils are damaged, releasing creatine kinase and resulting in pain. More severe injuries involve disruption of the extracellular matrix, fascia, and myotendinous architecture with the release of muscle enzymes, collagen and proteoglycan degradation, and local inflammation. When this damage involves the blood vessels supplying the muscle, this leads not only to increased bleeding and bruising but can result in a local ischemic environment, leading to additional muscle damage and impaired healing.

Various factors have been identified for their contribution to hamstring injuries, including but not limited to the following: high training volume, poor hamstring and quadriceps flexibility, poor muscle strength, improper or no warm-up, muscle fatigue and overexertion, and various anatomic imbalance of muscle strength and posture [3]. Many of these factors are especially applicable to the pediatric and adolescent athlete. For example, during periods of rapid growth, hamstring flexibility and muscle balance is lacking, potentially leading to increased risk of injury.

Specific Pointers

Epidemiology

A systematic review and meta-analysis of risk factors for hamstring injury in sport by Frecklton and Pizzari identified age as a significant risk factor for hamstring injury, with athletes over the age of 23 at an increased risk (OR:2.46, 95% CI 0.98 to 6.14, $p = 0.06$) [12]. Gabbe et al. attributed the increased risk with age to significant differences in hip flexor flexibility, hip internal rotation, and ankle dorsiflexion range of motion, total body weight, and body mass index, when comparing athletes older or younger than 20 years of age [13]. The majority of studies on hamstring injuries in athletes report highest incidence between 18 and 30 years of age. Valle et al. reported on 50 hamstring injuries among a large cohort of 1157 young athletes with an average age of 13.56 years and with the youngest hamstring injury occurring in a 9-year-old. They reported an age-related increased rate of injury with a peak incidence at age 17 [14]. Most commonly, hamstring injuries are seen in sports that involve explosive running, rapid acceleration and deceleration, kicking, and hurdling, including soccer, football, track and field, and dance.

Mechanism of Injury

The mechanism of hamstring injuries most commonly is an acute tensile overload. This can happen anywhere along the length of the hamstring from the proximal insertion on the ischial tuberosity, the proximal muscle tendon, the intramuscular area, the distal muscle tendon junction, or the distal insertions on the tibia and fibula [3]. Regardless of the location, acute hamstring injuries occur, most commonly, while sprinting full speed or attempting to overstride, immediately before or after foot contact. Distal hamstring injuries are often seen with hyperextension of the knee [15].

Hamstring injuries, less commonly, occur with chronic low-grade tensile overload forces, leading to microtear and tendinosis, or in the skeletally immature athlete apophysis at the bony origin.

Diagnosis: History and Exam Findings, Testing

History

With an acute hamstring injury, most athletes report a sudden sharp pain to the posterior thigh or knee. Injuries can occur with hip flexion and knee extension or hip extension with knee extension. The history may or may not include the report of a single identifiable stride as the cause of injury or an audible or palpable "pop." In a case series of professional soccer players with acute hamstring injuries, the timing of the injury was not discernible on video analysis [16]. Athletes who have sustained distal hamstring injuries often report a knee hyperextension moment and a sense of knee instability [15].

Physical Exam

After hamstring injury, most athletes present with a "stiff-legged" gait pattern in an attempt to avoid simultaneous hip flexion and knee extension [17]. While examining the patient in the prone position, there may or may not be swelling or ecchymosis to the posterior thigh or knee (Fig. 18.2). Ecchymosis can be an indication of a more severe injury, indicating significant macrotearing of the hamstring.

Despite the location of pain or bruising, the exam should include the entire hamstring from ischial tuberosity down to the distal insertions on the tibia and fibula. Palpatory exam may reveal a focal defect, secondary to muscle retraction, or, more consistently, focal tenderness over the muscle, tendon, or bony insertion.

In the prone position, hamstring strength should also be assessed with the knee flexed to 90 degrees against the examiner's forced extension to 30 degrees and compared to the contralateral side. This position reproduces an eccentric load to the hamstring and may help to identify the location of injury more precisely. Higher-grade injuries may demonstrate decreased knee flexion strength; however, diminished strength may also be a result of fear avoidance or guarding in more mild injuries.

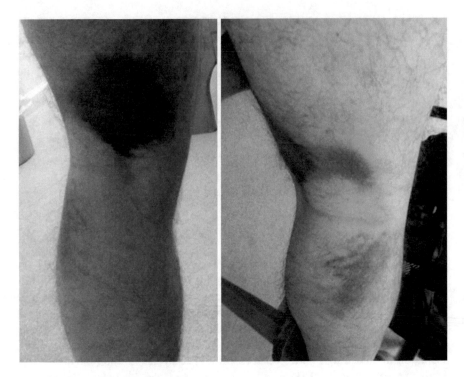

Fig. 18.2 Posterior thigh ecchymosis

Range of motion should be assessed in the supine position, assessing the popliteal angle with the hip and knee both flexed to 90 degrees and slowly extending the knee. This should be compared to the contralateral side.

Inspection, palpation, strength, and range of motion are often sufficient to identify a hamstring injury, but the Puranen-Orava test and bent-knee stretch test are specialized tests with moderate-to-high validity and reliability in identifying both proximal hamstring tendinopathy and strain; they may also be positive with a distal hamstring injury [18]. The bent-knee stretch test is performed in the supine position with the knee and hip placed into full flexion. The knee is then extended with reproduction of pain indicating a positive finding. The Puranen-Orava test is performed in a standing position with the knee fully extended and foot on a low-lying table. The spine is then flexed forward with a positive exam reproducing pain.

If a distal hamstring pathology is suspected, the physical exam should also include an evaluation of the other structures of the posterolateral corner. This should include a varus stress test of the lateral collateral ligament (LCL), a posterolateral drawer test (posterior drawer test with foot externally rotated to 15 degrees), and a dial test. Please refer to the chapter on posterolateral corner injury for more information.

Testing

The physical exam is the most beneficial diagnostic tool for most hamstring injuries; however, in skeletally immature athletes, and in those in which an insertional injury is suspected, radiographs should be obtained to evaluate for a bony avulsion. This includes an AP view of the pelvis to evaluate the ischial tuberosity or an AP and lateral view of the knee to evaluate for distal avulsion fractures.

To grade the extent of injury better, soft tissue imaging modalities can be very helpful, as well. Point-of-care musculoskeletal ultrasound (US) can be used to evaluate the hamstring from origin to insertion for convenient, timely, and reliable information in the clinic or training room. Detected abnormalities can range from a bony avulsion with displacement of the hyperechoic bony cortex, a tendon or muscle tear or rupture with hypoechoic signal within a muscle or tendon, or a more subtle partial tear or strain with loss of the normal muscle or tendon architecture and surrounding edema or hematoma. US can also be used to monitor interval healing of a hamstring injury. An added benefit of US is directly correlating a region of pain on palpation with pathologic changes. US has been shown to be as sensitive as magnetic resonance imaging (MRI) in imaging acute hamstring injuries, though it is important to mention that the diagnostic utility of US is highly operator dependent [19].

A noncontrast MRI of the thigh has been shown to be more reliable than US for deeper hamstring injuries and, therefore, frequently viewed as the modality of choice due, in part, to the reliability and availability across institutions [19]. A T2 hyperintense signal on MRI represents muscle or tendon edema or hemorrhage in the setting of acute injury. Sagittal and coronal sequences on MRI can also best longitudinally approximate the amount of muscle or tendon retraction in complete avulsions or ruptures. When there is a concern for a severe distal hamstring injury and knee instability, a noncontrast MRI of the knee is best to evaluate and differentiate the extent of a distal hamstring injury in the setting of concomitant posterior lateral corner injuries, as outlined above.

Management

Goals in managing hamstring injuries are focused on returning an athlete to his/her prior level of function while minimizing risk for reinjury.

Initial management strategies depend on the severity of the injury. In the most severe situation of a complete distal hamstring avulsion injury, surgical referral should be urgent [20], though the more common scenario of hamstring strains will follow a three-phase progressive rehabilitation protocol.

Phase 1 in rehabilitation, the acute phase, focuses on the reduction in pain and edema and on the prevention of excessive scar formation. The RICE (rest, ice, compression, elevation) protocol can be used during this phase of healing. Nonsteroidal anti-inflammatories (NSAIDs) or acetaminophen can be used for pain reduction during this phase. There lacks consensus around the use of NSAIDs during this early phase in recovery, as some data have shown NSAIDs impair muscle function and recovery, when used in this phase [21]. Immobilization can be considered but should be limited to less than 4 days to prevent excessive scar formation [22]. Short-term immobilization can also prevent excessive scar formation and contracture [23]. Range of motion during this phase is important but should be within a protected range of motion. A shortened stride with ambulation is recommended. The use of crutches is considered, when the injury is higher grade and the patient's functionally is limited. Avoidance of resistance training during this phase is also strongly recommended, and progressive agility and trunk stabilization exercises should be performed at only low-to-moderate intensity. Progression to phase II can occur when there is a normal, nonantalgic gait; the ability to jog pain free at low speed; and the ability to perform an isometric hamstring contraction in prone knee flexion at 90 degrees with at least 50–70% the total resistance force of the uninjured contralateral hamstring [24].

Phase II, the subacute phase, will focus on pain-free range of motion, correction of muscle imbalances, neuromuscular control, and low resistance eccentric loading of the hamstring. Emphasis is placed on a progressive increase in intensity and speed of exercises for neuromuscular control, agility, and trunk stability, based on tolerance. Strength should be maximized in mid ranges of motion. End range of motion loading should be limited during this phase in recovery. Pain medications during this phase can lead to overwork and further injury of the healing hamstring; therefore, they are generally not recommended during this phase of rehabilitation. Ice is the pain relief option of choice in this phase of recovery. Completion of this phase occurs with two specific parameters. The first is a pain-free isometric contraction with full resistance in a prone position and the knee flexed to 90 degrees. The second is the ability to jog both forward and backward at 50% maximum speed. This phase is the preparation phase for exercises specific for return to sport or activity [24].

Phase III will focus on higher level neuromuscular control and eccentric loading exercises. Multidirectional movement activities and an increase to full strength utilization at end ranges of motion should be emphasized during this phase. Return to activity criteria include lack of palpatory tenderness over the injury, full concentric and eccentric strength without pain, and absence of kinesiophobia [24].

Injectable Therapeutic Options

There is very limited data on the use of corticosteroids for the treatment of hamstring strains. Levine et al. looked retrospectively at a group of 58 professional football players, who received corticosteroid injection within 72 hours of hamstring strain onset. Their primary conclusion was that steroids did not cause any detrimental side effects and that there may be an accelerated recovery time for return to play [25]. Corticosteroids have been shown to be both myotoxic and tenotoxic [26], and data are lacking on a proven benefit.

Platelet-rich plasma, most commonly known as "PRP," is a regenerative medicine treatment that involves injecting a concentrated solution of platelets into a damaged area within the body to enhance the body's own ability to heal. It is considered to both accelerate healing early during injury recovery and to promote healing when rehabilitation efforts have not resolved pain and functional limitations. PRP has been shown to increase the expression of myogenic molecules within the body, thereby modulating anabolic and myogenic responses to injury [27]. Studies have both supported and refuted the efficacy of PRP injection for accelerated return to play after hamstring injury and prevention of injury recurrence. Rossi et al. used return to play and recurrence rate as outcome measures in a study comparing PRP injections (34 patients) to control (38 patients) with hamstring injuries [28]. Rehabilitation course post-injection was standardized [28]. Mean time to play was 4.9 days faster in the PRP versus control group ($p = 0.001$) [28]. In this study, the rate of recurrence did not show a statistical difference between the groups [28].

Sheth et al. published a systematic review looking at the benefit of PRP on a standard return-to-play rehabilitation program for a variety of muscle injuries. This study looked at 268 athletes across five studies with follow-up at 12 months [29]. When incorporating all muscle groups, there was a six-day decrease in return to sport noted in those who received a PRP injection; however, with a subgroup analysis focusing just on hamstrings, there was not a noted difference between control and PRP groups [29].

Another paper by Reurink et al. did not find a difference between hamstring reinjury rates in athletes who received PRP injections in acute hamstring strains versus those who did not [27].

Additional high-level randomized controlled trials that standardize for the intrinsic makeup of PRP being used are needed to confirm whether there is truly a benefit in using platelet-rich plasma injections for hamstring injuries.

Injury Prevention

Hamstring strains occur during excessive eccentric loading of the muscle tendon unit; therefore, eccentric strengthening has been proven to be the mainstay of hamstring injury prevention. Specifically, the Nordic hamstring lowering exercise has been shown to be effective in limiting recurrence of injury [22]. (Fig. 18.3) This exercise is performed with the athlete in an upright kneeling position. The feet and calves are stabilized by an assistant, and the patient maintains the hips and knees in parallel. The patient then lowers his body (from knees to chest) to the floor in a controlled fashion. Research has shown that use of the Nordic hamstring exercise reduces the rate of hamstring strains by more than 60% and reduces the rate of

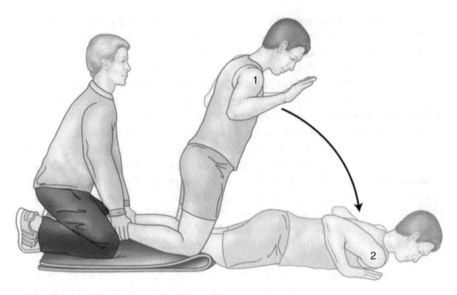

Fig. 18.3 Nordic hamstring exercise

recurrence by 85% [22]. The addition of neuromuscular control exercises of the lumbopelvic and lower extremity region have also been shown to help prevent injury [23]. Lastly, varying trunk positions for activity or sport-specific drills has been shown to reduce the hamstring injury occurrence rate [24]. Another key prevention strategy, especially in the pediatric athlete, is maintenance of good hamstring flexibility.

Demonstration Cases

Common Presentation

A 17-year-old female soccer player chases a ball to prevent it from going out of bounds. The sudden increase in speed causes a severe sharp pain with an associated snapping sensation in the posterior thigh. The player is able to limp off the field with support. There is no immediate bruising or ecchymosis. Tenderness is appreciated along the distal third of the posterolateral thigh. No palpable focal defects are appreciated. Knee range of motion incites pain over the region. Lachman maneuver, anterior drawer test, McMurray's, and dial test of the knee are all negative. There is reproducible pain with knee flexion strength testing. A point-of-care US performed in the locker room 3 hours post-injury shows small areas of hypoechogenicity involving 25% of the distal myotendinous junction of the hamstring.

A moderate distal hamstring strain of the biceps femoris is diagnosed. The player should be taken through a structured and graduated rehabilitation program as noted above, followed by a return-to-play protocol.

Uncommon Presentation

A 14-year-old male football player begins to develop posterolateral knee pain insidiously through the preseason football practices of his freshman year. He does not recall a specific event but rather a discomfort-like feeling that slowly becomes more noticeable. His only prior medical history is a history of Osgood-Schlatter disease 2 years ago. He feels the pain predominantly, when his foot is planted with the knee in full extension or hyperextension. The pain noticeably limits his ability to move at full speed.

He comes into the clinic for evaluation. On exam, he exhibits no focal defects in muscle structure, no visible knee effusions anterior or posterior, and no skin discoloration. He is tender over the posterolateral knee. He has full knee range of motion and strength testing. Popliteal angle is only 45 degrees bilaterally. He has a negative anterior drawer, Lachman, McMurray's, Thessaly's, and dial test. He does have a positive bent-knee stretch test and Puranen-Orava test. Simulated sprinting in the clinic reproduces pain. X-rays do not reveal any bony abnormalities or avulsion. No further imaging is indicated.

His diagnosis is consistent with a mild strain of the distal hamstrings, as a result of poor flexibility. Rehabilitation for this type of injury would focus on a progressive rehabilitation program of the hamstring (as noted above) and on hip flexor stretching, followed by return-to-play protocol.

Pearls and Pitfalls
- Acute isolated distal hamstring injuries are rare, and special consideration should be given to a full knee evaluation to rule out concomitant posterolateral corner injury.
- Hamstring injury recurrence rates are high and most often seen in the first 3 weeks of return to sport.
- The Nordic hamstring strengthening exercise has been proven to be beneficial in injury prevention.

Chapter Summary

Distal hamstring injuries are rare but an important injury consideration in the differential diagnosis of posterior thigh and knee pain in the adolescent patient. It is important to understand that the hamstring is a biarticular tendon-muscle complex that crosses both the hip and knee. This makes it susceptible to both stretch and eccentric load type injuries. Rehabilitation from distal hamstring injuries can be achieved with a graduated protocol and progressive return to play. Platelet-rich plasma injections have not been rigorously studied to prove efficacy in strain-like injuries, though safety of use has been identified in the available literature [27–29]. Prevention is aimed at maintaining flexibility and working on progressive eccentric loading exercises, with the Nordic hamstring lowering exercise proving to be superior in prevention management [23].

Chart/Table for Review

Condition	Hamstring Injuries
Description	Acute or chronic strain of biarticular muscle crossing the hip and knee at the posterior thigh
Epidemiology	Age-related increased rate with a peak incidence at age 17 Explosive sports involving rapid acceleration and deceleration, kicking, and hurdling
Mechanism (common)	Hyperextension of the knee Excessive eccentric load with hip flexed and knee extended
History and exam findings	Audible pop with inability to continue play Ecchymosis and/or palpable defect Pain with passive stretch of knee extended with hip flexed
Management	Graduated rehab protocol Focus on hamstring stretching and eccentric loading Progressive return to sport

References

1. Blackburn JT, Norcross MF, Cannon LN, Zinder SM. Hamstrings stiffness and landing biomechanics linked to anterior cruciate ligament loading. J Athl Train. 2013;48(6):764–72.
2. Beltran J, Matityahu A, Hwang K, Jbara M, Maimon R, Padron M, et al. The distal semimembranosus complex: normal MR anatomy, variants, biomechanics and pathology. Skelet Radiol. 2003;32(8):435–45.
3. Linklater JM, Hamilton B, Carmichael J, Orchard J, Wood DG. Hamstring injuries: anatomy, imaging, and intervention. Semin Musculoskelet Radiol. 2010;14(2):131–61.
4. Woodley SJ, Mercer SR. Hamstring muscles: architecture and innervation. Cells Tissues Organs. 2005;179(3):125–41.
5. Lieber RL, Friden J. Functional and clinical significance of skeletal muscle architecture. Muscle Nerve. 2000;23(11):1647–66.
6. De Smet AA, Best TM. MR imaging of the distribution and location of acute hamstring injuries in athletes. AJR Am J Roentgenol. 2000;174(2):393–9.
7. Terry GC, LaPrade RF. The biceps femoris muscle complex at the knee. Its anatomy and injury patterns associated with acute anterolateral–anteromedial rotatory instability. Am J Sports Med. 1996;24(1):2–8.
8. Ahmad CS, Redler LH, Ciccotti MG, Maffulli N, Longo UG, Bradley J. Evaluation and Management of Hamstring Injuries. Am J Sports Med. 2013;41(12):2933–47.
9. In Overlin AJFG. Madden CC, Putukian M, McCarty EC, young CC. Netter's sports medicine. 2nd edition. Philadephia: Elsevier; 2018. Table. 90:7.
10. Roe M, Murphy JC, Gissane C, Blake C. Hamstring injuries in elite Gaelic football: an 8-year investigation to indentify injry rates, time-loss patterns and players at increased risk. Br J Sports Med. 2018;53(15):982–8.

11. Crema MD, Guermazi A, Tol JL, Niu J, Hamilton B, Roemer FW. Acute hamstring injury in football players: association between anatomical location and extent of injury-a large single-center MRI report. J Sci Med Sport. 2016 Apr;19(4):317–22.
12. Freckleton G, Pizzari T. Risk factors for hamstring muscle injury in sport: a systematic review and meta-analysis. Br J Sports Med. 2013 Apr;47(6):351–8.
13. Gabbe BJ, Bennell KL, Finch CF. Why are older Australian football players at greater risk of hamstring injury? J Sci Med Sport. 2006 Aug;9(4):327:33.
14. Valle X, Malliaropoulos N, Parraga Botero JD, Bikos G, Pruna R, Monaco M, Maffulli N. Hamstring and other thigh injuries in children and young athletes. Scand J Med Sci Sports. 2018 Dec;28(12):2630–7.
15. Ropiak CR, Bosco JA. Hamstring Injuries. Bull NYU Hosp Jt Dis. 2012;70(1):41–8.
16. Andersen TE, Tenga A, Engebretsen L, Bahr R. Video analysis of injuries and incidents in Norwegian professional football. Br J Sports Med. 2004;38(5):626–31.
17. Cohen SB, Bradley J. Acute proximal hamstring rupture. J Am Acad Orthop Surg. 2007;15:350–5.
18. Cacchio A, Borra F, Severini G, et al. Reliability and validity of three pain provocation tests used for the diagnosis of chronic proximal hamstring tendinopathy. Br. J Sports Med. 2012;46:883Y7.
19. Connell DA, Schneider-Kolsky ME, Hoving JL, et al. Longitudinal study comparing sonographic and MRI assessments of acute and healing hamstring injuries. AJR Am J Roentgenol. 2004;183:975Y84.
20. Aldebeyan S, Boily M, Martineau PA. Complete tear of the distal hamstring tendons in a professional football player: a case report and review of the literature. Skelet Radiol. 2016 Mar;45(3):427–30.
21. Mishra D, Friden J, Schmitz M, Lieber R. Antiinflammatory medication after muscle injury. A treatment resulting in short-term improvement but subsequent loss of muscle function. J Bone Joint Surg Am. 1995;77:1510–9.
22. Mendiguchia J, Brughelli M. A return-to-sport algorithm for acute hamstring injuries. Phys Ther Sport. 2011;12:2–14.
23. Järvinen TA, Järvinen TL, Kääriäinen M, Äärimaa V, Vaittinen S, Kalimo H, et al. Muscle injuries: optimising recovery. Best Pract Res Clin Rheumatol. 2007;21(2):317–31.
24. Sherry MA, Johnston TS, Heiderscheit BC. Rehabilitation of acute hamstring strain injuries. Clin Sports Med. 2015;34(2):263–84.
25. Levine WN, Bergfeld JA, Tessendorf W, Moorman CT 3rd. Intramuscular corticosteroid injection for hamstring injuries. A 13-year experience in the National Football League. Am J Sports Med 2000; 28(3):297–300.
26. Scutt N, Rolf CG, Scutt A. Glucocorticoids inhibit tenocyte proliferation and tendon progenitor cell recruitment. Journal of orthopaedic research: official publication of the Orthopaedic Research Society. 2006;24(2):173–82.
27. Reurink G, Goudswaard GJ, Moen MH, Weir A, Verhaar JA, Bierma-Zeinstra SM, et al. Rationale, secondary outcome scores and 1-year follow-up of a randomised trial of platelet-rich plasma injections in acute hamstring muscle injury: the Dutch hamstring injection therapy study. Br J Sports Med. 2015;49(18):1206–12.
28. Rossi LA, Molina Rómoli AR, Bertona Altieri BA, Burgos Flor JA, Scordo WE, Elizondo CM. Does platelet-rich plasma decrease time to return to sports in acute muscle tear? A randomized controlled trial. Knee Surg Sports Traumatol Arthrosc. 2017 Oct;25(10):3319–25.
29. Sheth U, Dwyer T, Smith I, Wasserstein D, Theodoropoulos J, Takhar S, Chahal J. Does platelet-rich plasma lead to earlier return to sport when compared with conservative treatment in acute muscle injuries? A systematic review and meta-analysis. Arthroscopy. 2018;34(1):281–8.

Chapter 19
Gastrocnemius Injury

Lindsay W. Jones

Anatomy and Normal Function

The gastrocnemius or "calf muscle" consists of two heads and is located within the posterior fascial compartment of the leg. It spans two joints, the knee and the ankle. The medial and lateral heads of the gastrocnemius originate from their respective femoral condyles and join the soleus muscle at the mid to distal third of the posterior leg to form the common tendon, called the Achilles tendon. This tendon then inserts onto the calcaneus posteriorly. Another related muscle is the plantaris, running parallel to the gastrocnemii, originating just superior to the lateral gastrocnemius, and coursing between the two to the medial aspect of the Achilles, often joining it or occasionally inserting on the posterior medial calcaneus adjacent to the Achilles insertion. Occasionally, a sesamoid bone may be found in the lateral head of the gastrocnemius. This is often referred to as a "fabella." The function of these muscles is to plantar flex the foot and to flex the leg at the knee.

Pathology and Dysfunction

Injury pathology related to the gastrocnemius is typically a strain or small tear at the myotendinous junction or the muscle belly of the medial head of the gastrocnemius [6, 7]. Rarely, it may present with posterior medial knee pain, related to an avulsion injury at the proximal aspect of the medial head. This injury occurs more often in skeletally immature patients. Injury to this area results in an inability to ambulate with a normal heel-toe foot progression, due to pain at the injury site. Knee flexion

L. W. Jones (✉)
Orthopaedics, MedStar Union Memorial Hospital, Ellicott City, MD, USA
e-mail: Lindsay.W.Jones@medstar.net

© Springer Nature Switzerland AG 2021
N. Coleman (ed.), *Common Pediatric Knee Injuries*,
https://doi.org/10.1007/978-3-030-55870-3_19

beyond 30–45 degrees and terminal knee extension may be limited, secondary to pain. The chosen resting position is typically flexion to 20 or 30 degrees, as full extension causes pain, as well.

Specific Pointers

Epidemiology

While the gastrocnemius muscle is commonly injured in adults, it is less commonly associated with pediatric musculoskeletal injuries [6, 7]. Nonetheless, it does occur on occasion, typically in young adults rather than in children. There is no known gender propensity identified in the literature. Gastrocnemii injury occurs more commonly in basketball, soccer, lacrosse, football, or any other sport that involves rapid knee flexion and plantar flexion of the foot with change of direction and push off [7].

Mechanism of Injury

The typical mechanism of injury occurs during eccentric contraction of the gastrocnemius complex with resultant traction at the medial head of the gastrocnemius. The knee is typically flexed, and a sharp pain occurs at the posterior medial knee while planting the foot or pushing off with the foot to change to the contralateral direction. Alternative mechanisms of injury include forced dorsiflexion of the foot with the knee extended and knee hyperextension injuries with a planted foot [2, 3, 5–7].

Diagnosis

Components of history reported may include sudden onset of pain, followed by an antalgic gait; development of edema or ecchymoses at the level of the injury; and distal pain, improved with rest, ice, and/or nonsteroidal anti-inflammatory medications, and worsened with activity and ambulation [6]. Examination often demonstrates superficial edema, occasional ecchymoses, and invariable tenderness at the site of injury. Pain may be reproduced at the end-range of knee extension, with knee flexion beyond 45 degrees, with foot dorsiflexion, and/or with activation of the gastrocnemii in resisted knee flexion and resisted plantar flexion. Similarly, there may be pain with functional testing, including walking with a normal heel-toe progression; performing squats, both double and single leg; raising up on the toes; heel walking; and jumping. If pain is located near the origin of the gastrocnemius, at the knee, radiographs should be obtained to evaluate for an avulsion injury, typically at the medial head of the gastrocnemius [2, 3, 7]. This can be seen best on the lateral view. If pain is located at the belly of the muscle, not related to the knee, radiographs may not be warranted, unless there is concern for a tibial or fibular stress fracture/reaction. Advanced imaging, such as MRI, may be useful to evaluate the displacement of an avulsed bony fragment or to identify a radiographically occult medial gastrocnemius avulsion fracture [3–5]. MRI may also be considered if there is clinical suspicion for a proximal fibular stress fracture.

Management

Treatment of gastrocnemii myotendinous injuries is different from that for a bony avulsion injury. Strain pattern injury management generally consists of instituting a minimum of 10 days of rest from activity (with the affected leg); immobilizing the leg in a pneumatic walking boot, depending on severity of injury and difficulty with daily activities; applying ice 2 to 3 times per day for 20 minutes; and using NSAIDs regularly for 3–5 days. Return to normal walking, followed by gradual progression back to regular activities over a 4- to 6-week time-frame, is a typical recovery time-line for this injury. Occasionally, physical therapy is employed to regain baseline activity level and to prevent re-injury [7, 8].

Medial head of the gastrocnemius avulsion injury is typically managed nonoperatively; however, if there is displacement of the bony fragment on radiographs or MRI, surgical fixation should be considered [2, 3, 7, 8]. Treatment of the avulsion injury is similar to that of other fractures at tendon insertions, including nonweight bearing for 4–6 weeks, with gradual progression to weight bearing, as tolerated, after evidence of bony healing [8]. Medication management with an NSAID is recommended, as needed, for severe pain. Cryotherapy, elevation, and gentle compression may also be utilized for pain management. Full return to activity usually occurs within 3 months. Physical therapy is not always utilized, unless there is residual pain or range of motion limitation.

Demonstration Cases

Common Presentation

A 13-year-old male football player presents with acute onset of right posterior medial knee pain, while pushing off on the affected leg to cut around another player. He denies a notable popping sensation at time of injury. His pain was persistent, and he required assistance off the field, as he was unable to ambulate after the injury. Mild swelling developed in the calf region. He presented for evaluation at the specialist's office within 3 days of the injury. Examination was notable for an antalgic gait and limited knee range of motion, lacking 5 degrees of extension and 30 degrees of flexion, due to pain. Strength was intact with resisted knee and ankle motion. There was no appreciable knee effusion. He was neurovascularly intact. His radiographs were normal, without obvious fractures or abnormalities, and with open physes. His pain improved gradually and resolved by week 5 of rest and limited weight bearing. He had a full recovery without residual concern or limitations.

Uncommon Presentation

An18-year-old male football player presented after a direct blow by an opponent's shoulder to the anterior knee while the foot was planted. The athlete had immediate pain and inability to ambulate. The athletic trainer assessment on the field included no deformity and an intact neurovascular examination distal to the injury; however, given the concern for possible vascular disruption, based on the mechanism of injury, the patient was transported by emergency medical services (EMS) to the local trauma center for evaluation. Diagnosis of avulsion of the medial head of the gastrocnemius was made by radiographs, and an MRI ruled out associated injuries. Nonoperative management with nonweight bearing for 6 weeks was followed by a gradual return to activity.

Posterior knee dislocation has been reported in the literature as a rare mechanism for avulsion of the medial head of the gastrocnemius. It is more common in high velocity trauma, such as car accidents or skiing, than in team sports [2, 3]. When the mechanism for gastrocnemius avulsion includes dislocation, there are typically multiple associated injuries, including ligamentous and meniscal tears [2–4].

Pearls and Pitfalls

A key element of the injury history for gastrocnemius injury is acute onset. Patients typically recall the exact moment the injury occurred. Any reference to an insidious onset, progressive pain, or an overuse pattern of injury is less likely to be consistent with this diagnosis [2, 3, 6, 7].

Inspection may be normal; however, there is usually an area of tenderness on palpation and reproducible pain on activation of the gastrocnemius [2].

This injury can be confused with a few alternative conditions. The differential diagnosis list includes posterior medial or lateral meniscal tear, with or without a Baker's cyst; posterior medial or lateral corner injury; and distal hamstring injury, including medial- or lateral-sided, semimembranosus or semitendinosus, and biceps femoris, respectively.

Chapter Summary

Gastrocnemius injuries, causing posterior knee pain in the pediatric population, are rare and may be related to an avulsion at the origin of the muscle. Older pediatric patients may have muscle–tendon strain patterns of injury, typically seen in the adult population; however, those injuries present with posterior leg pain, rather than knee pain. Patients with a gastrocnemius avulsion present with acute onset pain after injury playing sports and usually describe an eccentric contraction at the knee with a planted foot. Pain is located posteromedially and is worse with full flexion and extension, as well as with ambulation. Nearly all gastrocnemius injuries, including avulsions, heal with nonoperative management. Despite the rarity of this condition, understanding the anatomy and presentation of the injury is necessary for the proper evaluation and management of patients presenting with posterior knee pain.

Condition	Knee-related gastrocnemius injury
Description	Avulsion injury at the bony origin of the medial head of the gastrocnemius muscle–tendon unit
Epidemiology	Exceedingly rare and often missed, when present
Mechanism (common)	Eccentric contraction of the muscle with a flexed knee and planted foot; may be more likely, if the tibia is externally rotated
History and exam findings	Acute onset posterior medial knee pain in a skeletally immature athlete, while playing sports; subsequent pain with movement. Exam notable for antalgic gait, tenderness over the posteromedial knee at the femoral origin of the medial gastrocnemius.
Management	3–6 weeks of conservative care, including rest from weight bearing; avoiding eccentric muscle activation; compression, elevation, icing, NSAIDs for a short course of treatment or as needed for pain management. Gradual return to sport using pain as a guide, once normal ambulation has resumed and full painless range of motion has returned.

References

1. Gottsegen CJ, Eyer BA, White EA, Learch TJ, Forrester D. Avulsion fractures of the knee: imaging findings and clinical significance. Radiographics. 2008;28(6):1755–70.
2. Maehara H, Sakaguchi Y. Avulsion fracture of the medial head of the gastrocnemius muscle: a case report. JBJS Case Connect. 2004;86(2):373–5.
3. Mio K, Matsuzaki K, Rikitake H, Nakaya T, Nemoto K, Chiba K. Avulsion fracture of the medial head of the gastrocnemius muscle associated with posterior knee dislocation: a case report. JBJS Case Connect. 2016;6(2):e241–5. https://doi.org/10.2106/JBJS.CC.00123. PMID: 29252618.
4. Patterson JT, Jokl P, Katz LD, Lawrence DA, Smitaman E. Case report isolated avulsion fracture at the medial head of the gastrocnemius muscle. Skelet Radiol. 2014;43:1491–4.
5. Yamazaki T, Maruoka S, Takahashi S, Saito H, Takase K, Nakamura M, et al. MRI findings of avulsive cortical irregularity of the distal femur. Skelet Radiol. 1995;24(1):43–6.

6. Armfield D, et al. Sports-related muscle injury in the lower extremity. Clin Sports Med. 2006;25:803–42.
7. Mueller-Wohlfahrt H, et al. Terminology and classification of muscle injuries in sport: the Munich consensus statement. Br J Sports Med. 2013;47:342–50.
8. Nsitem V. Diagnosis and rehabilitation of gastrocnemius muscle tear: a case report. J Can Chiropr Assoc. 2013;57(4):327–33.

Chapter 20
Posterolateral Corner Injury

Jeffrey M. Mjaanes

Anatomy and Normal Function

The lateral compartment of the knee is inherently unstable compared to the medial compartment, given the opposing convexities of the lateral femoral condyle and the lateral tibial plateau [1]. Several primary structures (Fig. 20.1) contribute to stability of the posterolateral knee: the lateral (fibular) collateral ligament (LCL), the popliteus muscle–tendon complex, the popliteofibular ligament (PFL), and the posterolateral capsule.

The LCL attaches proximally on the lateral femoral condyle and distally on the fibular head. This ligament serves as the primary restraint to varus opening of the knee, especially in the initial degrees of knee flexion.

The popliteus tendon attaches proximally on the lateral femoral condyle, and the muscle has its distal attachment on the posteromedial tibia. From the tendon originate three popliteomeniscal fascicles that attach to the lateral meniscus and confer stability. More distally, the popliteofibular ligament connects the popliteal myotendinous junction to the fibular styloid and aides in stabilizing the knee against external rotation forces.

Finally, the lateral portion of the joint capsule itself provides some stability to the knee. The dual-layered, thickened lateral joint capsule has confluences and connections with numerous lateral compartment structures. A Y-shaped thickening of the posterolateral capsule, which attaches the fibular styloid to the lateral gastrocnemius and the oblique popliteus ligament, is also referred to as the arcuate ligament. Related structures that confer dynamic stability include the biceps femoris, the iliotibial band (ITB), and the lateral gastrocnemius.

J. M. Mjaanes (✉)
Northwestern University, Evanston, IL, USA
e-mail: Jmjaanes@northwestern.edu

© Springer Nature Switzerland AG 2021
N. Coleman (ed.), *Common Pediatric Knee Injuries*,
https://doi.org/10.1007/978-3-030-55870-3_20

Fig. 20.1 Illustration of
posterolateral knee.
A. Popliteus muscle/
tendon. B. Popliteofibular
ligament (PFL). C. Lateral
gastrocnemius. D. Lateral
collateral ligament (LCL)

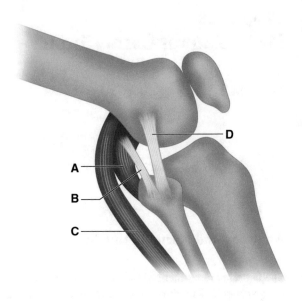

Pathology and Dysfunction

PLC structures act synergistically to resist external rotation of the tibia, posterior
translation of the tibia, and varus stress to the knee. Injuries to the PLC can,
therefore, result in instability in posterior and lateral directions. The extent of
disability often correlates with the specific structure(s) injured and/or the degree
of injury.

Isolated injury to the LCL may result in varus, but not posterior, instability especially at lesser degrees of knee flexion; however, injury to the popliteus complex and
PFL can result in posterolateral instability, especially at higher degrees of knee
flexion, due to diminished ability to withstand external tibial rotation.

Additionally, most PLC injuries do not occur in isolation. Studies indicate that
the majority of PLC injuries occur in combination with ruptures of the anterior
cruciate ligament (ACL), the posterior cruciate ligament (PCL), or both [2]. The
PCL serves to limit posterior translation of the tibia, especially with increased
degrees of knee flexion; the posterolateral corner (PLC), though, acts as the primary restraint to posterior translation as the knee nears full extension; therefore,
a high-grade injury to both the PCL and the PLC will result in a significantly
unstable knee at all degrees of flexion. In a combined injury, the clinician should
maintain a high index of suspicion for a knee dislocation, which spontaneously
reduced. This should prompt a thorough assessment of neurovascular structures,
especially the popliteal artery and common peroneal nerve. Evidence indicates
that 15–29% of PLC injuries have an associated common peroneal nerve
injury [4, 8].

Specific Pointers

Epidemiology

PLC injuries have been traditionally thought to be uncommon to rare; however, they are becoming increasingly recognized and studied in sports medicine. Given that these injuries are under-reported, their true incidence is unknown, but they are estimated to represent 5–9% of all knee injuries [3]. Typically, these injuries result from significant force, such as motor vehicle collisions, falls, and high-speed sports, including football and rugby. They can occur regardless of age and gender. Common mechanisms of injury to the PLC include a direct blow to the anteromedial tibia, contact and non-contact hyperextension, external rotation twisting injury, contact or non-contact varus force, or a direct blow to a flexed knee [6]. Injuries can also occur with dislocations of the knee joint [1].

Diagnosis: History and Physical Exam

The initial step in diagnosis is to obtain an accurate history of the injury and any symptoms present. The clinician should inquire about the manner the injury occurred and should suspect a PLC injury in cases with one of the common mechanisms described earlier. The clinician should inquire about feelings of instability in the joint, any associated numbness or tingling along the anterolateral lower leg and dorsum of foot, and any weakness, especially with ankle dorsiflexion and toe extension.

Acutely, the physical exam may reveal intra-articular swelling, as well as tenderness of the posterolateral structures. The patient may be unable to bear weight, or the gait will likely be significantly antalgic. In chronic cases of PLC injury, gait typically takes on a "varus thrust" pattern, in which the lateral compartment subluxes into varus on foot strike. A complete ligamentous exam, including assessment of the anterior and posterior cruciate ligaments, is imperative, due to the high frequency of concomitant injuries.

On exam, special testing can be utilized to evaluate the integrity of the various PLC structures.

The *varus stress test* is used to assess the LCL. The test is first performed by applying a varus stress on the knee at 0 degrees of flexion. Then, the examiner passively flexes the knee to 20–30 degrees and, using the exam table to stabilize the thigh, again applies a varus stress to the knee. In both cases, the clinician assesses the degree of laxity, or opening, on the lateral joint line. Comparison to the unaffected knee is advised. Greater laxity at 30 degrees often correlates with significant injury to the LCL, while positive varus stress at 0 degrees suggests injury to other posterolateral corner structures, in addition to the LCL.

A test of posterolateral rotation, the *dial test* can be done with the patient supine or prone. With the patient in the prone position and knees together, the examiner grasps the ankles and flexes the knees to 30 degrees of flexion (Fig. 20.2). Then the examiner externally rotates the feet. An increase in external rotation of 10 degrees or more on the affected side indicates a posterolateral knee injury. The clinician then repeats the test at 90 degrees of flexion. If external rotation increases at 90 degrees

Fig. 20.2 (**a**) Dial test at 90 degrees of knee flexion. (**b**) Dial test at 30 degrees of knee flexion

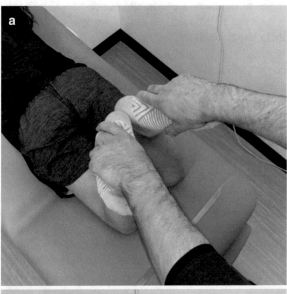

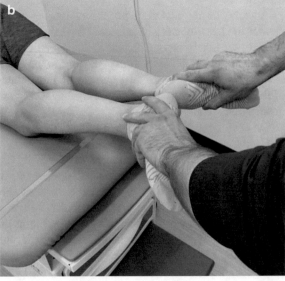

of flexion compared to at 30 degrees, this is highly suggestive of a combined PLC
and PCL injury.

Several other tests exist to assess for posterolateral instability. In the *posterolateral drawer test*, the patient is supine, and the clinician flexes the knee to 80–90 degrees, externally rotates the foot, and then applies a posterolaterally directed force on the tibia (Fig. 20.3). If the lateral tibial plateau rotates externally and posteriorly with respect to the medial plateau, the test is considered positive. In the *external recurvatum test*, the examiner holds the supine patient's great toes and lifts the heels off the table. In the PLC-deficient knee, the tibia will rotate into varus as the knee hyperextends compared to the unaffected side. Finally, one can also use the *reverse pivot shift test* to assess the PLC. In this test, the clinician passively takes the knee from 90 degrees of flexion to full extension, while applying a valgus load. At approximately 20–30 degrees of flexion, the lateral tibial plateau will abruptly sublux in the PLC-deficient knee, due to action of the iliotibial band.

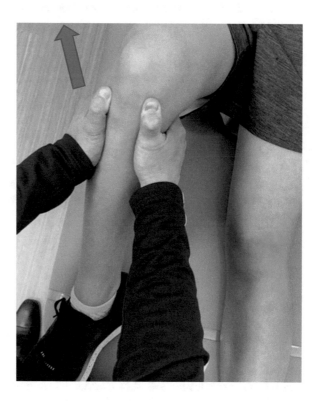

Fig. 20.3 Posterolateral drawer test. With the patient's knee flexed to 80–90 degrees, a posterior and laterally directed force (blue arrow) is applied to tibia and clinician assesses for external rotation and posterior motion

Imaging

Plain radiographs are indicated in cases of knee trauma. Often in PLC injuries radiographs will be normal; however, occasionally they may demonstrate tibial plateau or avulsion fractures. Avulsion injuries can involve the arcuate ligament off the fibular head (the "arcuate sign"), the popliteal tendon from its femoral attachment, the ITB from Gerdy's tubercle, or the lateral capsule from the lateral tibial plateau ("Segond fracture").

MRI is a useful modality for revealing the injured structures in the complex posterolateral corner. In addition to the standard sequences in the sagittal, axial, and coronal planes, thin-slice coronal oblique images through the fibular head and styloid may improve the accuracy, sensitivity, and specificity of identifying the LCL, PFL, popliteus tendon, and other PLC anatomy. One study suggests that early MRI (<12 weeks) is >90% accurate in diagnosing injuries to the posterolateral corner; however, this decreases to 27%, when performed more than 12 weeks after injury [3].

Classification/Grading

The most commonly used classification system for PLC injuries is the Hughston system. *Grade I* sprains have minimal-to-no (0–5 mm) laxity on varus stress, minimal-to-no (less than 5 degrees) rotational instability on dial test, and no evidence of capsule-ligamentous injury. *Grade II* injuries have moderate varus laxity (6–10 mm lateral opening), moderate rotational instability (6–10 degrees), and partial ligamentous injury. *Grade III* injuries have severe instability with >10 mm lateral opening on varus stress, >10 degrees external rotational instability on dial test, and complete ligament disruption [4].

Management

Non-operative

In low-grade PLC injuries, non-operative treatment may result in acceptable clinical outcomes. In grade I and many grade II injuries, non-surgical management consists of immobilization with a hinged knee brace in full extension and protected weight bearing with crutches for 3–6 weeks, during which time the patient may engage in isometric quadriceps strengthening. After the initial period of immobilization, the patient begins a program of progressive motion, weight bearing, and strengthening. Closed kinetic chain exercises, in which the distal end of the extremity is fixed on the ground, may begin around 6–8 weeks; however, many clinicians advise avoidance of hamstring strengthening exercises until 8–10 weeks post-injury. Resumption of full activity tends to occur around 3–4 months.

Operative

In grade III and some more severe grade II injuries, surgical intervention is often indicated. Operative management may consist of direct repair or primary reconstruction. Factors influencing surgical decision-making include the timing (acute or chronic) and the nature (isolated or combined) of the injury.

Some controversy exists as to whether PLC repair is preferred over reconstruction, although most authors agree that earlier intervention, repair or reconstruction, is favored over late reconstruction. Reasons cited for earlier intervention include increased risks of later soft-tissue stretching and capsular scarring; ultimately, scar formation may obscure the anatomy, especially the location and course of the common peroneal nerve [5]. Acute, isolated PLC injuries are often treated by direct, anatomic repair, ideally within the first 3 weeks. Nevertheless, as mentioned, some authors support early reconstruction over repair, citing increased failure rates with repair [7]. For the LCL, acute high-grade ruptures may be treated with repair of the intrasubstance tear and graft reconstruction. Avulsion and tibial plateau fractures should be stabilized either with internal fixation or suture anchors. In any case, many authors advocate postponing surgery by a week or two after injury to allow for the acute inflammation to subside; arthrofibrosis may result from surgery, particularly reconstructions, performed too early [2].

When the PLC is injured acutely along with other ligaments, surgical intervention to all involved structures can be performed at the same time or in staged procedures. At least one recent systematic review advocates for contemporaneous intervention, revealing that repair of acute grade III PLC injuries with staged cruciate ligament reconstruction is associated with a 38% failure rate; however, concurrent cruciate reconstruction results in a 9% mean failure rate [2]. Many surgeons now opt for repair and reconstruction at the same time. In cases of chronic PLC instability, reconstruction is performed with the goal of stabilizing the posterolateral corner but not necessarily reestablishing the normal anatomic relationships of the damaged structures.

Demonstration Cases

Common Presentation

A 19-year-old wrestler attempts to extend the left knee from flexed position in practice, when the opponent collides with the anteromedial knee forcing him into varus with external rotation. The athlete feels and hears a pop and has immediate pain over the posterolateral left knee.

On examination several days later, he has a mild effusion and tenderness along the left lateral collateral ligament proximally, as well as along the lateral aspect of the popliteal fossa. Range of motion and strength is normal. He has negative anterior and posterior drawer testing but has pain and 5 mm laxity with stress testing the left knee at 30 degrees of flexion, compared to a painless firm endpoint on the right. Varus stress testing at 0 degrees is symmetric. Dial test is negative.

MRI reveals a partial intrasubstance tear of the proximal fibers of the LCL, as well as intrasubstance fluid within the soleus muscle and surrounding the popliteus tendon distally (Figs. 20.4 and 20.5).

Fig. 20.4 Coronal MRI showing attenuation in signal of proximal LCL (A) consistent with partial tear

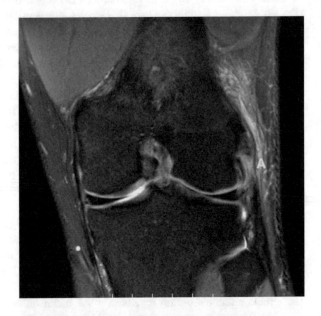

Fig. 20.5 Sagittal MRI showing strain of popliteus tendon (A) and fluid in soleus muscle (B)

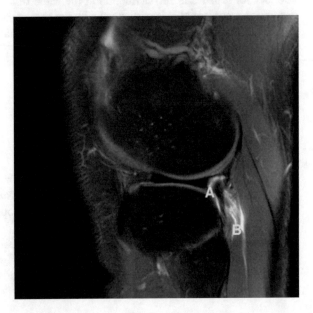

The athlete was diagnosed with a grade I–II LCL sprain and low-grade injury to the popliteus. He was treated with hinged knee brace immobilization for 3 weeks, followed by progressive rehabilitation, and was able to return to sport by 6 weeks post-injury.

Uncommon Presentation

An 18-year-old football player is running with the ball, when he is struck from the side and knocked off balance, forcing his extended right knee into varus, with resultant hyperextension and external rotation. He is unable to bear weight and is transported off the field. He has significant pain in the entire right knee and rapidly develops a hemarthrosis, as well as tingling along the dorsal aspect of his right foot.

On examination he has intraarticular swelling and tenderness along the lateral aspect of the knee. He has significant difficulty actively flexing the knee. He has a positive Lachman's and anterior drawer test and significantly positive varus stress testing at 30 degrees, with no firm endpoint noted on these tests. Dial test is positive on the right compared to the left. He has intact sensation along the right lower extremity distally, intact ankle dorsiflexion and great toe extension, and a normal dorsalis pedis pulse.

Plain radiographs are unremarkable. An MRI is obtained, which reveals a complete rupture of the anterior cruciate ligament (Fig. 20.6), partial tearing of the PCL (Fig. 20.7), a complete avulsion of the biceps femoris and lateral collateral ligament off the fibular head (Fig. 20.8), partial tearing of the popliteus tendon and arcuate

Fig. 20.6 Sagittal MRI showing complete rupture of the anterior cruciate ligament (A). Vacant normal anatomic location outlined in black

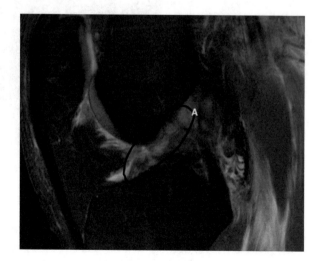

Fig. 20.7 Sagittal MRI of same patient showing thickened, tortuous posterior cruciate ligament (B), consistent with partial tearing

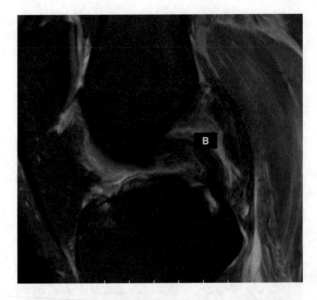

Fig. 20.8 Coronal view showing avulsion of the biceps femoris tendon and lateral collateral ligament off the fibular head (black arrow)

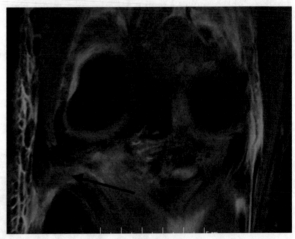

ligament (Fig. 20.9), tear of the posterolateral capsule, and a strain of the lateral gastrocnemius.

The athlete's knee was immobilized and a surgical consult obtained. Twelve days post-injury, he underwent surgical intervention, consisting of anterior cruciate reconstruction with patellar tendon autograft, primary repair of the LCL and biceps femoris, and repair of the posterolateral capsule.

Post-operatively he was kept non-weight bearing for 4 weeks, and then he began a progressive weight bearing, motion, and strengthening program. Full, pain-free return to sport was achieved in 10 months of post-injury.

Fig. 20.9 Partial tearing of popliteus muscle–tendon unit (C)

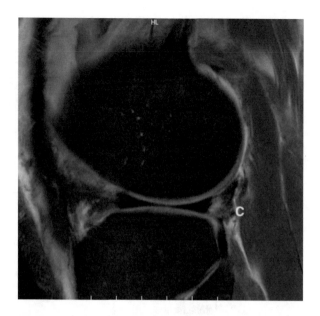

Pearls and Pitfalls
- Literature suggests that up to 70% of PLC injuries are misdiagnosed on initial presentation [3]. Based on mechanism of injury, the clinician should have a high index of suspicion for PLC injuries.
- Isolated PLC injuries are relatively rare entities. Combined injuries are being more commonly recognized.
- Remember to perform a complete ligamentous evaluation, as well as a neurovascular assessment to rule out concomitant injuries to the cruciate ligaments, popliteal artery, and common peroneal nerve.
- The clinician should become familiar with common tests for assessing the integrity of the PLC, such as the varus stress test and the dial test.
- Earlier use of MRI may be more accurate in identifying injured structures
- Most grade I and grade II injuries can be managed non-operatively. The general clinician should consider surgical consultation for all higher-grade injuries. In acute injuries, earlier surgical intervention appears to lead to improved outcomes.

Chapter Summary

The posterolateral corner is an often misunderstood anatomic region of the knee, yet it plays a critical role in conferring stability against varus, external rotation, and posterior forces. Injuries can span the spectrum from mild to severe and from

Table 20.1 Chapter Review

Condition	Posterolateral Corner (PLC) Injuries
Description	Injury to one or more of the following structures: lateral collateral ligament (LCL), popliteal muscle–tendon complex, popliteofibular ligament (PFL). Often seen with concurrent injury to ACL, PCL, or both
Epidemiology	High-energy injury: motor vehicle collisions, falls, high-energy sports
Mechanism (common)	1. Direct blow to the anteromedial tibia 2. Contact and non-contact hyperextension 3. External rotation twisting injury 4. Contact or non-contact varus force 5. Direct blow to flexed knee 6. Knee dislocation
History and exam findings	Posterolateral pain, intraarticular swelling, instability Positive varus stress test Positive dial test May have positive external rotation recurvatum, posterolateral drawer, and/or reverse pivot shift tests MRI useful in identifying injured structures
Management	Grade I and most grade II injuries can be managed non-operatively with early immobilization followed by progressive motion, weight bearing, and strengthening. Grade III and some grade II injuries require surgical intervention. In general, earlier intervention is preferred, and more commonly concomitant repair and/or reconstruction of involved structures leads to improved outcomes.

isolated to involving multiple structures. In general, isolated injuries are now recognized as rare, and the clinician should have a low threshold for suspecting concomitant injuries to structures, such as the anterior or posterior cruciate ligaments, lateral meniscus, popliteal artery, and peroneal nerve. Early diagnosis and management are the keys to improved clinical outcomes. While low-grade injuries can be managed non-operatively, higher-grade injuries, especially those involving multiple structures, should be treated surgically (Table 20.1).

References/Resources

1. Cooper JM, McAndrews PT, LaPrade RF. Posterolateral corner injuries of the knee: anatomy, diagnosis and treatment. Sports Med Arthrosc. 2006;14(4):213–20.
2. Geeslin AG, Moulton SG, LaPrade RF. A systematic review of the outcomes of posterolateral corner knee injuries, Part 1. Am J Sports Med. 2015;44(5):1336–42.
3. Pacheco RJ, Ayre CA, Bollen SR. Posterolateral corner injuries of the knee: a serious injury commonly missed. J Bone Joint Surg. 2011;93-B:194–7.
4. Shon O-J, Park J-W, Kim B-J. Current concepts in posterolateral corner injuries of the knee. Knee Surg Relat Res. 2017;29(4):256–68.
5. Ranawat A, Baker CL III, Henry S, Harner CD. Posterolateral corner injury of the knee: evaluation and management. J Am Acad Orthop Surg. 2008;16:506–18.

6. Schweller EW, Ward PJ. Posterolateral corner knee injuries: review of anatomy and clinical evaluation. J Am Osteopath Assoc. 2015;115:725–31.
7. Stannard JP, Brown SL, Farris RC, McGwin G Jr, Volgas DA. The posterolateral corner of the knee: repair versus reconstruction. Am J Sports Med. 2005;33(6):881–8.
8. Chahla J, Moatshe G, Dean CS, LaPrade RF. Posterolateral corner of the knee: current concepts. Arch Bone Jt Surg. 2016;4(2):97–103.

Chapter 21
Popliteal Cyst

Joseph M. Powers and Tracy Ray

Anatomy

The popliteal fossa is bounded superomedially by the semimembranosus and semi-tendinosus and superolaterally by the biceps femoris. The two heads of the gastrocnemius create the inferior border. The popliteal fascia forms the roof of the fossa, and the floor is formed by the posterior aspect of the distal femur [1, 2]. Popliteal cysts, also known as the eponymously named Baker's cyst, originate from the bursa between the medial head of the gastrocnemius and the semimembranosus. There may be occasional involvement of the subgastrocnemius bursa, as well [3].

In children, the majority of these cysts have no communication with the joint capsule, may arise spontaneously, and may be referred to as primary popliteal cysts [3–5]. In the adult population, popliteal cysts are frequently associated with a joint effusion and internal derangement, and 70% of cysts communicate with the knee joint [1, 6]. Popliteal cysts in children with communication to the joint via associated effusions from trauma or inflammatory conditions resemble those seen in adults and may be termed secondary popliteal cysts [5].

Epidemiology

Popliteal cysts occur approximately twice as often in males compared to females [4, 7]. The peak prevalence is 4–7 years of age, but they have been reported in children as young as 2 [8, 9]. On retrospective review of pediatric knee MRIs, the

J. M. Powers (✉)
Sports Medicine, Northside Hospital, Orthopedic Institute, Atlanta, GA, USA

T. Ray
Sports Medicine, Piedmont Healthcare, Watkinsville, GA, USA

© Springer Nature Switzerland AG 2021
N. Coleman (ed.), *Common Pediatric Knee Injuries*,
https://doi.org/10.1007/978-3-030-55870-3_21

prevalence of popliteal cysts has been estimated at 6.3%, considerably lower than the adult population [10].

Associated Conditions

The majority of popliteal cysts in children arise spontaneously and are usually an incidental finding on exam. There has been speculation that, in some cases, repeated trauma to the popliteal fossa, such as swinging legs against the front a chair, may lead to inflammation and bursal distension [5]. In most instances, however, there is no clear precipitating event.

Intraarticular pathology, such as meniscal or ligamentous tears, chondral lesions, or osteochondritis dissecans, may result in effusions; thus, popliteal cysts may be observed with these conditions.

Children with juvenile idiopathic arthritis (JIA) may develop popliteal cysts, which can become symptomatic. These are typically associated with underlying joint effusions. Popliteal cysts may be noted in up to 61% of children with JIA [11].

Infectious causes of popliteal cysts are rare. There have been reports of Lyme arthritis causing popliteal cyst development. Additionally, brucellosis, tuberculosis, candidiasis, and aspergillosis have been implicated [12].

Rupture of a popliteal cyst may create inflammation and swelling of surrounding soft tissues, mimicking thrombophlebitis. If swelling extends beyond the popliteal fossa, consideration should be given to the diagnosis of deep venous thrombosis [13].

Other conditions rarely associated with popliteal cysts include connective tissue disorders, such as Ehlers Danlos [4]. There has been one case report in the literature of a ruptured popliteal cyst in a child with hemophilia A [14]. Additionally, there has been one case of synovial sarcoma in a 13-year-old girl with bilateral popliteal cysts [15].

Diagnosis

The majority of popliteal cysts will present with a history of fullness or mass in the popliteal fossa without associated pain. Primary popliteal cysts may rarely be observed bilaterally. If a history of trauma is elicited, a thorough examination of the knee to evaluate for internal derangement should be undertaken. If other systemic symptoms or additional joint involvement is suggested (i.e. effusion), a workup for an underlying inflammatory condition should be considered.

On exam, the clinician will notice a fullness or mass arising behind the knee in the popliteal fossa, typically involving the posteromedial aspect [5]. Physical exam alone may be sufficient for diagnosis in many cases. For secondary popliteal cysts, Foucher's sign may be present as follows: when the knee is in full extension, the gastrocnemius and semimembranosus muscles occlude passage of fluid from the cyst into the intraarticular space, making the cyst more prominent and firm; when the knee is partially flexed, the cyst becomes more compressible and softer [16]. Transillumination has been described as one technique to investigate this area further, as well [4].

Radiographs are frequently normal, when obtained in the workup of popliteal cysts, although soft tissue swelling may be observed on the lateral view. The addition of a tunnel view may reveal irregularity of the chondral surface of the femoral condyles that can be seen with osteochondritis dissecans. This condition may produce an effusion, causing a secondary popliteal cyst.

With the increasing availability of ultrasound, this modality may be considered an excellent option for evaluating popliteal cysts. Serial exams may be conducted to monitor changes in the appearance of the cyst. Ultrasound is also helpful for differentiating a cyst from other soft tissue masses, such as soft tissue tumors [4]. Additionally, Doppler may be utilized to confirm the absence of blood flow to the cyst, which may be seen with a popliteal artery aneurysm [13]. Ultrasound has also been used to observe Foucher's sign, in secondary popliteal cysts in the adult population [16].

Under ultrasound, popliteal cysts will appear as a well-defined anechoic mass. Occasionally, septations and synovial proliferation and thickening may be present. Debris may be identified within the cyst, as well. With hemarthrosis, seen with trauma or hemophilia, it may be possible to identify layering of the components with ultrasound. Hemarthrosis may also produce synovial hypertrophy, secondary to associated irritation. As previously mentioned, popliteal cysts may rupture, and, in these cases, ultrasound will reveal a fluid collection with indistinct margins [13].

If there is concern for internal derangement, magnetic resonance imaging (MRI) may be considered to evaluate further. Additionally, if atypical extension of the cyst is suspected, the high-resolution and multiplanar imaging with MRI can help to delineate the popliteal cyst further. For an isolated primary popliteal cyst, obtaining an MRI is likely unnecessary [4, 13].

Vascular lesions, ganglion cysts, parameniscal cysts, synovial chondromatosis, and soft tissue tumors should be considered in the differential diagnosis of popliteal cysts [5].

Management

Observation alone is typically recommended for primary popliteal cysts. The presence of an associated effusion should prompt the clinician to probe for other pathology. If underlying inflammatory disorders are identified, treatment may lead to eventual resolution of the cyst. Similarly, if underlying structural pathology is present, the cyst should resolve upon treatment of the causative condition.

There is no consensus in the literature regarding frequency of monitoring with serial ultrasounds. Mean time to resolution has been reported from 28 to 35 months with a wide range. Unless there is a change in clinical status, infrequent monitoring is sufficient. If the cyst is enlarging or long standing, consider workup of JIA [5].

Ultrasound can be used to guide aspiration of popliteal cysts, if more aggressive treatment is desired. This may be considered in those with discomfort or if the cyst is exerting mass effect on surrounding structures. There are no studies identified in the literature in the pediatric population regarding aspiration of primary popliteal cysts. Once again, if the popliteal cyst is secondary to underlying joint pathology, treatment should be directed at the primary condition. If aspirating, care should be taken to avoid the neurovascular structures within the popliteal fossa. Recurrence of the cyst may occur after aspiration.

It has been suggested that popliteal cysts with involvement of the subgastrocnemius bursa may be more likely to persist on serial exams than those exclusive to the gastrocnemio-semimembranosus bursa [3]. If asymptomatic, continued watchful waiting may be all that is required.

Surgical intervention for primary popliteal cyst may be considered for those patients with pain, restricted motion, or restricted activity after other secondary causes have been ruled out and a sufficient period of observation has been undertaken.

Demonstration Cases

Common Presentation

A 6-year-old male presents for evaluation of fullness in the right popliteal fossa. He denies pain. His parents noticed the fullness approximately 1 month ago. They have not observed a limp or other limitation in activity. There are no systemic symptoms.

On exam there is no evidence of effusion. There is fullness and the suggestion of swelling in the posteromedial aspect of the popliteal fossa, but there is no tenderness to palpation. The area of swelling is non-pulsatile. There is slightly restricted end range flexion on the affected knee, which is pain free. Extension is full. Strength is full bilaterally. There is a normal, non-antalgic gait.

Consideration could be given to ultrasound at this point to confirm the presence of primary popliteal cyst. If the clinician is confident in the diagnosis of a primary popliteal cyst, watchful waiting and observation until resolution of cyst would be recommended.

Uncommon Presentation

An 8-year-old male presents for evaluation of fullness in the right popliteal fossa. He notes occasional pain but has difficulty describing the quality of the pain. His parents noticed the fullness approximately 1 month ago. They feel as though there may be some mild swelling of the knee and an occasional limp. Teachers and other caregivers have also noticed the limp. There is no history of witnessed trauma, and the child cannot recall any trauma. There is no significant family history for rheumatologic conditions.

On exam there is trace swelling and effusion. There is fullness and the suggestion of swelling in the posteromedial aspect of the popliteal fossa. The area of swelling is non-pulsatile. There is slightly restricted end range flexion on the affected knee, which is pain free. Extension is full, as is strength bilaterally. There is a mild limp appreciated, favoring the affected side.

Given the presence of an associated effusion, this is likely a secondary popliteal cyst. At this point, further investigation of underlying inflammatory condition would be warranted.

Pearls and Pitfalls

Most popliteal cysts in children are incidental, isolated findings that do not cause pain or disability and have an excellent prognosis. Typically unilateral and more frequently seen in males, primary popliteal cysts are expected to resolve spontaneously. Diagnosis is based upon history and physical exam, and may be supplemented by ultrasound or, occasionally, MRI. If a primary popliteal cyst is identified, reassurance may be provided and watchful waiting undertaken with repeat exams until resolution of the cyst is documented.

If other systemic symptoms are present or if there is associated joint effusion or a history of trauma, a more thorough investigation is required to identify the causative source of the popliteal cyst. Resolution of the cyst would be expected upon treatment of the underlying condition.

Condition	Popliteal cyst
Description	Primary—painless swelling over the posteromedial knee Secondary—due to intraarticular pathology, inflammatory, or infectious causes
Epidemiology	More commonly seen in males (2:1), typically observed in early school age years
Mechanism	Primary—usually no associated trauma or mechanism. Speculation that mild repetitive trauma may be implicated
History and exam findings	Primary popliteal cysts may be incidental findings or brought to attention by parents. Exam reveals fullness in the popliteal fossa. If other systemic symptoms are present or there is a history of trauma, suspect secondary popliteal cyst.
Management	Primary—reassurance, watchful waiting, consider serial ultrasound Secondary—treat the underlying condition

References

1. Nichols JS, et al. Surgical anatomy & pathology of the popliteal fossa. Orthop Trauma. 2013;27:113–7.
2. Dagur G, et al. Anatomical approach to clinical problems of the popliteal fossa. Curr Rheumatol Rev. 2017;13(2):126–38.
3. Akagi R, et al. Natural history of popliteal cysts in the pediatric population. J Pediatr Orthop. 2013;33:262–8.
4. Harcke HT, et al. Popliteal cysts in children: another look. J Pediatr Orthop. 2016;25:539–42.
5. Shapira M, et al. Visual diagnosis: bilateral posterior swelling of the knees in a 12-year-old boy. Pediatr Rev. 2011;32:169.
6. De Maeseneer M, et al. Popliteal cysts in children: prevalence, appearance and associated findings at MR imaging. Pediatr Radiol. 1999;29:605–9.
7. Dinham JM. Popliteal cysts in children. J Bone Joint Surg. 1975;57:69–71.
8. Gristina AG, et al. Popliteal cysts in adults and children: a review of 90 cases. Arch Surg. 1964;88:357.
9. Pandey PK, et al. Baker's cyst in a 2 year old child. IOSR JDMS. 2015;14:59–61.
10. De Maeseneer M, et al. Popliteal cysts in children: prevalence, appearance and associated findings at MR imaging. Pediatr Radiol. 1999;29:605–9.
11. Lan IM, et al. MRI appearance of popliteal cysts in childhood. Pediatr Radiol. 1997;27:130–2.
12. Magee TH, et al. Lyme disease presenting as popliteal cyst in children. J Pediatr Orthop. 2006;26:725–7.
13. Alessi S, et al. Baker's cyst in pediatric patients: ultrasonographic characteristics. J Ultrasound. 2012;15:76.
14. Rodriguez V, et al. Haemorrhage into a popliteal cyst: an unusual complication of haemophilia A. Haemophilia. 2002;8:725–8.
15. Ayoub KB, et al. Synovial sarcoma arising in association with a popliteal cyst. Skelet Radiol. 2000;29:713–6.
16. Blome A, et al. Ultrasonographic characteristics of Baker's cysts: the sonographic Foucher's sign. J Emerg Med. 2017;53(3):753–5.

Chapter 22
Medial Collateral Ligament Injury

Reno Ravindran

Introduction

The medial collateral ligament (MCL) is one of several ligaments of the knee. Its main function is to provide stability to the medial knee against valgus, internal, and external torque loads. The MCL is the most commonly injured ligament in the knee. MCL injury can occur in isolation or in conjunction with anterior cruciate ligament (ACL) and meniscal injuries.

Anatomy

The MCL is composed of three layers, including a thin layer that overlies the gastrocnemius, the superficial medial collateral ligament (sMCL), and the deep medial collateral ligament (dMCL). The sMCL has a barbell configuration, a single point of femoral insertion, and two distal tibial insertions. The first tibial insertion is more proximal, inserts just anterior to the semimembranosus tendon, and is approximately 12 mm distal to the joint line. The second tibial insertion is more distal and is, on average, 61 mm distal the joint line. It inserts just anterior to the posteromedial crest of the tibia. The two distal insertions of the sMCL have different biomechanical properties. The proximal insertion stabilizes against valgus forces in all degrees of knee flexion, while the distal insertion is responsible for stability in external rotation at 30 ° and 60 ° of knee flexion and in internal rotation [1].

R. Ravindran (✉)
Sports Medicine, Nationwide Children's Hospital and The Ohio State University College of Medicine, Dublin, OH, USA
e-mail: reno.ravindran@Nationwidechildrens.org

© Springer Nature Switzerland AG 2021
N. Coleman (ed.), *Common Pediatric Knee Injuries*,
https://doi.org/10.1007/978-3-030-55870-3_22

The dMCL is closely related to the joint capsule below the sMCL. Its main function is to help stabilize against valgus forces along with controlling internal and external rotation. The dMCL has two components: the meniscofemoral and meniscotibial ligaments. The meniscofemoral ligament has its first insertion immediately distal to the insertion of the sMCL in the femur approximately 15.7 mm proximal to the femoral joint line. The second is shorter and thicker and inserts on average 3.2 mm distal to the joint line and 9 mm proximal to the sMCL [1].

Epidemiology

The MCL is the most commonly injured ligament in an athlete's knee. The annual incidence of MCL injuries among high school football players is 24.2 per 100,000 athletes [1]. Contrary to historic teaching that ligamentous injury is rare in skeletally immature athletes, MCL injuries represent 26% of all knee injuries in high school athletes [2]. Approximately 10% of isolated MCL injuries will be bony avulsion injuries rather than purely ligamentous sprains. Nearly 78% of patients who sustain a grade III MCL injury can have an injury to another associated structure. MCL injuries are most commonly seen in skiing, football, soccer, rugby, wrestling, and ice hockey. Football and soccer injuries tend to be higher grade, while injuries from skiing and wrestling tend to be lower grade. Male athletes are 2.62 times more likely than female athletes to sustain an MCL injury [3].

Mechanism of Injury

Although MCL injuries can occur after contact and noncontact valgus forces, the majority of MCL injuries are contact injuries. Most athletes with an MCL injury will describe an impact to the lateral side of the knee, while the foot was planted. Patients may say the knee "popped" or felt like it was "collapsing" or "buckling inward." They will pinpoint their pain to the medial aspect of the knee, anywhere along the MCL. Some will complain of pain with weight-bearing or of loss of knee motion, due to pain; others may feel the knee collapse or "wobble" with each step. Most MCL injuries involve the sMCL at the proximal insertion on the femur [4].

Diagnosis

An initial thorough physical exam should consist of inspection for swelling, effusion, or any open wounds and any signs of neurovascular compromise. Significant deformity or neurovascular compromise can suggest a fracture or dislocation of the knee, which should prompt reduction (if neurovascular compromise is suspected or evident), immobilization, and transport to the hospital. Ecchymosis can be seen on the medial aspect of the knee in the context of grade II and III injuries. Localized swelling may be present on the medial aspect of knee and may help differentiate a femoral-area MCL injury versus a tibial-area MCL injury. Palpation around the knee, including along the course of the MCL, can also help to localize the area of injury. As the MCL is extra-articular, the presence of an effusion should clue the examiner into an associated intra-articular or other concomitant injury [4].

Laxity stress testing of the MCL is the mainstay of the ligament's examination. Valgus stress of the knee at various degrees will help determine the extent of the injury. Based on the exam, MCL injuries are graded as grade I, II, and III injuries. Grade I injuries are stretch injuries or microscopic tears to the ligament with no significant disruption. With Grade I injuries the patient may elicit pain with valgus stress but no increased laxity. Grade II injuries show partial tears of the ligament. Patients with these injuries will have pain with valgus stress and have increased laxity, as compared to the contralateral side. Grade III injuries are full, or near full, thickness tears of the ligament. Grade III injuries are associated with gross laxity and pain with valgus stress [4].

Stress testing of the ligament begins with the patient lying supine and his/her leg resting in extension on the table. The examiner will place his/her contralateral hand at the medial ankle or lower leg, while the ipsilateral hand supports the posterolateral knee. The examiner will then apply a valgus force by pushing on the medial ankle/lower leg at 0 °and at 30 ° and pay attention to any amount of laxity (comparing to the patient's contralateral side). Grade I laxity is 0–5 mm opening with pain and a firm endpoint. Grade II laxity is 5–10 mm opening with a less firm endpoint. Grade III laxity is >10 mm opening with no endpoint. A functional grading system involves laxity at specific degrees of the exam. Minimal laxity seen at 30 ° with minimal pain is a grade I. Laxity at 30 ° but stable at 0 ° is a grade II injury, and laxities at both 30 ° and 0 ° suggest a grade III injury (Fig. 22.1) (Table 22.1).

Fig. 22.1 Valgus examination of medial collateral ligament

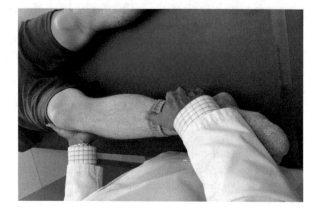

Table 22.1 Functional grading system

	0 ° of flexion	30 ° of flexion
Grade I	Stable	0–5 mm
Grade II	Stable	5–10 mm
Grade III	>10 mm	>10 mm

Fig. 22.2 X-ray Notch view demonstrates Salter–Harris III fracture of the distal femoral condyle

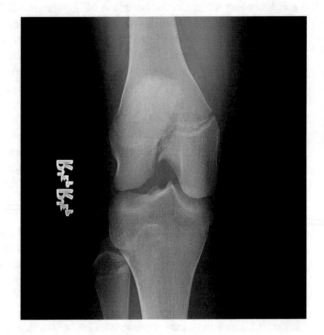

Imaging

X-rays are the first-line imaging tests to evaluate a knee injury. X-rays are not always necessary for isolated MCL injuries but are of benefit to assess for associated bony fractures or avulsion injuries that may occur along with an MCL injury. Standard anteroposterior (AP) and lateral views, along with a notch view and sunrise view, are sufficient views in the pediatric patient. These views will also assess the physis to rule in or out a Salter–Harris fracture that may present as laxity on valgus stress testing [4] (Fig. 22.2).

Magnetic resonance imaging (MRI) is the gold-standard imaging test to assess for MCL injury, as it allows for the best evaluation of the degree and location of the injury. It can also depict any concomitant injuries to other ligaments, the physis, the menisci, and cartilage. If a grade I MCL injury is noted on exam and no other injury is suspected, an MRI is not necessary to manage the patient. In the setting of an effusion, questionable physeal injury, chondral defect, or other ligamentous injury, an MRI is warranted [4].

Fig. 22.3 Coronal MRI images demonstrates grade III tear of medial collateral ligament with surrounding edema (blue arrow)

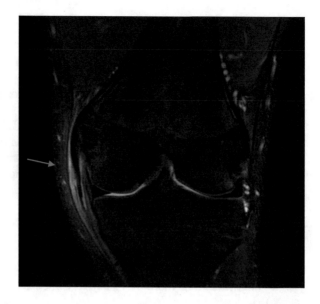

The coronal images (i.e. images obtained in an anterior-to-posterior direction) using T-1 and T-2 weighted sequences will demonstrate edema along the MCL in the setting of a grade I injury and disruption of fibers with grades II and III injuries (Fig. 22.3). Axial plane images (i.e. images obtained in a superior-to-inferior direction) can demonstrate edema along the posteromedial corner and suggest dMCL involvement. The sagittal plane images (i.e. images obtained in a right-to-left direction) evaluate the posterior meniscofemoral and meniscotibial ligament attachments [4]. With a valgus mechanism a lateral femoral condyle bone contusion may also be evident on MRI.

An MRI can also suggest which medial-sided knee injuries should be considered for surgical intervention. Injuries with medial structures entrapped in the knee, also known as a stener-like lesion, should be surgically repaired. A stener lesion is when the sMCL detaches off the tibial insertion and entraps above the pes anserinus tendons, which would also require surgical repair [4].

Computed tomography (CT) is useful for evaluating bony ligament avulsion injuries, as well as for assessing fractures and osteochondral injuries.

Ultrasound (US) has gained momentum in the past few years as an imaging modality for soft-tissue injury around the knee. As US machines are becoming more available and affordable, more clinicians are becoming better skilled at evaluating injuries, such as MCL injuries. US can assess the location of the tear and, in expert hands, the degree of the tear. Practical use of US is still restricted at this time, given the limited US experience and training for sports medicine and orthopedists [4].

Management

MCL injuries can oftentimes be managed non-surgically. Isolated grade I and II MCL injuries are almost always managed non-surgically, as are grade III injuries at the femoral insertion. Grade III tears at the tibial insertion have been shown to have better outcomes with surgical intervention [3].

Non-operative management for grade I and II MCL injuries includes the use of a hinged knee brace and a prescription for physical therapy (PT). Therapy goals are broken down into three phases. Phase 1 focuses on protecting the injury in a hinged knee brace and resting. The therapist will help to reduce inflammation and swelling via ice, cold whirlpool and other modalities, such as electrical-stimulation, ultrasound, and other compressive units. The therapist will also help the athlete regain full knee motion, strengthen surrounding muscles, and normalize gait. Phase 2 focuses on increasing strength; initiating regional therapy, including work on the core, hip abductors, external rotators, and biomechanics; and starting aerobic activity, like jogging in a straight line. Phase 3 focuses on functional progression, including running, agility, plyometrics, and sport-specific movements [3].

The timeline for return to sport varies and depends on the extent of the injury, the athlete's sport and position, and associated injuries. Grade I injuries, on average, typically take 1–2 weeks to return to sport, whereas grade II injuries can take 4–6 weeks. The criteria for returning to sport include being pain free with full range of motion, having no instability on exam, and displaying symmetric muscle strength. Grade III injuries can average 6–8 weeks before return to sport and may require a period of bracing and absolute rest before rehabilitation. For example, management may include using a hinged knee brace locked in 10 degrees of flexion and maintenance of non-weight bearing with crutches for 2 weeks, as this author prescribes; there is no consensus at this time. After the 2 weeks, rehab can begin, if the clinical examination demonstrates less laxity [3].

Upon returning to sport, some providers might prescribe a hinged knee brace with activity; however, this practice is debated and not supported by evidence.

Outcomes for grade I and II MCL injuries managed non-operatively are typically good to excellent. Athletes can often return to sport at their previous level of activity with no concerns.

Non-operative treatment for grade III injuries remains controversial with some showing good results and others showing chronic laxity and early arthritis. MCL injuries at the tibial insertion have been shown to have less healing capacity than those at the femoral origin; therefore, grade III MCL injuries at the tibial insertion have been shown to have better outcomes with surgical intervention [3].

Demonstration Cases

Common Presentation

A 16-year-old male soccer player came into the office with a right knee injury, which he sustained three days prior at his playoff game. The other team's midfielder slide tackled him on his lateral side, while he was running. He felt his knee buckle "inwards" and heard a pop. He went to the ground immediately with pain. Initially, he was unable to bear weight and had to be helped off the field by his teammates. He had been icing his knee and using crutches since the injury. He noted feeling better but was scared to bear his full weight on that leg. He ambulated into the office on crutches and was non-weight bearing.

On examination, he had a mild swelling noted on the medial aspect of his proximal knee. His range of motion was full in extension and slightly limited in flexion, due to pain. He was tender to palpation on the medial distal femur and mildly in the medial joint line. Valgus stress at 0 ° elicited pain but no laxity. Valgus stress at 30 ° elicited pain and mild laxity. The rest of his exam was benign. He had a four-view X-ray series done in the office, which was normal.

He was diagnosed with a grade II MCL sprain. He was then placed in a hinged knee brace and told to wean off the crutches as tolerated over the next few days and to ice 15–20 minutes at a time as often as every hour with precautions not to keep it on longer than that timeframe. He underwent physical therapy for range of motion, strength, and functional progression and was seen in follow-up in clinic after 3–4 weeks.

At follow-up in 4 weeks, he looked great with full, painless ROM. He was progressing well in PT. The goal was for him to return to soccer over the next 1–2 weeks.

Uncommon Presentation

A 14-year-old female soccer player came into the office after being "trucked" by an opposing player the night before. She was not quite sure what happened to her knee, but she had been tackled and fallen to the ground. She had tried to stand up, but she had felt a sharp pain in her knee and fallen back to the ground. The athletic trainer covering the game had run onto the field to assess. The athletic trainer had performed a valgus test and noticed gross laxity and had been unable to complete any other testing, due to pain. The player had been helped off the field and placed on crutches and advised to follow up in the sports medicine clinic with concerns for an MCL injury.

She ambulated into clinic on crutches and was non-weight bearing. Upon examination, she was noted to have a large effusion. Her knee ROM was limited to 70 ° of flexion and lacked the last 20 ° degrees of extension. She had a very difficult exam, prompting X-rays to be obtained before the rest of the exam was completed. She had a four-view of X-ray series, which showed a Salter–Harris III fracture of her distal femur, which was only seen on the notch view (Fig. 22.2). She was then placed in an immobilizer brace for stability, scheduled for an emergent CT scan, and referred to Orthopedic Surgery for surgical planning.

She went on to have an arthroscopically assisted open reduction and internal fixation of a right distal medial femoral condyle physeal intra-articular fracture. She was non-weight bearing for 4 weeks in a hinged knee brace locked in extension. She started PT at 8 weeks post-op and progressed well back to soccer and basketball 4 months later.

> **Pearls and Pitfalls**
> - Always be aware of growth plate injuries in the setting of a valgus injury in a skeletally immature athlete.
> - An effusion in the knee likely indicates a concomitant intra-articular or patellar injury in the setting of a valgus injury and should be investigated accordingly.
> - Most MCL injuries can be managed non-operatively.

Chapter Summary

The MCL is one of the most commonly injured knee ligaments. Most MCL injuries can be managed conservatively, but some require surgical intervention. A thorough history and a solid physical exam, combined with imaging, can help determine the best course of treatment. Treatment for MCL injuries ranges from conservative treatment, with bracing and rehab, for incomplete tears to surgical repair for complete tears. Clinical outcomes are generally favorable, with most patients returning to baseline activity levels.

Condition	MCL Injury
Description	Stretch/tear of the MCL, leads to instability at medial aspect of knee
Epidemiology	Most commonly injured knee ligament. MCL injuries represent 26% of all knee injuries in high school athletes
Mechanism (common)	Valgus stress
History and exam findings	Valgus injury. Pain and swelling on medial aspect of knee. Laxity at the medial knee when a valgus stress is applied.
Management	Conservative management for Grade I and II injuries. Surgical management for Grade III, if the MCL is torn off of the tibia insertion

References

1. Encinas-Ullan CA, Rodriguez-Merchan E. Isolated medial collateral ligament tears: an update on management. EFORT Open Rev. 2018;3(7):398–407.
2. Kramer DE, Miller PE, Berrahou IK, Yen YM, Heyworth BE. Collateral ligament knee injuries in pediatric and adolescent athletes. J Pediatr Orthop. 2020;40:71.
3. Kim C, Chasse PM, Taylor DC. Return to play after medial collateral ligament injury. Clin Sports Med. 2016;35(4):679–96.
4. Craft JA, Kurzweil PR. Physical examination and imaging of medial collateral ligament and posteromedial corner of the knee. Sports Med Arthrosc Rev. 2015;23(2):e1–6.

Chapter 23
Pes Anserine Pain Syndrome

Larry M. Cowles and Anthony I. Beutler

Anatomy and Normal Function

The pes anserinus is a multilayered complex, which lies on the inferior medial aspect of the knee. This complex is comprised of three tendons, which are normally arranged in two layers, with the partially overlapped gracilis and semitendinosus tendons laying inferior to the sartorius tendon. This arrangement of tendons gives the appearance of a goose foot, *pes anserinus* in Latin (Fig. 23.1) [1–3]. Between the tibia and tendon structures lies the anserine bursa, which originates at the tibial joint line and extends to the insertion of the pes anserinus. This bursa acts as a buffer

Fig. 23.1 Pes Bursa and associated pes anserine tendons

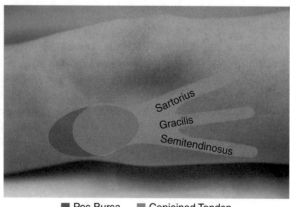

Sartorius

Gracilis

Semitendinosus

■ Pes Bursa ■ Conjoined Tendon

L. M. Cowles · A. I. Beutler (✉)
Department of Family Medicine, Uniformed Services University, Bethesda, MD, USA
e-mail: Anthony.beutler@usuhs.edu

© Springer Nature Switzerland AG 2021
N. Coleman (ed.), *Common Pediatric Knee Injuries*,
https://doi.org/10.1007/978-3-030-55870-3_23

or cushion that allows the pes anserine tendons to glide over the tibia and medial collateral ligament [2, 3].

The main function of the sartorius is to flex, adduct, and internally rotate the hip. In addition, it functions as a secondary knee flexor. The gracilis is responsible for hip adduction and also assists with knee flexion. The semitendinosus works collectively with the semimembranosus and biceps femoris to flex the knee and extend the hip.

Pathophysiology

The pathophysiology of Pes Anserine Pain Syndrome (PAPS) is not well defined. Historically, pain was thought to be due to inflammation of the pes anserine bursa, but studies have rarely shown inflammation of the bursa [4]. More current pathogenesis models suggest that PAPS is due to tendinopathy of one or more of the above tendons. Our clinical experience shows that the semitendinosus is most commonly the culprit. In the rare cases of true anserine bursitis, the patients experience visible swelling, more than pain [5]. Because tendinopathy is very rare in the pediatric population, PAPS in children would likely be due to either direct trauma or a combination of highly abnormal biomechanics and overuse [6].

Specific Pointers

Author's note: In over 20 years of clinical sports medicine practice, we do not remember seeing a case of PAPS in a pediatric athlete with open growth plates. If we have missed one or two, there is no harm done as PAPS is not life/limb threatening. In that same 20+-year span, we have, however, seen several pediatric patients who have been misdiagnosed with PAPS, when what they really have is a tibial growth plate fracture. Missing a tibial growth plate fracture can have severe consequences (growth arrest, leg length discrepancy, permanent disability, etc.). Hence, we recommend that pediatric evaluation of medial knee/proximal tibial knee pain should first rule out the more common and much more serious tibial growth plate fracture before entertaining the rare and rather inconsequential diagnosis of PAPS.

Epidemiology

No current epidemiological information exists for PAPS in the pediatric population. Some studies of epidemiology have been done in the adult population, including a large, population-based study in Mexico, which had a prevalence of 0.34 percent in

13,000 surveyed individuals [7]. Another study had a prevalence of 0.54 percent of males and 0.7 percent of females out of 4240 subjects from three indigenous groups from Mexico and one from Argentina [8]. In all cases, there was a higher prevalence in middle-aged overweight women, who also had knee osteoarthritis.

Mechanism of Injury

The vast preponderance of information on the mechanism of injury is related to the adult patient, as PAPS in the pediatric patient is rare. Extrapolating from adult cases, it is likely that PAPS in the pediatric patient would be caused by improper knee mechanics, overuse, direct impact to the area, or a combination of these factors. As stated above, patients with improper mechanics, such as varus (Fig. 23.2) or valgus (Fig. 23.3) deformities, as well as true leg length discrepancies are likely predisposed to a pes anserine injury.

Fig. 23.2 Demonstration of varus deformity

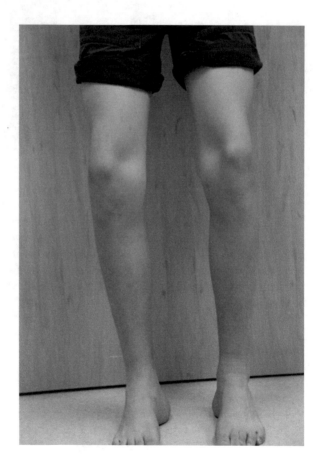

Fig. 23.3 Demonstration
of valgus deformity

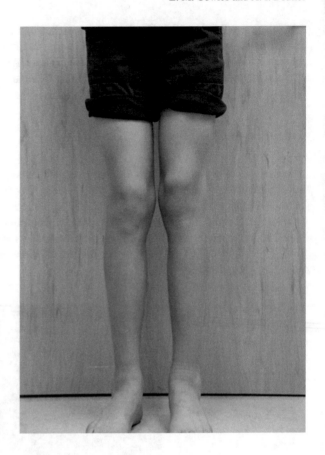

Diagnosis

The diagnosis of PAPS in the pediatric population is rare, and care should be taken
to rule out other potentially harmful conditions that can present as PAPS. Clinical
presentation of PAPS features medial knee pain, often worse with exertion, and
tenderness to palpation over the upper posteromedial tibia between the tibial joint
line and pes anserine insertion (Fig. 23.4) [9]. In most cases, there will be an absence
of swelling [10].

Physical Exam

- Visual inspection—assessment of knee alignment may reveal a valgus or varus
  deformity.
- Palpation—palpation over the medial knee should reveal localized pain over the
  conjoined tendons of the pes anserinus and/or pes anserine bursa (Fig. 23.4).

Fig. 23.4 Palpation of pes
bursa and associated pes
anserine tendons

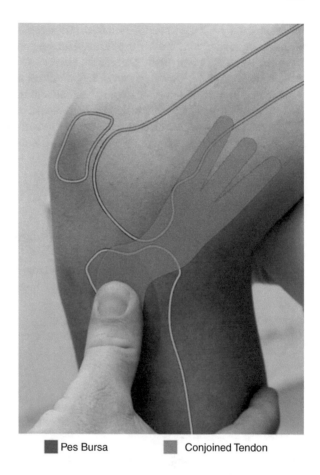

■ Pes Bursa   ■ Conjoined Tendon

Tenderness at the medial joint line may suggest a different diagnosis, such as a meniscal tear, meniscal cyst, or osteosarcoma. To distinguish between joint line tenderness and pes tenderness, we recommend that examiners palpate the semitendinosus tendon as it runs from the pes anterior to posterior, 1–2 cm below the joint line. Since semitendinosus tendinopathy is a common culprit in PAPS, tenderness at this point below the joint line suggests PAPS as a primary pain generator. Conversely, minimal tenderness over the semitendinosus tendon would suggest a joint line source of pathology.

- Range of motion—a normal range of motion with possible increased pain at full extension would be expected.
- Strength—a decrease in effort may be seen, due to pain, otherwise a normal strength test should be seen.
- Neurovascular—no abnormalities should be present.
- Provocative tests—there are no specific provocative tests for this condition; however, pain may be expected with both varus and valgus stress testing.

- Radiography—X-rays are not indicated, if true pes anserine bursitis is suspected; however, x-rays with follow-up advanced imaging are recommended in the pediatric patient with bony tenderness at the knee.
- Ultrasonography—If available in office, an ultrasonic examination of the knee could be used to obtain more detailed anatomical information. An obvious fluid collection in the bursa or thickened heterogeneous tendon insertions suggest PAPS; however, as stated above, in many cases no fluid collection exists and tendinopathy is very uncommon in pediatric patients, especially those with open growth plates.

Differential Diagnosis

- Tibial growth plate fracture versus proximal tibial stress fracture
- Tibial osteomyelitis
- Other masses in the medial knee (i.e. hemangioma, lipoma, bursal cysts)
- Snapping pes anserinus and medial friction syndrome
- Other bursitis in the medial knee
- Medial meniscus tear
- Medial meniscus cyst
- Medial collateral ligament sprain
- Fat pad tenderness

Management

Initial therapy—Although diagnosis of PAPS in the pediatric population is rarely seen, treatment would be similar to what is commonly accepted in the adult population. The initial treatment of PAPS includes use of an analgesic and/or short-term nonsteroidal anti-inflammatory drugs (NSAIDs), quadriceps-strengthening exercises, and, if indicated, core, gluteal, and short hip rotator strengthening. Weight-reduction programs can also be effective in the overweight patient. Since PAPS is thought to be related to an underlying knee condition, such as an angulation deformity (e.g. valgus or varus), local treatment measures typically provide only transient relief. Strengthening exercises are preferred, as they strengthen the muscles acting on the knee, as well as improve the patient's overall fitness. Given the rarity of the condition, no long-term studies of exercise for PAPS in the pediatric population have been published.

Persistent symptoms—PAPS in the pediatric patient should resolve with proper rest and rehab, as their young bodies have amazing healing potential. In patients who have difficulty performing strengthening programs, due to pain, or fail to improve with initial therapy, a local glucocorticoid injection can be considered. However, in the rare pediatric patient where steroid injection may be indicated, it should be a one-time event. The need for repeated steroid injections in a pediatric athlete indicates that the correct culprit causing the pain has not been identified. Anecdotal evidence and clinical experience suggest that one-time steroid injections are safe for pediatric patients of any age. Because they are performed so rarely, there are no large studies confirming this experience-based recommendation. For the procedure, the patient is positioned in a supine position with slight flexion of the affected knee. For landmark-guided injections, trace the medial thigh muscles as they become tendinous, cross the medial joint line, and insert into the pes anserine. Find the point of maximal tenderness along the tendons, usually 1–2 cm inferior to the medial joint line and slightly anterior from medial collateral ligament. The needle is kept parallel to the tibia and inserted into the point of maximal tenderness down to the bone then withdrawn slightly before the injection is performed [6]. The preferred injected solution is 2 mL of lidocaine 1 percent without epinephrine and 40 mg methylprednisolone or triamcinolone acetonide [6, 11].

Demonstration Cases

Classic Presentation

A 17-year-old right arm/leg dominant female high school soccer player presented to your clinic describing painful swelling of her medial left knee for approximately 2 weeks. The athlete reported that she has had similar pain in the past but was not seen for it. This time the pain seems to be lasting longer and worsening over time. She also noted that the coach has been running them a lot lately, as the team has been having a bad season.

Physical Examination

The athlete was well developed, well nourished, and presented in no acute distress. Inspection of the left knee showed moderate swelling of the posteromedial knee without erythema, ecchymosis, or obvious effusion. Observation of stance revealed mild genu valgum of the knees. Inspection of the feet, while weight bearing, demonstrated a flattening of arches and marked pronation bilaterally. Physical examination of the left knee demonstrated exquisite tenderness to palpation over the posteromedial knee with underlying sponginess. Normal range of motion with approximately −5 ° of extension and 130 ° of flexion was noted; however, pain increased at the ends of motion. Bilateral hip examination was also pain free and demonstrated normal full range of motion. Strength testing revealed 5/5 strength symmetrically in the lower extremities to manual muscle test. A Trendelenburg test was performed, and a sagging of the right pelvis was noted, when in left single leg stance. A single leg squat was performed, and medial deviation of the knees L > R was also noted. McMurray test, Lachman test, and varus/valgus stress test were all normal.

Diagnostic Evaluation

Dynamic real-time ultrasound evaluation was performed, and evaluation of the medial and proximal tibia demonstrated no bony abnormalities. There was no evidence of medial meniscus pathology or parameniscal cysts. A moderate hypoechoic fluid signal was seen within the pes anserine bursa.

Nonclassic, but More Common Pediatric Presentation

A 15-year-old male high school wrestler presented to your clinic describing an achy pain of the left posteromedial knee. The athlete reported that approximately 2 weeks ago, before the onset of symptoms, during a wrestling match, he noted a sharp pain in the posteromedial aspect of the knee, when his leg was forcefully placed into a valgus strain. This event caused the wrestler to terminate participation in the wrestling competition that day, due to pain. The sharp pain lasted 48 hours and then decreased to a dull ache.

Physical Examination

The athlete was well developed, well nourished, and presented in no acute distress. Inspection of the left knee showed slight swelling of the posteromedial knee without erythema, ecchymosis, or obvious effusion. Physical examination of the left knee demonstrated tenderness to palpation over the posteromedial knee with slight underlying sponginess. Pain free, normal range of motion with approximately −5 ° of extension and 130 ° of flexion was noted. Bilateral hip examination was also pain free and demonstrated normal full range of motion. Strength testing revealed 5/5 strength symmetrically in the lower extremities to manual muscle test. McMurray test, Lachman test, and varus/valgus stress test were all normal.

Diagnostic Evaluation

Dynamic real-time ultrasound evaluation was performed, and evaluation of the medial and proximal tibia demonstrated no bony abnormalities. There was no evidence of medial meniscus pathology or parameniscal cysts. No hypoechoic fluid signal was seen within the pes anserine bursa. As per protocol, with bony knee tenderness to palpation in the pediatric population, bilateral knee radiographs demonstrated open growth plates but no obvious abnormality. Advanced imaging with MRI demonstrated increased fluid signal in the proximal tibial growth plate, most evident on T2 images, consistent with a Salter–Harris type 1 growth plate injury.

Pearls and Pitfalls
As with many periarticular joint injuries in the pediatric population, one must keep a broad differential. A complete history to include red flag symptoms, such as night pain, fever, weight loss, and limp, may direct the diagnosis to infection, occult fracture, or malignancy. As outlined above, this is especially important in suspected PAPS, since occult fracture is actually more common than PAPS in the pediatric athlete with open growth plates.

Chapter Summary

In pediatric cases with medial knee pain, the differential is broad. It may include Pes Anserine Pain Syndrome; however, PAPS should be low on the differential and may be safely omitted, if the child has open growth plates. In a skeletally mature pediatric athlete with overuse and/or anatomic risk factors and pain located directly over the pes anserine and bursa, with or without swelling—if X-rays are negative for bony involvement, and red flag symptoms (such as night pain, fever, and weight loss) are negative—then PAPS can be considered. Treatment should include physical therapy to strengthen any core, hip, and or knee weakness. Corticosteroids can be considered, if the pain persists or as an adjunct to provide a pain-reduced window for the patient to engage in therapy.

Suggested helpful websites, videos, etc.
https://www.physio-pedia.com/images/b/b0/Pes_anserinus_bursitis.pdf
   https://www.youtube.com/watch?v=tBly3_faKOA – *patient surface anatomy of pes and injection technique*

Chart/table for review

Condition	Pes Anserine Pain Syndrome
Description	Pain at the insertion of the conjoined tendons of sartorius, gracilis, and semitendinosus
Epidemiology	Exceptionally (possibly nonexistent) rare in pediatric athlete with open physes. Rare in skeletally mature pediatric athletes
Mechanism (common)	Overuse pathology combined with abnormal anatomic alignment (i.e. knee varus or valgus)
History and exam findings	In skeletally mature athlete: Pain at the pes anserinus, point tenderness over the semitendinosus tendon, negative knee radiographs, and absence of red flag symptoms. Diagnostic ultrasound may demonstrate fluid collection in bursa and/or hypoechoic tendinopathy
Management	Mainstay of treatment is rehabilitation to include core, hip, and or knee-strengthening exercises

References

1. LaPrade RF, Engebretsen AH, Ly TV, Johansen S, Wentorf FA, Engebretsen L. The anatomy of the medial part of the knee. J Bone Joint Surg Am. 2007;89(9):2000–10.
2. Lee JH, Kim KJ, Jeong YG, Lee NS, Han SY, Lee CG, et al. Pes anserinus and anserine bursa anatomical study. Anat Cell Biol. 2014;47(2):127–31.
3. Ridley WE, Xiang H, Han J, Eidley LJ. Pes anserinus: normal anatomy. J Med Imaging Radiat Oncol. 2018;62(Suppl 1):148.
4. Uson J, Aguado P, Bernad M, Mayordomo L, Naredo E, Balsa A, et al. Pes anserinustendino-bursitis: what are we talking about? Scand J Rheumatol. 2000;29:184–6.
5. Voorneveld C, Arenson AM, Fam AG. Anserine bursal distention: diagnosis by ultrasonography and computed tomography. Arthritis Rheum. 1989;32:1335–8.
6. Cardone DA, Tallia AF. Diagnostic and therapeutic injection of the hip and knee. Am Fam Physician. 2003;67:2147–52.
7. Alvarez-Nemegyei J, Peláez-Ballestas I, Rodríguez-Amado J, Sanin LH, Garcia-Garcia C, et al. Prevalence of rheumatic regional pain syndromes in adults from Mexico: a community survey using COPCORD for screening and syndrome-specific diagnostic criteria. J Rheumatol Suppl. 2011;86:15–20.
8. Alvarez-Nemegyei J, Peláez-Ballestas I, Goñi M, Julián-Santiago F, García-García C, et al. Prevalence of rheumatic regional pain syndromes in Latin-American indigenous groups: a census study based on COPCORD methodology and syndrome-specific diagnostic criteria. Clin Rheumatol. 2016;35(Suppl 1):63–70.
9. Wolf M. Knee pain in children, part III: stress injuries, benign bone tumors, growing pains. Pediatr Rev. 2016;37(3):114–9.
10. Klontzas ME, Akoumianakis ID, Vagios I, Karantanas AH. MR imaging findings of medial tibial crest friction. Eur J Radiol. 2013;82(11):e703–6.
11. Sarifakioglu B, Afsar SI, Yalbuzdag SA, et al. Comparison of the efficacy of physical therapy and corticosteroid injection in the treatment of pes anserine tendino-bursitis. J Phys Ther Sci. 2016;28:1993–7.

Chapter 24
Fibular Injury (Proximal)

Nathaniel S. Nye, Korey Kasper, and Jacquelyn Hale

Anatomy and Normal Function

The fibula is a long bone comprised of a tubular diaphysis of cortical bone with cancellous regions at the proximal and distal ends. Sixty percent of the linear growth of the fibula comes from the proximal epiphysis, which remains open for 18–20 years in males and 16–18 years in females [1]. The proximal fibula serves a critical role in static and dynamic knee stability as the attachment site of the posterolateral corner complex, which consists of the lateral collateral ligament (LCL), the biceps femoris tendon, the popliteus tendon, and the arcuate complex (the arcuate complex consisting of the arcuate ligament, popliteofibular ligament, and the fabellofibular ligament when present) [2]. The proximal fibula also serves as the origin of the soleus, extensor digitorum longus, tibialis posterior, and fibularis (peroneus) longus muscles. It provides rotational stability to the knee and ankle, while supporting 7–16% of body weight during walking [3].

The fibular head articulates with the lateral tibial condyle at the proximal tibiofibular joint (PTFJ); this synovial joint space communicates with that of the tibiofemoral joint in 10% of the population [4–7]. PTFJ stability is provided by the anterior and posterior proximal tibiofibular ligaments; by fibular attachment to the lateral collateral ligament (LCL), the interosseous membrane, and the distal PTFJ; and by the surrounding musculature (including biceps femoris and popliteus) [8–11]. The tibia and fibula are tethered throughout their length by the interosseous membrane until they meet again distally at the distal tibiofibular joint.

N. S. Nye (✉)
Sports Medicine Clinic, Fort Belvoir Community Hospital, Ft. Belvoir, VA, USA
e-mail: Nathaniel.s.nye.mil@mail.mil

K. Kasper · J. Hale
Sports Medicine Clinic, 559th Medical Group, JBSA-Lackland, TX, USA

© Springer Nature Switzerland AG 2021
N. Coleman (ed.), *Common Pediatric Knee Injuries*,
https://doi.org/10.1007/978-3-030-55870-3_24

The primary functions of the PTFJ include the following: (1) act as a buttress for tibial bending, (2) dissipation of torsional forces applied to the ankle, and (3) tensile weight bearing [8, 12, 13]. To accommodate rotation of the talus with ankle dorsiflexion, the fibula rotates externally. During knee extension, the fibular head is pulled posteriorly as the biceps femoris and LCL become taut [8].

Just distal to the fibular head is the fibular neck, where the common fibular (peroneal) nerve wraps around the fibula, posterolaterally to anteromedially, before dividing into its superficial and deep divisions [14]. Via its divisions, this nerve ultimately provides sensation to the posterolateral lower leg and knee joint and innervates muscles of the anterior and lateral lower leg compartments.

Pathology and Dysfunction

Injuries to the proximal fibula may include the dislocation or subluxation of the PTFJ, a contusion, and a fracture (acute or stress). These may also result in injury to the common fibular nerve or compromise the muscular, tendinous, or ligamentous attachments to that area. Though rare, the most commonly reported PTFJ injury is anterolateral dislocation of the proximal fibula [5, 7, 15]. The mechanism usually involves high-energy twisting motions, often with force applied through a flexed knee with concurrent foot inversion, plantar flexion, and lower leg external rotation [6, 8, 15–17].

Ogden et al. [13] classified PTFJ instability into four types:

- Type I: subluxation or ligamentous laxity without dislocation (atraumatic hypermobility)
- Type II: anterolateral dislocation involving the anterior and posterior tibiofibular ligaments (most common injury, 85% of cases)
- Type III: posteromedial dislocation resulting from a direct trauma and often disrupting the common fibular nerve
- Type IV: superior dislocation typically resulting from a high energy ankle injury and occasionally associated with a tibial shaft fracture

Just as PTFJ injury is rare in children, so are isolated fractures of the proximal fibula. Acute proximal fibular fractures can result from direct blows to the lateral lower leg, as well as from excessive varus stress, and may be associated with concurrent fracture of the distal tibia or rupture of the interosseous membrane and distal tibiofibular joint (Maisonneuve fracture). Bone stress injury of the proximal fibula is also uncommon but has been reported in children and adolescents [18]. These injuries typically present with an atraumatic onset of progressive, exertional pain localized to the lateral knee or proximal lower leg in the setting of increased activity or exercise, often involving distance running or pivoting/agility sports, such as soccer or basketball.

Due to the common fibular nerve's superficial positioning and proximity to the fibula, it is predisposed to traction or transection with PTFJ dislocation/subluxation and with a proximal fibula fracture. Nerve injury can also result from direct compression or entrapment, such as with sitting cross-legged, resting against a desk or car door while seated, or being compressed by an adjacent ganglion cyst [14].

Specific Pointers

- Anteroposterior and lateral X-rays of the tibia and fibula are usually sufficient to rule out acute fracture or dislocation. Comparison to X-rays of the contralateral fibula or axial CT scan can increase sensitivity and specificity when initial films are inconclusive.
- If an acute fracture or PTFJ dislocation is confirmed, obtain plain films of the ankle to evaluate for a Maisonneuve fracture or Maisonneuve-equivalent injury [19].
- If a stress fracture is suspected, but plain films are negative, consider magnetic resonance imaging (MRI) for increased sensitivity.
- Evaluate suspected common fibular nerve injury with strength and sensation testing of the lower leg and perform Tinel's test at the fibular neck. Diagnosis can be further evaluated and confirmed with MRI, ultrasound, and/or electromyography (EMG).
- Uncomplicated fractures of the proximal fibula may be treated with a short-leg walking cast or stirrup splint for 3–4 weeks.
- Both-bone fractures and Maisonneuve injuries require urgent orthopedic referral.

Epidemiology

Proximal fibula injuries are uncommon to rare in the pediatric population, and data on epidemiology is limited [4, 15, 18, 20]. As described above, these injuries may occur in a wide variety sports or trauma, owing to the wide variety of mechanisms of injury which can cause them (e.g., high energy collision, rapid torsion of a flexed knee, congenital laxity with atraumatic instability, or repetitive loading and overuse). It is unknown whether there are sex biases for this injury [5].

Diagnosis: History and Examination Findings, Testing

Patients with proximal fibular injuries may report a sudden onset of pain and/or swelling following a specific mechanism of injury (i.e., acute fracture or dislocation), or, conversely, symptoms may develop insidiously (i.e., stress fracture, nerve entrapment) following a recent increase in activity or repetitive movements. Pain and swelling are typically well-localized to the lateral knee or lower leg; however, global knee pain and swelling may be reported when important knee stabilizers have been injured, such as with acute PTFJ dislocation, posterolateral corner rupture, or arcuate fracture. Foot drop or lower leg weakness and numbness may be reported if the common fibular nerve or its branches are involved.

On examination, asymmetric lateral knee contours may be apparent upon inspection and comparison to the contralateral knee. The patient often presents with an antalgic gait. While proximal fibula tenderness and pain with knee flexion may indicate any proximal fibular injury, patients with acute proximal fibula fracture or dislocation are likely to have limited knee flexion and extension, localized swelling, and severe tenderness to palpation. A bone stress injury should be suspected in the setting of an overuse history with mild-to-moderate focal bony tenderness to palpation, reproduction of pain with a single leg hop, or pain from application of a vibrating tuning fork to the fibular head. The patient may also experience pain with ankle inversion, eversion, and dorsiflexion and may obtain relief from plantar flexion [4, 5, 17]. If an acute proximal fibula fracture or dislocation is diagnosed, the provider should also evaluate the ankle for tenderness, swelling, or other signs of distal fibula injury [21]. In cases of common fibular nerve injury, examination may reveal weakness with ankle dorsiflexion and eversion and sensory loss along the lateral leg, lateral ankle, and dorsolateral foot. Tinel's test at the fibular neck may recreate or exacerbate symptoms.

Anteroposterior and lateral X-rays of the knee are first-line imaging for diagnosis of proximal fibula injury. Sensitivity for subtle PTFJ dislocation may be enhanced with comparison X-rays of the contralateral side. Although axial computed tomography (CT) is more sensitive to this injury, plain films are preferred in pediatric patients because of its lower radiation exposure [15]. If a proximal fibular fracture or dislocation is confirmed on X-ray, an ankle and tibia–fibula series (if not already done) should be obtained to rule out Maisonneuve fracture or Maisonneuve-equivalent injury [19]. The distal tibia and fibula should be evaluated for fracture, and the ankle mortise (i.e., the medial and lateral malleoli articulating with the talus) should be evaluated for any widening, which would indicate disruption of the distal tibiofibular syndesmosis and/or deltoid ligament. If initial X-rays are negative but a bone stress injury is suspected, a period of impact restrictions with or without crutches and follow-up in 1–3 weeks with repeat X-rays should be considered [22]. If X-rays remain negative and the patient's condition is not improving, MRI is recommended for further evaluation of suspected fibular stress injury. If a common fibular nerve injury is suspected, MRI or ultrasound may be utilized to confirm and evaluate the extent of injury [17]. While both MRI and ultrasound provide excellent soft tissue visualization, including nerves, ultrasound offers greater spatial resolution but is more operator skill dependent.

Management

Since it is not the primary weight-bearing bone of the lower leg, most fractures of the proximal fibula in children may be treated with a short-leg walking cast or stirrup splint for 3–4 weeks. Referral to orthopedic surgery is recommended when there is fracture displacement or a concomitant injury to the PTFJ, knee, or tibia [23]. Both-bone fractures, including Maisonneuve fractures, warrant immediate orthopedic referral.

There is no widely accepted standard of care for PTFJ dislocations; however, they are often treated nonoperatively with full recovery [16]. Approximately 8–10% of cases reduce spontaneously, while 90% require closed reduction. Usual nonoperative treatment consists of a period of immobilization, generally for 3–4 weeks in either a cast or knee immobilizer [7, 24], followed by 2–3 months of physical therapy. In approximately 75% of cases, patients are able to return to pain-free activity by 9–12 months with nonoperative treatment [4, 16, 17, 24]. A 2017 systematic review showed that 9 of 35 patients (25.7%) treated nonoperatively had persistent symptoms, and 8 of these proceeded to surgical stabilization procedures [16]. Relatively high rates of complications are seen with PTFJ stabilization surgeries (18–36%, depending on technique), including hardware-related pain, wound infections, stress fractures, and fibular nerve palsy. Without treatment, PTFJ dislocation or subluxation can result in reduced knee and PTFJ stability, abnormal gait, limited tolerance of pivoting movements, common fibular nerve dysfunction, and reduced quality of life [11, 16, 25].

Bone stress injuries of the proximal fibula are considered low risk, as they exhibit high rates of success with nonoperative treatment [26]. They are managed primarily through activity modification and impact restriction. If walking is painful or antalgic, a 2–4-week period of nonweight bearing with crutches is generally sufficient to allow the bone to heal enough to resume pain-free ambulation. Underlying contributing factors for bone stress injury must be addressed, such as hormonal abnormalities (i.e., female athlete triad), iron or vitamin D deficiency, poor gait mechanics, or training errors. Once the patient is pain free with ambulation and activities of daily living, rehabilitation can progress and a gradual return to running program can be considered. Patients generally return to full activity, including sports participation, in 6–12 weeks, depending on injury severity, timeliness of diagnosis, and degree of contributing factors [22, 26].

Common fibular neuropathy may be self-limited or require physical therapy for soft tissue mobilization and nerve glide exercises. Refractory cases may be treated with corticosteroid or 5% dextrose injections. If these treatments fail or if the nerve has been severely injured or transected by trauma or fracture, surgical neuroplasty may be required.

Demonstration Cases

Common Presentation

A 14-year-old female soccer player presented with left lateral leg pain just distal to the knee after getting kicked in that area during a game. She reported pain with weight bearing and stated, "I can't lift my foot when I walk." Examination revealed visible ecchymosis and abrasion in the region of the proximal fibula, tenderness to palpation along the proximal fibula, and obvious weakness (4/5) with ankle dorsiflexion, compared to the right. X-ray revealed a nondisplaced fracture of the fibular neck. The patient was immobilized in a short-leg walking cast for 4 weeks. At follow-up, the patient denied pain, numbness, and tingling. The cast was removed. On exam, she was nontender and exhibited full ankle range of motion; strength was mildly decreased, consistent with disuse from immobilization. Sensation over the lateral lower leg, ankle, and foot was full and normal. Repeat X-ray showed stable alignment with callus formation around the nondisplaced fracture site. Following an uncomplicated course of physical therapy, the patient successfully returned to soccer 3 months after the injury.

Uncommon Presentation

A 16-year-old boy was tackled, while carrying the ball during a football game. With his right foot planted, he twisted his ankle, as he was taken down. He was unable to bear weight thereafter and complained of pain in his right lower leg. He was taken to the emergency room, where an ankle effusion was noted, and he had diffuse tenderness of his anterior ankle. Ankle radiographs showed a widened ankle mortise but no fracture. After seeing this, the Emergency Room physician ordered tib-fib plain films, which revealed a displaced oblique fracture of the proximal fibula. The on-call orthopedic surgeon was consulted, who confirmed the diagnosis of a Maisonneuve fracture and placed the patient in a bulky short-leg posterior splint. The patient was taken to the operating room the next morning for open reduction and internal fixation of the distal tibiofibular syndesmosis and displaced fibular fracture.

Pearls and Pitfalls
- Examination of ankle and knee injuries should always also include examination of the proximal fibula for tenderness/injury; if suspicious, obtain films of the entire tibia–fibula in addition to the ankle.
- Injury at the proximal fibula can also result in injury to the common fibular nerve, which may lead to pain, paresthesias, and/or foot drop.
- When examining body parts that are uncommonly injured (such as the proximal fibula), examining the contralateral side for comparison is invaluable.
- Consider obtaining an axial CT, if a PTFJ dislocation is suspected, despite unrevealing bilateral (comparison) radiographs.

Chapter Summary

The proximal fibula is often neglected during knee examination; however, because of its importance in stabilizing the knee and ankle joints, the proximal fibula must be assessed following knee and ankle injuries. Proximal fibula injuries may include dislocation or subluxation of the PTFJ, acute fibular fracture, bone stress injury, and common fibular nerve injury. Imaging should begin with plain films, which may be followed by advanced imaging, when the diagnosis remains unclear. Nondisplaced proximal fibula fractures and PTFJ dislocations most often heal uneventfully with 3–4 weeks of immobilization and nonweight bearing, while bone stress injuries generally require restrictions from running and sports participation and crutch use, if walking is painful. Orthopedic Surgery should be urgently consulted for cases of Maisonneuve injury, displaced fracture, or both-bone fractures.

References

1. Rathjen KE, Kim HKW. Physeal injuries and growth disturbance. In: Beaty JH, Kasser JR, editors. Rockwood and Wilkins' fractures in children. 7th ed. Philadelphia: Lippincott Williams & Wilkins; 2014. p. 103–4.
2. Cohen BH, DeFroda SF, Hodax JD, Johnson D, Kristopher Ware J, Fadale PD. The arcuate fracture: a descriptive radiographic study. Injury. 2018;49(10):1871–7.
3. Boulton C, O'Toole RV. Tibia and fibula shaft fractures. In: Court-Brown CM, Heckman JD, McQueen MM, Ricci WM, Tornetta P, editors. Rockwood and Green's fractures in adults. 8th ed. Philadelphia: Lippincott Williams & Wilkins; 2014. p. 2465–8.
4. Almeida Silvares PR, Fernandes Guerreiro JP, Müller SS, Pereira RV, Vannini R. Acute isolated anterolateral dislocation of the proximal tibiofibular joint. Rev Bras Ortop. 2015;45(4):460–4.
5. Iosifidis MI, Giannoulis I, Tsarouhas A, Traios S. Isolated acute dislocation of the proximal tibiofibular joint. Orthopedics. 2008;31(6):605.
6. Ashraf MO, Jones HM, Kanvinde R. Acute traumatic fracture dislocation of proximal tibiofibular joint: case report and literature review. Injury. 2015;46(7):1400–2.
7. Cunningham NJ, Farebrother N, Miles J. Review article: isolated proximal tibiofibular joint dislocation. Emerg Med Australas. 2019;31(2):156–62.
8. Alves-da-Silva T, Guerra-Pinto F, Matias R, Pessoa P. Kinematics of the proximal tibiofibular joint is influenced by ligament integrity, knee and ankle mobility: an exploratory cadaver study. Knee Surg Sports Traumatol Arthrosc. 2019;27(2):405–11.
9. Martin B, Corbett J, Littlewood A, Clifton R. Proximal tibiofibular dislocation: a case report of this often overlooked injury. BJR Case Rep. 2016;28(3):20150372.
10. Marchetti DC, Moatshe G, Phelps BM, et al. The proximal tibiofibular joint: a biomechanical analysis of the anterior and posterior ligamentous complexes. Am J Sports Med. 2017;45(8):1888–92.
11. Bathala EA, Bancroft LW, Peterson JJ. The case: arcuate fracture of the knee. Orthopedics. 2008;31:200–3, 290–3.
12. Espregueira-Mendes J, Vieira da Silva M. Anatomy of the proximal tibiofibular joint. Knee Surg Sports Traumatol Arthrosc. 2006;14(3):241–9.
13. Ogden J. Sublaxation and dislocation of the proximal tibiofibular joint. J Bone Joint Surg Am. 1974;56(1):145–54.
14. Marciniak C. Fibular (peroneal) neuropathy: electrodiagnostic features and clinical correlates. Phys Med Rehabil Clin N Am. 2013;24(1):121–37.

15. Sekiya JK, Kuhn JE. Instability of the proximal tibiofibular joint. J Am Acad Orthop Surg. 2003;11(2):120–8.
16. Kruckeberg BM, Cinque ME, Moatshe G, Marchetti D, DePhillipo NN, Chahla J, LaPrade RF. Proximal tibiofibular joint instability and treatment approaches: a systematic review of the literature. Arthroscopy. 2017;33(9):1743–51.
17. NieuweWeme RA, Somford MP, Schepers T. Proximal tibiofibular dislocation: a case report and review of literature. Strategies Trauma Limb Reconstr. 2014;9(3):185–9.
18. Lehman TP, Belanger MJ, Pascale MS. Bilateral proximal third fibular stress fractures in an adolescent female track athlete. Orthopedics. 2002;25(3):329–32.
19. Bissuel T, Gaillard F, Dagneaux L, Canovas F. Maisonneuve equivalent injury with proximal tibiofibular joint dislocation: case report and literature review. J Foot Ankle Surg. 2017;56(2):404–7.
20. Prada-Cañizares A, Auñon-Martin I, Pretell-Mazzini J, Quintana-Plaza J, Resines-Erasun C. Pediatric maisonneuve: case report of a rare pattern of injury. J Pediatr Orthop B. 2013;22(5):470–4.
21. Taweel NR, Raikin SM, Karanjia HN, Ahmad J. The proximal fibula should be examined in all patients with ankle injury: a case series of missed maisonneuve fractures. J Emerg Med. 2013;44(2):e251–5.
22. Nye NS, Covey CJ, Sheldon L, Webber B, Pawlak M, Boden B, Beutler A. Improving diagnostic accuracy and efficiency of suspected bone stress injuries. Sports Health. 2016;8(3):278–83.
23. Eiff M, Hatch R. Tibia and fibula fractures. In: Fracture management for primary care. 3rd ed. Philadelphia: Saunders/Elsevier; 2012. p. 180.
24. Semonian R, Denlinger P, Duggan R. Proximal tibiofibular subluxation relationship to lateral knee pain: a review of proximal tibiofibular joint pathologies. J Orthop Sports Phys Ther. 1995;21(5):248–57.
25. Borgohain B, Saikia B, Sarma A. Proximal tibiofibular joint: rendezvous with a forgotten articulation. Indian J Orthop. 2015;49(5):489–95.
26. Boden BP, Osbahr DC, Jimenez C. Low-risk stress fractures. Am J Sports Med. 2001;29(1):100–11.

Chapter 25
Lateral Collateral Ligament Injury

Rajat K. Jain

Anatomy and Normal Function

The lateral collateral ligament (LCL) is part of the posterolateral corner, a large complex of structures on the lateral aspect of the knee. Specifically, the lateral knee is comprised of 28 individual static and dynamic stabilizers, with the primary stabilizers including the LCL, the popliteofibular ligament (FCL), and the popliteus muscle [1, 2] (Fig. 25.1). The LCL originates on the lateral aspect of the femur and inserts onto the fibula. On the femoral attachment, the LCL is proximal and posterior to the origin of the popliteus, while the fibular attachment is distal and anterior to the popliteofibular ligament.

The LCL plays a significant role in the static stability of the posterolateral corner of the knee. Specifically, the LCL is the primary varus stabilizer of the knee. Studies with cadavers have shown that creating a complete tear in the LCL results in the greatest amount of varus instability at 30 ° of knee flexion [3]. Furthermore, the LCL has been shown to have a role in stabilizing external rotation of the tibia, with the greatest effect being seen at more than 30 ° of knee flexion [3].

R. K. Jain (✉)
Northwestern University Health Service, Evanston, IL, USA
e-mail: rajat.jain@northwestern.edu

© Springer Nature Switzerland AG 2021
N. Coleman (ed.), *Common Pediatric Knee Injuries*,
https://doi.org/10.1007/978-3-030-55870-3_25

Fig. 25.1 The primary static stabilizers of the posterolateral corner include the lateral collateral ligament, popliteofibular ligament, and popliteus tendon. (Adapted from LaPrade et al. [2])

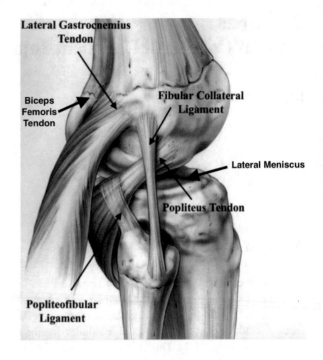

Specific Pointers

Epidemiology

LCL injuries can occur in athletes of all ages and genders. Grawe et al. [4] summarize a study of 20,000 knee injuries across various sporting activities and found that isolated LCL pathology occurs in <2% of injuries [5]. The authors also describe a study, in which tennis and gymnastics had the highest risk for LCL injury [4, 6]. While the study describes the epidemiology of LCL injuries in specific club sports, this author's experience has shown that the nature of wrestling lends itself to a significant risk of LCL injury.

Mechanism of Injury

Typically, injuries to the LCL occur after trauma to the knee. Specifically, the most common mechanism is a varus directed blow to the anteromedial aspect of the knee. Less commonly, hyperextension and non-contact varus stress injuries can also cause damage to the LCL [7].

Diagnosis

After sustaining an injury to the LCL, patients can present with a myriad of complaints. They might describe pain at the site of trauma (i.e. the medial knee) or lateral knee; perceived instability with side-to-side or "cutting" movements that occur, while the knee is in extension; or a sensation of walking "bow-legged," due to the increase in laxity. Furthermore, patients may complain of foot drop or paresthesias in the common peroneal nerve distribution, as common peroneal nerve injuries can occur in up to one-third of posterolateral corner injuries [7].

When examining a patient who may have sustained an LCL injury, swelling around the lateral soft tissue of the knee may be noted, given the relatively superficial position of the LCL. The amount of swelling may correlate with the degree of injury to the posterolateral corner complex. Additionally, the subcutaneous position of the LCL provides an opportunity for palpation during examination. Specifically, palpation can be assisted by placing the patient in the figure-of-four position, during which an intact LCL can be palpable as a discrete cord-like structure [4] (Fig. 25.2).

As previously described, the LCL serves as the primary restraint to varus forces at 30 ° of knee flexion. The varus stress test can and should be performed at full extension and 30 ° of flexion. The test is performed by holding the patient's foot or ankle with one hand and using the contralateral hand to stabilize the femur and apply a varus force (Fig. 25.3). Increased varus laxity only at 30 ° of flexion would indicate an isolated LCL injury; however, varus laxity in full extension frequently denotes injury to other structures of the posterolateral corner [7]. Traditionally, the

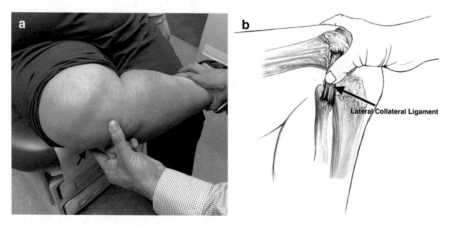

Fig. 25.2 (**a, b**) Photographs of the physical examination with the patient's lower extremity in the figure-of-four position. The figure-of-four position (**a**) allows the examiner to directly palpate (arrow) the lateral collateral ligament (**b**). (Illustration adapted from Grawe et al. [4])

Fig. 25.3 Demonstration of the varus stress test performed at 30 ° of knee flexion

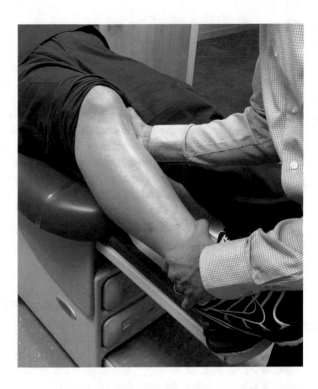

Table 25.1 Classification of LCL knee injuries based on physical examination

Grade	Sprain type	Varus opening
Grade I	Minor	≤5 mm
Grade II	Moderate	6–10 mm
Grade III	Severe	≥10 mm

amount of varus opening, as compared to the contralateral side, can classify the grade of injury to the LCL (Table 25.1).

The posterolateral corner should also be assessed when an LCL injury is suspected. The Dial test is another helpful tool for the examiner, measuring external rotation of the tibia relative to the femur. While the patient lays prone on the examination surface and both knees flexed to 30 °, the provider externally rotates the tibia at the foot and ankle level (Fig. 25.4). An increase of more than 10 ° of external rotation compared with the contralateral side suggests an injury to the posterolateral corner.

When an LCL injury is suspected after examination, imaging of the affected knee should begin with dedicated weight-bearing x-rays that include standard anteroposterior (AP), lateral, and bent knee patellofemoral (sunrise) view radiographs [7]. When possible, obtaining varus stress radiographs can provide objective diagnosis of LCL injuries. Lateral compartment opening is determined by measuring the shortest distance between the most distal aspect of the lateral femoral condyle and the associated tibial plateau [3]. MRI is considered the imaging modality

Fig. 25.4 Demonstration of the dial test being performed with the patient prone on the examination table and knees flexed to 30 °

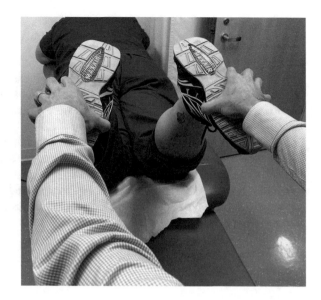

Table 25.2 Classification of LCL knee injuries based on MRI results

Grade	MRI findings
Grade I	Subcutaneous fluid surrounding the mid-substance of the ligament at one or both insertions
Grade II	Disruption of the ligament with partial tearing of ligament fibers at either one of the insertions or mid-substance, with increased edema
Grade III	Complete tearing of ligament fibers at either the mid-substance or one of the insertions with increased edema

of choice for evaluating LCL and posterolateral corner injuries. The LCL can be best appreciated on the axial and coronal views [4]. Common findings on MRI can include a medial compartment bone bruising pattern, related to the commonly seen hyperextension-varus mechanism [4]. Varying amounts of peri-ligamentous edema and intra-substance signal can be seen with increased edema and discontinuity of LCL fibers in higher-grade tears (Table 25.2) [8].

Management

The decision to proceed with conservative or surgical management of LCL tears is determined by the grade of injury and, especially, the presence of injuries to other structures. Typically, in the setting of knee dislocation, where other ligamentous structures are likely to be injured, early surgical intervention is recommended. According to Grawe et al. [4], a torn LCL does not heal as well as medial collateral ligament injuries, thereby lowering the threshold for surgical intervention.

Non-surgical

Isolated LCL grade I and II tears can often be managed with non-surgical manage-ment; however, literature on non-operative management of grade I and II is sparse [7]. While good results have been reported for non-surgical management for grade I and II injuries [9, 10], sample sizes for those with isolated grade I and grade II injuries were 7 and 11 patients, respectively.

Non-surgical treatment can involve use of early immobilization, either with a knee immobilizer or hinged knee brace that restricts varus motion but allows flexion and extension of the knee during ambulation. After pain and the sensation of varus instability have resolved, the brace can be discontinued, with return to sports as tolerated by the athlete. In cases of prolonged immobilization, physical therapy may be necessary to return strength and proprioception to pre-injury levels.

Surgical

Repair and reconstructions can be used for isolated acute LCL grade III tears. Repairs are typically performed when the ligament is avulsed from an attachment site and an anatomic reduction remains possible with the knee in full extension [4].

In the setting of a complete mid-substance tear or intra-substance stretch injury, ligamentous reconstruction is necessary. Furthermore, LCL reconstruction is rec-ommended in chronic injuries and when anatomic reduction is not possible [4].

Demonstration Cases

Common Presentation

A 21-year-old male wrestler presents with 1 month of lateral knee pain. He recalls a match during which his opponent made repeated wrestling moves that resulted in trauma to the anteromedial knee. He had no swelling and continued wrestling with a knee brace for 2 weeks. During subsequent matches, he would feel episodes of lateral instability without enduring further trauma. Since the culmination of wres-tling season, the athlete described lateral knee pain with ambulation and episodes of instability with side to side movements. Physical examination revealed tenderness to palpation along the mid and distal LCL with a positive varus stress test at 30 ° knee flexion. Despite initial immobilization, the athlete continued to have knee dis-comfort and instability and, therefore, underwent an MRI (Fig. 25.5). He was man-aged non-surgically with a hinged knee brace and physical therapy for 6 weeks and was able to return to sports without any limitations.

Fig. 25.5 Coronal MRI of the knee, arrow directed at a thickened proximal to mid LCL with a high-grade tear of the distal ligament from the fibular head

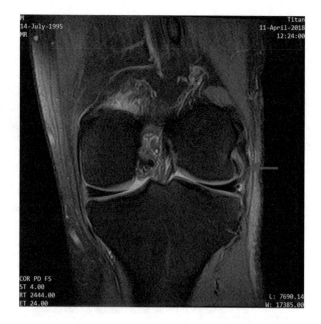

Uncommon Presentation

A 15-year-old female presents with medial and lateral knee pain after an injury in which her younger brother jumped on the medial aspect of her knee while she was sitting on the sofa in a figure-of-four position. She has not seen any swelling but notes medial and lateral knee pain with ambulation. Physical examination reveals tenderness to palpation over the medial femoral condyle and along the proximal LCL. She has a positive varus stress test at 30 ° flexion. She was treated with a hinged knee brace for 1 week and was able to return to activities of daily living without limitation.

> **Pearls and Pitfalls**
> LCL injuries rarely occur in isolation and should prompt the provider to examine for injuries to other structures in the posterolateral corner. Associated injuries lead to poor outcomes with non-surgical management and may result in chronic pain.

Chapter Summary

The LCL is part of a greater group of structures known as the posterolateral corner, is an essential varus stabilizer for the lateral aspect of the knee, and acts as a secondary restraint to external rotation of the tibia. Typically, LCL injuries occur in the setting of traumatic varus forces and in conjunction with other knee pathology. Grade I and II injuries can be treated non-surgically, while grade III injuries can be treated with either repair or reconstruction.

Condition	LCL injury
Description	Lateral knee ligament that restricts varus forces and external rotation of tibia
Epidemiology	Athletes, especially wrestling, tennis, and gymnastics
Mechanism (common)	Varus force to the anteromedial knee
History and exam findings	Lateral knee pain and possible varus instability with ambulation. Physical exam with lateral knee swelling, positive varus stress test, possible positive dial test with other posterolateral corner injuries
Management	Non-surgical treatment for grade I and II injuries with early immobilization. Surgical treatment for grade III injuries.

References

1. James EW, LaPrade CM, LaPrade RF. Anatomy and biomechanics of the lateral side of the knee and surgical implications. Sports Med Arthrosc Rev. 2015;23(1):2–9.
2. LaPrade RF, Ly TV, Wentorf FA, Engebretsen L. The posterolateral attachments of the knee: a quantitative and qualitative morphologic analysis of the fibular collateral ligament, popliteus tendon, popliteofibular ligament, and lateral gastrocnemius tendon. Am J Sports Med. 2003;31:854–60.
3. Song Y, Watanabe K, Hogan E, D'Antoni AV, Dilandro AC, Apaydin N, et al. The fibular collateral ligament of the knee: a detailed review. Clin Anat. 2014;27(5):789–97.
4. Grawe B, Schroeder AJ, Kakazu R, Messer MS. Lateral collateral ligament injury about the knee: anatomy, evaluation and management. J Am Acad Orthop Surg. 2018;26(6):e120–7.
5. Bushnell BD, Bitting SS, Crain JM, Boublik M, Schlegel TF. Treatment of magnetic resonance imaging-documented isolated grade III lateral collateral ligament injuries in National Football League athletes. Am J Sports Med. 2010;38(1):86–91.
6. Majewski M, Susanne H, Klaus S. Epidemiology of athletic knee injuries: a 10-year-study. Knee. 2006;13(3):184–8.
7. Chahla J, Moatshe G, Dean CS, LaPrade RF. Posterolateral corner of the knee: current concepts. Arch Bone Jt Surg. 2016;4(2):97–103.
8. Sikka RS, Dhami R, Dunlay R, Boyd JL. Isolated fibular collateral ligament injuries in athletes. Sports Med Arthrosc Rev. 2015;23(1):17–21.
9. Kannus P. Nonoperative treatment of Grade II and III sprains of the lateral ligament compartment of the knee. Am J Sports Med. 1989;17(1):83–8.
10. Krukhaug Y, Molster A, Rodt A, Strand T. Lateral ligament injuries of the knee. Knee Surg Sports Traumatol Arthrosc. 1998;6(1):21–5.

Chapter 26
Iliotibial Band Syndrome

Chelsea Backer and Matthew Sedgley

Anatomy and Normal Function

The iliotibial band (IT band, ITB) is a thick band of fascia that extends distally from the lateral iliac crest to insert at the proximal tibia at Gerdy's tubercle. The IT band fascia is formed proximally by the tensor fascia lata and gluteus maximus [1]. Distally, the IT band passes over the lateral femoral condyle (LFC) to insert onto the tibial plateau at Gerdy's tubercle, about 2 cm inferior to the lateral joint line. With attachments at the lateral hip and knee, the IT band connects the hip extensors and abductors to the lower leg, providing stability at the knee. There are fibrous attachments distally from the IT band to the femur [1, 2]. The IT band is connected to the linea aspera by an intermuscular septum and to the supracondylar region of the femur (including the epicondyle) by coarse, fibrous bands (which are not pathological adhesions) that are clearly visible by dissection or on MRI [1, 2].

The IT band assists with knee extension and flexion, as well as with lateral knee stability. When the knee is in 30 degrees of flexion, the IT band lies posterior to the LFC, and, when in terminal extension, lies anterior to the LFC. Proximally, the IT band contributes to extension, abduction, and external rotation of the hip. The IT band is used primarily during walking, running, cycling, or any activity that requires flexion and extension of the knee.

C. Backer
Family Health Center, MedStar Franklin Square Medical Center, Rosedale, MD, USA

M. Sedgley (✉)
MedStar Union Memorial Hospital, Westminster, MD, USA
e-mail: matthew.d.sedgley@medstar.net

© Springer Nature Switzerland AG 2021
N. Coleman (ed.), *Common Pediatric Knee Injuries*,
https://doi.org/10.1007/978-3-030-55870-3_26

Pathology and Dysfunction

Previously, Iliotibial band syndrome (ITBS) was thought to be caused by repetitive flexion and extension of the knee. This friction of the IT band at the lateral femoral condyle was thought to contribute to distal irritation and inflammation, triggering lateral knee pain [3]. The IT band can also become inflamed at the proximal insertion, causing lateral hip pain. It is now recognized that ITBS etiology is weakness in endurance of the hip abductor muscle. This leads to compression of sensitive tissues below the IT band. Overtraining and failure to develop hip abductor muscle endurance produces this condition [4–6].

During the early stance, or foot strike, phase of running, the knee is in approximately 30 degrees of flexion. Repeated flexion can lead to IT band strain. While there is some debate, studies have suggested that ankle, knee, and hip kinetic chain malalignment can lead to increased tension of the IT band over the lateral femoral condyle [7]. Anatomically, weak hip abductors can lead to increased hip adduction, causing genu valgum and internal rotation at the knee, placing increased tension on the IT band [4, 6]. Extrinsic factors, like running on a track or banked surface, a sudden increase in mileage, and even cold weather have been shown to increase the risk for ITBS [3, 8]. Overstriding, taking short steps, and having a leg length discrepancy of >0.5 cm [9] are gait factors than can also lead to ITBS.

Epidemiology: Age, Gender, and Common Sports

Iliotibial band syndrome has not been reported in sedentary individuals. Rates among those that do exercise are variable and generally range from 7% to 14% of runners [9]. Iliotibial band syndrome is the second most common cause of knee pain after patellofemoral pain syndrome [9]. IT band syndrome is more common in women than men and is frequently seen in runners, cyclists, and military recruits. Iliotibial band syndrome usually presents unilaterally.

Mechanism of Injury: Common/Likely, Uncommon/Less Likely

While the direct mechanism of injury leading to iliotibial band syndrome is unknown, the cause is likely multifactorial. Iliotibial band syndrome is an injury due to lack of endurance of hip abduction strength. Previously, it was generally thought to occur from the IT band sliding anteriorly and posteriorly over the lateral femoral condyle during repetitive knee flexion and extension. While this repetitive motion can cause friction, irritation, and inflammation of the distal IT band, iliotibial band syndrome is more a direct consequence of hip drop from hip abductor weakness [4]. Newer theories suggest that symptoms are not caused by friction but rather by compression of fatty tissue and nerve endings (the Pacinian corpuscles) by the IT band [2]. The IT band can also impinge at the lateral femoral condyle (LFC), when the knee is flexed to 20–30 degrees; however, the main contributor to the syndrome is weak hip abductors. Weak hip abductors can lead to hip adduction in stance phase and increased rotational strain on the IT band [10]. Tightness of the tensor fascia lata and gluteus muscles can also play a role.

Long distance running and increases in activity, especially on uneven ground or downhill, can contribute to the development of IT band syndrome [11]. Running or walking on a track and exercising in cold weather are also potential risk factors for IT band syndrome. Fatigue in runners has interestingly not been thought to contribute to the condition [11].

Diagnosis: History and Exam Findings, Testing

Iliotibial band syndrome is a running injury, diagnosed based on history and clinical exam findings. IT band syndrome occurs in athletes, particularly runners, and has rarely been described in the sedentary population. The predominant complaint is diffuse lateral knee pain, sometimes with swelling. Pain can become sharp or burning and more localized over time. There is no knee instability. Symptoms usually start after or during exercise at a specific distance.

Tenderness can be localized to the lateral aspect of the knee about 2 cm above the lateral joint line. Pain is generally worse with the knee in extension, while standing, or with the knee flexed to 30 degrees. There may a popping sensation felt or heard from irritation of the IT band as it slides over the LFC. Pain can be felt at any point from the hip to the calf. Pain tends to be worse with running, especially on a track or going downhill. A positive Ober's test and Noble compression test can help with the diagnosis [3, 7]. The Ober's test is completed with the patient lying on the non-painful side. The unaffected hip and knee should be flexed at 90 degrees. The ipsilateral leg should be extended and abducted with the knee flexed to 90 degrees. If unaffected (i.e. no IT band tightness), the leg will adduct fully with gravity (i.e., the knee will lower to the exam table) and the patient will not experience any pain. If the IT band test is positive, the leg will remain abducted, and the patient may experience lateral knee pain. The Noble test is completed with the patient supine or lying on the unaffected side. While the ankle is held, the knee is repeatedly flexed, while palpating the lateral femoral condyle. Snapping, crepitus, or tenderness to palpation is a positive test. A Trendelenburg gait can be observed when a runner is in stance phase; the pelvis of the non-weight bearing extremity tilts downward and, to compensate, the trunk tilts away. This sign can also demonstrate hip abductor weakness.

Radiographs are not particularly useful in IT band syndrome and not recommended, if that is the sole concern. Magnetic Resonance Imaging (MRI) can highlight a thickened distal IT band with deep fluid collection [12]. MRI can also be used to rule out other causes of lateral knee pain, if suspected, such as lateral collateral ligament pathology, a stress fracture, or a lateral meniscus tear. Less costly, point-of-care imaging can be easily done with ultrasound (US). Musculoskeletal US can be useful to view the dynamic motion of the IT band in knee flexion and extension [13, 14]. While diagnosis is often clinical, musculoskeletal US may be of primary use, if any imaging is considered [15].

Management

ITBS can be challenging to treat, as most of those affected by the condition are highly motivated to continue exercising. ITBS does, however, respond well to conservative management. Treatment protocols should include activity modification, stretching, hip strengthening, and massage.

Rest, ice massage, and over-the-counter pain medications, such as acetaminophen or an NSAID, like ibuprofen, can, when combined with physical therapy, decrease pain during the acute phase of iliotibial band syndrome [16]. Decreasing mileage, changing shoes, altering the course, and cross-training may also minimize pain. When resuming training, mileage should be increased slowly and only when the athlete is pain free. Cross-training should include activities during which the knee is not repetitively placed in 30 degrees of flexion. Some physical therapists recommend running on a treadmill at an elevated incline of 3–5 degrees to minimize irritation of the Pacinian structures [17]. Running up an incline or hill may have a similar effect in rehabilitation.

Stretching and foam rolling are popular treatments, although there is a paucity of evidence in the literature to support their use. Strengthening the surrounding musculature (ex. gluteus medius and hip abductors) can increase hip stability and decrease hip adduction. Increasing hip abduction strength is the key to treating this condition. Skilled physical therapists and a home exercise program can focus on muscle weakness to increase hip abduction endurance and strength.

Corticosteroids can also be utilized, although there is little evidence they provide long-term relief [18]. Injections should be targeted over the LFC. While rare, there was one case study of IT band tendon rupture after repeated injections [19].

Dry needling, kinesiology taping, IT band straps, biologics (ex. platelet rich plasma), and prolotherapy have not been well studied in IT band syndrome. If the aforementioned conservative measures are unsuccessful, an orthopedic consult for surgical release or lengthening, via surgical fenestration of the distal IT band tissue, may be indicated.

Demonstration Cases

Common Presentation

A 14-year-old boy has recently started his cross-country season. His training plan was to increase his mileage by one mile each week. Instead, he decided to increase by 3 miles each week. He now has had pain on the outside of his right knee for

3 weeks. Every time he reaches 9 miles into a run, and not before, the pain occurs. Stretching and icing only give temporary relief. He went to urgent care and had a full lower extremity exam. He had full range of motion of his hips and knees without pain. There was no pain elicited at the greater trochanteric bursa. He had negative Lachman, McMurry, and Thessaly tests. There was no laxity with anterior or posterior drawer or with varus or valgus stress testing. He did, however, have tenderness of the lateral knee with 30 degrees of flexion, as well as hip abductor weakness. Ober's test was positive. X-rays were unremarkable. He was told to follow up with the athletic training staff at his high school. His school athletic trainer switched his training to inside on a treadmill with a 5-degree incline, allowing him to maintain cardiorespiratory fitness and to work on his form. He was also given core therapeutic exercises to increase his hip abduction and gluteal strength. After 6 weeks, he was able to progress past 10 miles and had complete resolution of his symptoms.

Uncommon Presentation

A 19-year-old girl presented to her sports medicine physician with a four-year history of knee pain with running. Every time she attempts to go for long distance runs, she experiences right lateral knee pain. She has sought care at orthopedic clinics in the past and was given corticosteroid injections around the distal iliotibial band at the lateral femoral condyle. She noted only temporary relief. She has worked with a physical therapist twice in the past and has felt no improvement.

Her physical examination demonstrated a normal right lower extremity on inspection. She was tender to palpation at her lateral femoral condyle. The range of motion of the knee was full. She had pain when Ober's test was performed. The knee ligaments were normal on exam. Thorough neurological muscle strength testing revealed that her knee flexion and extension were 5 out of 5; however, her extensor hallucis longus (EHL) and gluteus medius on the right were 4 out of 5, as was her right hip abduction. X-rays of the right knee and spine were normal. Due to her weakness of the EHL, an MRI of the lumbar spine was obtained to identify any disk pathology or nerve impingement and showed a large L1–2 disc herniation, impinging the transversing L5 nerve root. Since disk herniation is a common finding on MRI, an electromyogram (EMG) was performed to assess for any neuromuscular abnormalities and to confirm or refute the presence of radiculopathy. The EMG showed no peripheral nerve damage and confirmed mild radiculopathy of the L5 nerve root. An epidural steroid injection was performed to reduce inflammation, due to the L1–2 disc herniation, and, after the third injection, the EHL and hip abduction strength returned to normal. She returned to running, but, after increasing her distance once again, there was right knee pain laterally at the LFC. She underwent MRI of the right knee that showed fluid under the distal iliotibial band. The patient was referred to orthopedic surgery for an ITB lengthening procedure and made a complete recovery.

Pearls and Pitfalls

ITBS is a common reason for knee pain in active adolescents; however, it should not be the sole consideration. Knee pain in the youth athlete requires initial consideration of a broader differential diagnosis list. Careful evaluation of the hip is recommended to exclude slipped capital epiphysis of the hip. Since ITBS is commonly seen in runners, alternative diagnoses that are commonly seen in runners, like stress fracture, should also be considered. Due to the location of ITBS, exam of the all the lateral knee and connecting structures is essential to rule out the following, which may cause pain to radiate to the lateral knee: flabella friction syndrome; lateral collateral ligament (LCL) sprain; tibial plateau stress fracture; gastrocnemius, soleus, and biceps femoris strain; and referred pain from a pars defect, herniated disk, or spondylolisthesis [9, 20].

ITB syndrome, while frustrating for the young athlete, is benign. Systemic symptoms or night pain should prompt evaluation and a more extensive workup for other causes of knee pain. ITB syndrome rarely requires imaging. The key to diagnosis is noting ITB tenderness with an otherwise normal knee exam and hip abductor weakness and lack of muscle endurance [6, 21, 22].

A careful history may reveal a training error, such as rapid increases in distance and/or a neglect of core muscle strengthening. Physical examination will often demonstrate weak hip abduction and deficits in abduction endurance. Ober's test and Noble test will be positive, although there is no specific evidence to determine the diagnostic accuracy of either exam. Athletes often demonstrate a Trendelenburg gait, which can be noted on exam and on video gait analysis. There is also often increased internal rotation and hip adduction on the video analysis [6, 21, 22].

Chapter Summary

ITBS is a common cause of lateral knee pain in runners, cyclists, and other athletes that participate in activities that require repetitive flexion and extension of the knee. This overuse-related pain usually presents about 2 inches superior to the lateral joint line. Diagnosis is primarily clinical. With the history of lateral knee pain and by using special exam tests, such as Ober's and Noble test, a clinician may narrow a broad differential diagnosis list. Imaging may be useful to exclude other diagnoses but is not absolutely necessary. If other diagnoses are suspected and imaging is obtained, a fluid collection at the distal ITB insertion site might be noted on US or MRI. ITBS generally responds to conservative treatment, which should be targeted at strengthening the hip abductors and modifying training (ex. decreasing mileage) until the athlete is pain free. If needed, one can consider interventions, like steroid injections and surgical intervention.

Condition table

Condition	Iliotibial band syndrome
Description	Pain at the lateral knee near the lateral femoral condyle from weakness in hip abductor endurance strength causing compression of soft tissues compressed by the distal IT band structure.
Epidemiology	Iliotibial band syndrome is more common in runners; it may be seen in other sports including cycling.
Mechanism (common)	Running increasing distances without concomitant strengthening of hip abductors leads to fatigue and overuse. This causes hip adduction and compression of nerve rich tissue at distal IT band.
History and exam findings	Runner with lateral knee pain after a recent increase in volume and with a lack of core training; exam is normal except for pain at the lateral femoral condyle, made worse with extension of the knee in the last 30 degrees.
Management	Success is seen with hip abductor strengthening. NSAIDs may give temporary relief. Rarely, does stretching the iliotibial band help. In more challenging cases, corticosteroid injection at the LFC may be used. In severe cases, fenestration or lengthening surgery may be considered.

Suggested websites

1. http://www.runningwritings.com/2012/02/injury-series-biomechanical-solutions.html
2. https://www.aafp.org/afp/2005/0415/p1545.html

References

1. Fairclough J, Hayahshi K, Toumi H, Lyons K, Bydder G, Phillips N, Best TM, Benjamin M. The functional anatomy of the iliotibial band during flexion and extension of the knee: implications for understanding iliotibial band syndrome. J Anat. 2006;208(3):309–16. https://doi.org/10.1111/j.1469-7580.2006.00531.x.
2. Fairclough J, Hayashi K, Toumi H, Lyons K, Bydder G, Philips N, Best TM, Benjamin M. Is iliotibial band syndrome really a friction syndrome? J Sci Med Sport. 2007;10(2):74–6. https://doi.org/10.1016/j.jsams.2006.05.017.
3. Noble C. The treatment of iliotibial band friction syndrome. Br J Sports Med. 1979;13(2):51–4. https://doi.org/10.1136/bjsm.13.2.51.
4. Fredericson M, Cookingham CL, Chaudhari AM, Dowdell BC, Oestreicher N, Sahrmann SA. Hip adductor weakness in distance runners with iliotibial band syndrome. Clin J Sport Med. 2000;10:169–75.
5. Ferber R, Noehren B, Hamill J, Davis IS. Competitive female runners with a history of iliotibial band syndrome demonstrate atypical hip and knee kinematics. J Orthop Sports Phys Ther. 2010;40(2):52–8.
6. Noehren B, Davis I, Hamill J. Prospective study of the biomechanical factors associated with iliotibial band syndrome. Clin Biomech. 2007;22:951–6.
7. Louw M, Deary C. The biomechanical variables involved in the aetiology of iliotibial band syndrome in distance runners – a systematic review of the literature. Phys Ther Sport. 2014;15(1):64–75. https://doi.org/10.1016/l.ptsp.2013.07.002.

8. Messier SP, Edwards DG, Martin DF, Lowery RB, Cannon DW, James MK, Curl WW, Read HM Jr, Hunter DM. Etiology of iliotibial band friction syndrome in distal runners. Med Sco Sports Exerc. 1995;27(7):951–60.
9. Taunton JE, Ryan MB, Clement DB, McKenzie DC, Lloyd-Smith DR, Zumbo BD. A retrospective case-control analysis of 2002 running injuries. Br J Sports Med. 2002;36:95–101. https://doi.org/10.1136/bjsm.36.2.95
10. Mucha MD, Caldwell W, Schlueter EL, et al. Hip abductor strength and lower extremity running related injury in distance runners: a systematic review. J Sci Med Sport. 2017;20(4):349–55. Epub 20 Sept 2016
11. Brown AM, Zifchock RA, Hillstrom HJ, Song J, Tucker CA. The effects of fatigue on lower extremity kinematics, kinetics and joint coupling in symptomatic female runners with iliotibial band syndrome. Clin Biomech (Bristol, Avon). 2016;39:84–90. https://doi.org/10.1016/j.clinbiomech.2016.09.012. Epub 30 Sep 2016.
12. Nishimura G, Yamato M, Tamai K, Takahashi J, Uetani M. MR findings in iliotibial band syndrome. Skelet Radiol. 1997;26(9):533–7. https://doi.org/10.1007/s002560050281.
13. Jelsing EJ, Finnoff J, Levy B, Smith J. The prevalence of fluid associated with the iliotibial band in asymptomatic recreational runners: an ultrasonographic study. PM R. 2013;5(7):563–7; Epub 27 Feb 2013. https://doi.org/10.1016/j.pmrj.2013.02.010.
14. De Maeseneer M, Marcelis S, Boulet C, Kichouh M, Shahabpour M, de Mey J, Cattrysse E. Ultrasound of the knee with emphasis on the detailed anatomy of anterior, medial, and lateral structures. Skelet Radiol. 2014;43(8):1025–39; Epub 13 Mar 2014.
15. Chang K, Cheng Y, Yu-Hsuan W, Wu C-H, Levent O. Dynamic ultrasound imaging for the iliotibial band/snapping hip syndrome. Am J Phys Med Rehabil. 2015;94(6):e55–6. https://doi.org/10.1097/PHM.0000000000000299.
16. Schwellnus MP, Theunissen L, Noakes TD, Reinach SG. Anti-inflammatory and combined anti-inflammatory/analgesic medication in the early management of iliotibial band friction syndrome: a clinical trial. S Afr Med J. 1991;79(10):602–6.
17. Willy R. Mythbusting iliotibial band with Dr. Rich Willy – "It is not friction". British Journal of Sports Medicine Blog, 9 Aug 2019. https://soundcloud.com/bmjpodcasts/mythbusting-iliotibial-band-itb-pain-with-dr-rich-willy-pt-phd-its-not-friction-393. Accessed 21 Aug 2019.
18. Gunter P, Schwellnus MP. Local corticosteroid injection in iliotibial band friction syndrome in runners: a randomized control trial. Br J Sports Med. 2004;38(3):269–72. https://doi.org/10.1136/bjsm.2003.000283.
19. Pandit SR, Soloman DJ, Gross DJ, Golijanin P, Provencher MT. Isolated iliotibial band rupture after corticosteroid injection as a cause of subjective instability and knee pain in a military special warfare trainee. Mil Med. 2014;179(4):e469–72. https://doi.org/10.7205/MILMED-D-13-00438.
20. Khaund R, Flynn S. Iliotibial band syndrome: a common source of knee pain. Am Fam Physician. 2005;71(8):1545–50. https://www.aafp.org/afp/2005/0415/p1545.html. Accessed on 24 Aug 2019.
21. Hamill J, Miller R, Noehren B, Davis I. A prospective study of iliotibial band strain in runners. Clin Biomech. 2008;23:1018–25.
22. Davis J. Injury series: biomechanical solutions for iliotibial band syndrome. Running Writings. 10 Feb 2012. http://www.runningwritings.com/2012/02/injury-series-biomechanical-solutions.html. Accessed on 24 Aug 2019.

Chapter 27
Femoral Injury (Distal)

Thomas L. Pommering

Anatomy and Normal Function

The distal femur physis is a morphologically complex structure that has only recently been studied in detail [1]. It is characterized by a series of five important ridges, notches and peaks that change and evolve as the child approaches skeletal maturity [1]. Its undulating shape lends protection to this important structure, but when its complex anatomy is disrupted by shearing forces, the resulting traumatic epiphysiodesis lends to relatively high growth arrest rates [1, 2]. From a cellular aspect, the physis is composed primarily of cartilage that is made up of three distinct zones of maturation, making the physis inherently vulnerable to shearing forces.

The distal femur physis is important, as it contributes to 70% of growth from the femur and contributes to 35–40% of the entire length of the lower limb [2, 3] . The medial and lateral collateral ligaments attach distal to the physis [4]. The distal femur physis contributes an average of 1 cm of annual growth to the lower limb, making it the fastest growing physis in a child [2, 3]. Lower limb growth occurs until approximately 14–16 years old in girls and 16–18 years old in boys [3, 4].

Pathology and Dysfunction

As mentioned earlier, the complex morphology of the physis is both protective to its integrity and a contributing factor to the degree of injury that the physis sustains. In addition, the physis may be two to five times weaker than the surrounding fibrous

T. L. Pommering (✉)
Departments of Pediatrics and Family Medicine, Nationwide Children's Hospital Division of Sports Medicine, The Ohio State University College of Medicine, Columbus, OH, USA
e-mail: Thomas.pommering@nationwidechildrenshospital.org

© Springer Nature Switzerland AG 2021
N. Coleman (ed.), *Common Pediatric Knee Injuries*,
https://doi.org/10.1007/978-3-030-55870-3_27

Salter harris classification

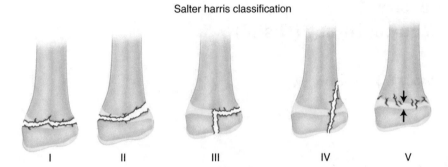

I	II	III	IV	V

Fig. 27.1 Salter–Harris classification. (Reprinted with permission from Cepela et al. [6])

soft tissue, making it the "weak link in the chain" and vulnerable to forces that produce unique injuries in kids compared to adults [5]. Physeal fractures are most commonly classified using the Salter–Harris (SH) Classification as demonstrated in Fig. 27.1 [6].

Specific Pointers

Epidemiology

Distal femoral physeal fractures account for 2–5% of all physeal fractures [7]. One large retrospective study found an 80% predilection toward males for this injury [3]. In general, the SH II fracture is the most common type of fracture, accounting for 75–80% of distal femur physeal fractures [2, 3]. Salter–Harris I and II fractures are most commonly associated with sports. Altogether, motor vehicle accidents, car versus pedestrian accidents and sports, particularly American football, are the most common activities associated with this injury [3, 5, 7].

Mechanism of Injury (MOI)

The most common mechanisms are a direct blow to the distal femur with some degree of rotation or a direct valgus/varus force to the knee [2, 4, 7]. It should be noted that this is a common MOI for other types of acute intra-articular knee injuries, so physeal injuries should always be considered in the differential diagnosis of a skeletally immature child.

Diagnosis

History and Physical Exam A high index of suspicion for this injury should be considered, if the MOI is as described above. Pain will be usually localized over the medial physis and can be circumferential about the distal physis. An examination pearl is that the distal femoral physis can be palpated by dropping a perpendicular line from the mid-axis of the patella posteriorly to the femur, while the knee is fully extended. This line will fall in the plane of the distal femoral physis [8]. An effusion can be present, especially if the fracture is intra-articular or if a concomitant internal knee injury has occurred, but lack of an effusion does not rule out the injury. If there is no effusion, there can be soft tissue swelling over the injured physis. Range of motion is limited by pain, and the knee may be held in slight flexion from hamstring muscle spasm [4]. The patient will limp or be unable to bear any weight. Valgus stress to the knee will be painful and often demonstrate laxity compared to the contralateral side but should be done only after obtaining radiographs to avoid unintentionally displacing a fracture and should not be done, if a fracture is confirmed. Swelling in the popliteal space may indicate a concomitant vascular injury [4].

Imaging: Radiographs A minimum of 2 orthogonal radiographic views of the knee should be obtained (anteroposterior and lateral). A sunrise view will help identify a patellar fracture or dislocation, and a tunnel view will identify a tibial spine fracture or an osteochondral lesion in the femoral intercondylar notch. The radiographic findings can be subtle in minimally displaced fractures, showing only a small fleck of bone next to the physis or slight asymmetric widening of the physis. Nondisplaced fractures will look normal on radiograph during the acute phase but may show subtle periosteal reaction along the metaphysis within 3 weeks of the injury [8]. Radiographic stress knee views obtained by placing valgus or varus force across the knee are highly discouraged, since they are extremely painful to the patient and can displace a fracture causing further physeal injury [4, 8]. A high index of suspicion should be maintained, if the mechanism of injury and the physical exam suggest a distal physeal injury, even in the setting of normal radiographs, whereby advanced imaging should be obtained.

Imaging: Magnetic Resonance Imaging (MRI) MRI is indicated for patients with radiographically normal or subtle findings, nondisplaced fractures, or if other intra-articular injuries are suspected [4, 7, 9–12]. Nondisplaced, vertical fractures through the sagittal plane of the distal femur are accurately visualized on MRI, when often missed on radiographs [9]. Computed Tomography scans are sometimes needed with comminuted, angulated SH III and IV fractures to aid in surgical planning [4, 7, 13]. Common MRI findings for SH I fractures will be widening and increased signal within the physis [9, 10]. Figure 27.2 demonstrates this finding, plus a subperiosteal hematoma originating from and tracking proximal to the medial physis.

Management

Nondisplaced SH I and II Fractures Most experts agree that nondisplaced SH I and II fractures can be treated with a nonweight-bearing, long leg casting for 4–6 weeks [2, 4, 7, 8, 13, 14]. Repeat radiographs should be obtained within the first week to be sure displacement has not occurred [7, 8]. Younger, obese children may require hip spica casting [8].

Any displaced SH Fracture Achieving excellent alignment of a displaced fracture is essential for proper healing and for reducing the likelihood of growth arrest. Any displaced SH fracture should be referred to a pediatric orthopedist for treatment. Displaced fractures that cannot be reduced will not maintain proper reduction or have been deemed unstable must undergo operative fixation. The fracture pattern determines if fixation requires using percutaneous pins versus cannulated screws via techniques that spare the physis [7, 8, 13]. Open reduction is required for fractures that cannot be reduced or for unstable SH III and IV fractures that require visualized anatomic reduction [2, 7, 14].

Demonstration Cases

Common Presentation

A 12-year-old football player sustains a valgus force to the knee, causing him to be unable to continue playing or to bear weight. Another common presentation would be a 10-year-old female is riding her bike and puts her leg down on the ground to

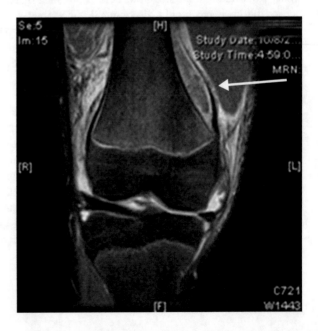

Fig. 27.2 Coronal T2 knee MRI showing increased signal in the distal femoral physis and a subperiosteal hematoma (arrow) tracking proximal from an SH I fracture

stop, forcing her knee into hyperextension. You note an effusion on exam and limited range of motion and ability to bear weight. The patient is tender at the distal femoral physis, and you consider the possibility of a collateral ligament injury. As the diagnosis is evident on radiographs with widening, but no displacement, of the physis, an MRI will be needed. Treatment for this patient will be 4–6 weeks of reliable long leg immobilization, preferably a long leg cast with a radiograph obtained through the cast after the first week of immobilization to confirm fracture stability. After immobilization is completed and follow-up radiographs demonstrate healing and/or lack of complications, the patient will need physical therapy to regain range of motion, strength, and functional ability.

Uncommon Presentation

The original mechanism by which this injury was historically described was when a child riding a horse-drawn wagon got their leg caught in the moving wheel and hyperextended their knee [2]. Though less relevant today, there are still societies that rely on this mode of transportation. So, keep this in mind if you care for patients, such as The Amish, or if you spend time practicing in a Third World country, where this mechanism of injury is still relevant. The physical exam and radiographic findings will be similar to the more common mechanisms of injury. It is still important to keep this injury in your differential diagnosis, when it presents in an atypical way.

Pearls and Pitfalls
- Children having a knee hemarthrosis in the setting of an acute knee injury will have a serious intra-articular injury, which could include an SH fracture, 70% of the time [12]. Normal radiographs in this setting should not preclude further imaging.
- Remember that the physical exam may suggest a collateral ligament injury; however, the physis is often more vulnerable to injury than the ligament [4, 5].
- To locate the physis, drop a perpendicular line down the center axis of the patella. It will intersect the femur at the level of the distal femoral physis [8].
- Avoid obtaining stress radiographic views, due to the risk of further physeal injury. Instead, obtain an MRI, if your index of suspicion is high [4, 7, 8].
- Physeal arrest is the most common complication of this injury, occurring in about 50% of all distal physeal femoral fractures, especially if displaced [3, 13]. This is demonstrated by bony bridges seen on radiograph or MRI [14, 15]. More specifically, the rate of growth disturbance for the following types of SH fractures is as follows: SH I (36%), SH II (58%), SH III (49%), and SH IV fractures (64%) [4, 8].

- A good neurovascular exam is important to rule out peroneal nerve injury, compartment syndrome, or vascular injury to the popliteal artery [2–4, 7, 8].
- Other complications from this injury are knee stiffness, posttraumatic arthritis, angular limb deformities, and leg length discrepancy [2, 7, 13].

Chapter Summary

Distal femur physeal injuries are most often seen with sports activities but can also be seen with high energy injuries, such as motor vehicle impact. The exam may suggest a collateral ligament injury, but a physeal injury should always be suspected, if a valgus, varus, or hyperextension mechanism is described. Radiographs are usually diagnostic, but nondisplaced SH I fractures may require an MRI to confirm the diagnosis. A CT is indicated for displaced, comminuted fractures, requiring surgery. Anatomic alignment is essential for healing. Despite good reduction, casting, and fixation techniques, growth arrest is a common complication. Uncommon but serious complications that should not be missed include popliteal artery and peroneal nerve injury.

Condition	
Description	Distal femur physeal injury
Epidemiology	Accounts for 2–5% of all physeal fractures. Salter–Harris II fractures are the most common type accounting for 75–80% of all distal femur physeal injuries. 80% predilection for males. The distal femur physis is fastest growing physis in a child contributing to 70% of growth from the femur and 40% of growth from the entire lower limb which amounts to about 1 cm of growth per year.
Mechanism (common)	In the sports setting—valgus force to the knee. In the recreational setting—bicycling accident where the knee is hyperextended while trying to stop of get off of the bicycle.
History and exam findings	A high index of suspicion should be maintained in the setting of high-risk mechanisms and medial knee pain in a skeletally immature patient. Localized medial knee pain over the physis. Presence of localized swelling or effusion is variable. Limited range of motion. Limping or unable to bear weight. Medial knee pain and laxity with valgus stress. When the injury is suspected, care should be exercised with valgus stress testing, especially before obtaining knee films, so as not to damage the physis further.
Management	*Nondisplaced SH I/II*—long leg cast × 4–6 weeks. *Any displaced SH fracture*—anatomic reduction important to minimize risk of growth arrest, which is relatively high for any type of SH fracture involving this physis. Reduction can be achieved by closed or operative methods. *SH III/IV fractures*—require a visualized reduction so are often managed with open reduction.

References

1. Liu RW, Armstrong DG, Levine AD, Gilmore A, Thompson GH, Cooperman DR. An anatomic study of the distal femoral epiphysis. J Pediatr Orthop. 2013;33:743–9.
2. Moran M, Macnicol MF. Paediatric epiphyseal fractures around the knee. Curr Orthopaed. 2006;20:256–65.
3. Arkader A, Warner WC, Horn BD, Shaw RN, Wells L. Predicting outcome of physeal fractures of the distal femur. J Pediatr Orthop. 2007;27:701–8.
4. Shaath K, Shirley E, Skaggs D. Distal femoral physeal fractures – pediatric. In: Orthobullets. Updated 16 Oct 2018. Pediatric Orthopaedic Society of North America. https://www.orthobullets.com/pediatrics/4020/distal-femoral-physeal-fractures%2D%2Dpediatric. Accessed 1 Oct 2019.
5. Caine D, DiFiori J, Maffulli N. Physeal injuries in children's and youth sports: reasons for concern? Br J Sports Med. 2006;40:749–60. https://doi.org/10.1136/bjsm.2005.017822.
6. Cepela DJ, Tartaglione JP, Dooley TP, Patel PN. Classifications in brief: Salter-harris classification of pediatric physeal fractures. Clin Orthop Relat Res. 2016;474:2531–7.
7. Mayer S, Albright JC, Stoneback JW. Pediatric knee dislocations and physeal fractures about the knee. J Am Acad Orthop Surg. 2015;23:571–80.
8. Wall EJ, May MM. Growth plate fractures of the distal femur. J Pediatr Orthop. 2012;32:S40–6.
9. Gufler H, Schulze CG, Wagner S, Baumbach L. MRI for occult physeal fracture detection in children and adolescents. Acta Radiol. 2013;54:467–72.
10. Pai DR, Strouse PJ. MRI of the pediatric knee. Am J Radiol. 2011;196:1019–27.
11. McKissick RC, Gilley JS, DeLee JC. Salter-Harris type III fractures of the medial distal femoral physis – a facture pattern related to the closure of the growth plate. Am J Sports Med. 2008;36:572–6.
12. Askenberger M, Ekstrom W, Finnbogason T, Janarv P. Occult intra-articular knee injures in children with hemarthrosis. Am J Sports Med. 2014;42:1600–6.
13. Parikh SN, Wells L, Mehlman CT, Scherl S. Management of fractures in adolescents. J Bone J Surg Am. 2010;92:2947–58.
14. Brousil J, Hunter JB. Femoral fractures in children. Curr Opin Pediatr. 2013;25:52–7.
15. Ecklund K, Jaramillo D. Patterns of premature physeal arrest: MR imaging of 111 children. Am J Radiol. 2002;178:967–72.

Chapter 28
Tibial Injury (Proximal)

Jessica Heyer and L. Kaleb Friend

Anatomy and Normal Function

The proximal aspect of the tibia articulates with the femur; along with the patella, these three bones form the knee joint. The soft tissues that surround the knee confer most of the stability of the knee, including ligaments, tendons, muscles, and the menisci. Since the pediatric patient has immature/developing bone, injuries to the knee often affect the bone instead of the ligaments or tendons, leading to avulsion injuries, in which the tendon–bone interface fails by avulsing bone at an attachment site. The knee is surrounded by a thick capsule; posteriorly, the level of the trifurcation of the popliteal artery lies at the level of the proximal tibial physis [1, 2].

The proximal tibia has two ossification centers, the proximal tibia physis, which contributes to longitudinal growth, and the tibial tubercle physis. The tibial tubercle physis is an apophysis, meaning that it does not contribute to the length of the bone but is an attachment site of a tendon (the patellar tendon). The average growth from the proximal tibia physis is 9–10 mm per year [3]. The proximal tibia physis appears by 2 months of age and closes between 16 and 19 years [4]. The tibial tubercle appears around 10–12 years of age and closes between 16 and 19 years [1, 4, 5].

J. Heyer
Orthopedic Surgery, George Washington University Hospital, Washington, DC, USA

L. K. Friend (✉)
Orthopedic Surgery and Sports Medicine, Children's National Hospital, George Washington University, Washington, DC, USA
e-mail: kfriend@childrensnational.org

© Springer Nature Switzerland AG 2021
N. Coleman (ed.), *Common Pediatric Knee Injuries*,
https://doi.org/10.1007/978-3-030-55870-3_28

The extensor mechanism of the knee involves the quadriceps muscle leading to the quadriceps tendon, to the patella, to the patellar tendon, and to the patellar tendon's attachment on the tibia. All of these components are required to be intact for extension of the knee [1].

Intraarticularly, the cruciate ligaments provide anterior/posterior stability to the knee, as well as some rotational stability. The anterior cruciate ligament (ACL) runs from the medial aspect of the lateral femoral condyle and inserts into the anterior tibial spine (or the tibial intercondylar eminence), which is a ridge on the proximal tibial plateau [1]. Surrounding the knee are many other smaller ligaments that contribute to the global stability of the knee.

Pathology and Dysfunction

There are several relevant injuries, when discussing the proximal tibia. These include tibial tubercle, tibial spine, Segond, proximal tibial metaphyseal, and proximal tibia physeal fractures. Risk of these fracture patterns varies by age, and prototypical mechanisms have been described [6].

Tibial tubercle fractures involve an avulsion of the patellar tendon, leading to a fracture through the apophysis of the tibial tubercle. These fractures can also propagate through the proximal tibial physis. With a displaced tibial tubercle injury, the extensor mechanism of the knee will not function [1].

Tibial spine fractures involve an avulsion of the ACL; in the pediatric population, injuries that would cause an ACL tear may cause this avulsion fracture of the tibial spine instead, due to the incomplete ossification of the epiphysis [1]. An injury that sometimes accompanies ACL tears is a tear of the anterolateral ligament (ALL). A Segond fracture is an avulsion fracture of the ALL off of the proximal aspect of the lateral tibia. When a Segond fracture is seen, a practitioner should consider a concurrent ACL injury [7].

Metaphyseal fractures are injuries of the proximal aspect of the tibia, just distal to the epiphysis. These injuries are often seen in younger patients and can either be complete or greenstick injuries [6].

Proximal tibial physeal injuries are injuries through the physis of the proximal tibia and can be akin to knee dislocation events. They are more frequently associated with acute neurovascular injury and compartment syndrome, which may not always be obvious, based on the absence of significant displacement on injury films, as the initial displacement may have been reduced since the time of injury [6]. These unstable injuries require prompt recognition of the injury pattern, so that appropriate testing for more complex neurologic and vascular injury and monitoring for compartment syndrome can be accomplished.

Specific Pointers

Tibial Tubercle Fractures

Epidemiology (Age, Gender, Common Sports)

Tibial tubercle fractures are more frequently encountered in males and are usually seen around ages 14–16, as the tibial tubercle physis is starting to close from posterior to anterior [1]. These are most often seen in patients who were participating in jumping sports, like basketball [1]. Tibial tubercle avulsion fractures account for less than 3% of all pediatric fractures [5].

Mechanism of Injury

Tibial tubercle fractures are often the result of indirect injury and usually transpire during jumping activities/sports. The avulsion occurs during an eccentric firing of the extensor mechanism, while the leg is about to leave the ground or during landing [5].

Some patients may have a history of Osgood–Schlatter disease, although the connection between the injury and Osgood–Schlatter disease is still unclear [8].

Diagnosis (History and Exam Findings, Testing)

The patient will describe attempting to jump up or landing, feeling immediate pain in the knee, and sometimes a pop, and then falling to the ground. On exam, there will be swelling and tenderness over the tibial tubercle and a knee effusion [9, 10]. The patient will often be unable to perform a straight leg raise, and attempting to extend the knee actively will cause significant pain. Some patients may maintain the ability to extend actively, due to an intact retinaculum, but an extensor lag will often still be present.

Plain radiographs of the knee (AP and lateral) will demonstrate increased gapping between the tibial tubercle physis and the proximal tibia. There may be propagation of the fracture posteriorly through the proximal tibia physis, as well, or the fracture may exit through the proximal tibia epiphysis into the joint.

Management

Tibial tubercle fractures can cause injury to the anterior tibial recurrent artery, which is draped over the anterior tibia, leaving the patient at risk for compartment syndrome [1, 11]. The risk of compartment syndrome following a tibial tubercle injury can be as high as 5% [8, 11]. Patients with this injury are admitted and monitored for possible signs of compartment syndrome preoperatively.

Tibial tubercle fractures can be treated with closed reduction and casting in extension if a patient can actively extend the knee. Most often, these injuries require treatment with closed versus open reduction and internal fixation to stabilize the fracture [5]. Open reduction may be necessary, due to periosteal or soft tissue interposition at the fracture site, preventing closed reduction. These fractures can be stabilized with cannulated screws. Post-operatively, patients are placed in a long-leg cast or knee immobilizer and can be weight bearing as tolerated [1, 5, 10].

Tibial Spine Fractures and Segond Fractures

Epidemiology (Age, Gender, Common Sports)

Tibial spine fractures are rare, with an incidence of 3 per 100,000 pediatric trauma cases per year [12]. Male and females have approximately equal incidence [12], and it occurs in children ranging from ages 8 to 14 [9, 10].

Mechanism of Injury

Typically these injuries occur via indirect injury, in which there is a twisting injury to the knee. The knee hyperextends and internally rotates, causing an ACL avulsion, or the knee is forcefully rotated while flexed [10, 12]. Direct injuries can cause an avulsion of the ACL, although this would be more common in a multiple injured patient with multiple injured knee ligaments. Approximately 50% of these injuries occur in falls from bicycles [1, 10].

Diagnosis (History and Exam Findings, Testing)

Often patients present with a history of knee pain after pivoting and difficulty bearing weight on the affected leg. The knee will be swollen, and, if aspirated, hemarthrosis would be present. A patient may have a block to full extension from the fracture fragment [1]. On exam, there will be a positive Lachman test without an endpoint and a positive anterior drawer test [1, 13]. The medial and lateral collateral ligaments and the menisci should also be assessed for concurrent injury, via varus/valgus stress tests and McMurray/joint line palpation testing, respectively; however, due to patient cooperation or guarding, the knee examination maneuvers may be futile [10, 13].

With a tibial spine fracture, imaging will demonstrate a fleck of bone off the center of the tibial plateau that appears to have been avulsed. An AP with 5 degrees caudad tilt, matching the slope of the proximal tibia, may be better suited to visualize a tibial spine fracture [14]. With a Segond fracture, imaging will demonstrate a fleck of bone off the lateral aspect of the proximal tibia, just above the fibular head. Both should raise suspicion for an ACL injury. Computed tomography (CT) better assesses the fracture and displacement, while an MRI is better for assessing the integrity of the ligaments in the knee, e.g., whether the ACL fibers remain intact, and the menisci [12].

Management

A tibial spine fracture can be of varying degrees. With minimal displacement, non-operative treatment can be pursued [1]. The knee is immobilized in extension in a long-leg cast for 4–6 weeks. If there is displacement greater than 1–2 mm, the fracture requires fixation. This can be done either with open reduction and internal fixation or with arthroscopic reduction and fixation. Post-operatively, the patient is placed in a long-leg cast or knee brace for 4–6 weeks and often requires significant rehabilitation with outpatient physical therapy to return to sport [1, 9, 10, 12].

Proximal Tibial Metaphyseal Fractures

Epidemiology (Age, Gender, Common Sports)

Tibial metaphyseal injuries are often seen in the 3–6-year-old population [6]. This type of proximal tibia injury is the only type, in which females predominate [6].

Mechanism of Injury

Most frequently, these injuries occur due to the indirect injury of landing on the knee in hyperextension with a varus or valgus force. Most commonly, there is a valgus deformity at the fracture site. Trampoline jumping is a common mechanism of injury [6].

Diagnosis (History and Exam Findings, Testing)

Patients will have immediate inability to bear weight after the injury. There will be swelling and possible deformity of the proximal tibia and tenderness over the fracture site. Plain radiographs of the tibia will demonstrate the fracture.

Management

Non-displaced fractures may be treated non-operatively with a long-leg cast for 4–6 weeks. If there is a greenstick valgus fracture, a reduction is performed and the leg is subsequently placed in a long-leg cast. Displaced fractures are taken to the operating room and are generally able to be closed reduced, although occasionally interposition of soft tissue will require an open reduction [6].

Non-operative treatment of minimally displaced fractures is at risk for Cozen's phenomenon [15]. Cozen's phenomenon is a minimally displaced greenstick fracture that goes on to develop increased valgus deformity approximately 6–12 months after injury that then usually resolves within 3 years [15–17]. These are treated with observation and reassurance to parents. If a valgus deformity persists as the patient nears skeletal maturity, guided growth or a varus-producing osteotomy may be considered [17, 18].

Proximal Tibial Physeal Injuries

Epidemiology (Age, Gender, Common Sports)

Proximal tibial physeal injuries account for <1% of all pediatric fractures [1, 2]. They can occur in all age groups, but those with physeal injuries tend to be older than those with metaphyseal fractures; peak incidence is between 10 and 16 years old [6].

Mechanism of Injury

Approximately 50% of these injuries occur in sporting events, which is often due to an indirect injury, in which there is a hyperextension force on the knee [1]. This injury can also be seen with emergent breaking of a bicycle with one leg in hyperextension and forcefully striking the ground with forward momentum [6].

A less common cause of injury is high energy direct trauma, like being struck by the bumper of a car [1, 6].

Diagnosis (History and Exam Findings, Testing)

As mentioned above, a proximal tibia physeal injury can mimic a knee dislocation, and approximately 7% have peroneal or popliteal injuries [2, 6]. A thorough neurovascular exam is important, when this type of injury is suspected. The neurovascular exam should include ankle-brachial indices (ABIs); however, there have not been any studies that correlate ABIs with vascular injury in the pediatric population, so the threshold for "normal" ABI is not defined [3]. In the adult population, ABIs >0.9 and palpable dorsalis pedis and posterior tibial pulses have been found to have 100%

sensitivity for detecting a vascular injury after knee dislocations [19]. In the pediatric population, ABIs have been found to have high inter-observer reliability and can eliminate the need for unnecessary CT angiograms and their inherent radiation [20].

As noted previously, with radiographic imaging, it is important to remember that the fracture may have been more displaced at the initial injury and subsequently reduced, giving the appearance of a less significant injury.

Management

These injuries may be treated with either closed or open reduction and stabilization with pins and require close monitoring for vascular compromise or compartment syndrome. If there is concern for a vascular injury, it is recommended that a vascular surgery consultation be made and that a vascular surgeon be present for possible exploration and/or repair, as needed [6]. After reduction, it is important to perform a thorough neurovascular exam to ensure that the peroneal nerve or popliteal artery did not become entrapped in the fracture site [3].

Demonstration Cases

Tibial Tubercle Fracture

A 14-year-old boy presented to the Emergency Department with left knee pain after attempting a layup in a basketball game. He noticed pain mid-jump and fell to the ground. He was unable to ambulate after his injury. On exam, he has a palpable defect inferior to the tibial tubercle and associated tenderness. He is unable to perform a straight leg raise, and his leg is held in flexion.

Radiographs of the knee were obtained (Figs. 28.1 and 28.2), which are an AP and lateral of the left knee in a skeletally immature individual. There is a fracture through the tibial tubercle, extending posteriorly through the tibial physis. The fracture appears extraarticular. He was admitted for compartment checks overnight, and a tibial tubercle open reduction internal fixation was performed the next morning (Figs. 28.3 and 28.4).

Tibial Spine Fracture

The patient is a 10-year-old male with a right knee injury secondary to falling off the back of his bicycle. He presents unable to bear weight and with a large knee effusion. X-rays demonstrate a displaced tibial spine fracture (Figs. 28.5 and 28.6). The knee joint was aspirated, and local analgesia injected after 45 mL of blood was removed from the knee. The knee was then extended with persistent displacement of the fracture. The patient was placed in a knee brace locked in extension, trained

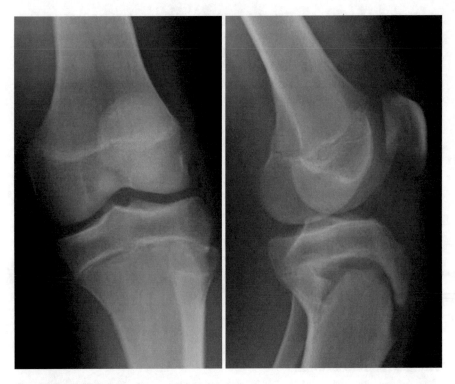

Figs. 28.1 and 28.2 Injury images, tibial tubercle fracture

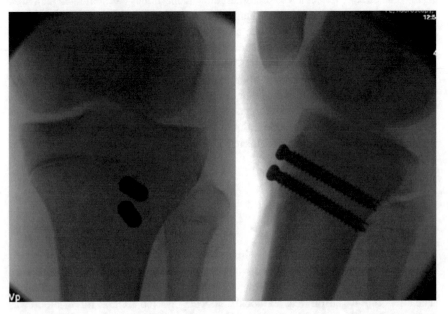

Figs. 28.3 and 28.4 AP and lateral of the left knee with two cannulated screws in the tibial tubercle with reduction of the fracture that was seen in Figs. 28.1 and 28.2

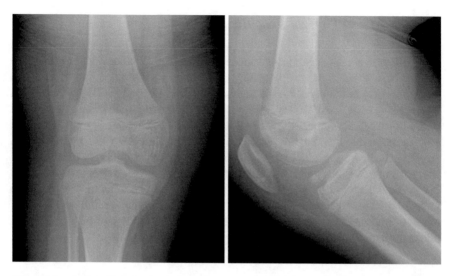

Figs. 28.5 and 28.6   Right knee AP, lateral showing the displaced tibial spine avulsion fracture

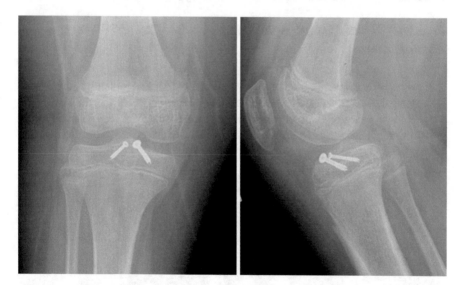

Figs. 28.7 and 28.8   Right knee AP, lateral 6 weeks post-operatively following arthroscopic-assisted reduction and internal fixation

on crutches, and discharged home. The patient was scheduled as an outpatient for surgery 10 days after the injury and underwent arthroscopic reduction and screw fixation (Figs. 28.7 and 28.8) after diagnostic arthroscopy determined that ACL fibers were largely intact and menisci were without evidence of tear. He underwent appropriate outpatient physiotherapy and returned to sport 6 months after injury.

Proximal Tibia Physeal Fracture

The patient is an 8-year-old male involved in a motorbike accident on the race course. He presented to the emergency department with knee pain, swelling, and mild deformity at the knee. X-rays revealed a Salter–Harris type IV proximal tibia fracture (Figs. 28.9 and 28.10). Ankle-brachial index was significantly diminished in the injured limb. Interventional radiology performed an arteriogram in the OR after closed reduction and pinning of the physeal fracture. He was found to have a popliteal artery intimal tear that necessitated vein interposition graft, external fixation spanning the knee, and fasciotomies for compartment syndrome prophylaxis (Figs. 28.11 and 28.12). The injured proximal tibial physis went on to experience growth arrest at that physis. To maintain the normal tibiofibular relationship and to achieve limb parity, further surgery was needed. The ipsilateral proximal fibula and contralateral tibia and fibula phases were arrested surgically.

Additional Cases of Proximal Tibia Physeal Fracture

Proximal Tibial Metaphyseal Fracture with Cozen's Phenomenon

The patient is a 28-month-old female who sustained an incomplete proximal tibia metaphyseal fracture that was relatively non-displaced (Figs. 28.13 and 28.14). She was treated in a cast without reduction needed, and the cast was removed at 4 weeks with a clinically and radiographically healed fracture. The patient was briefly lost to

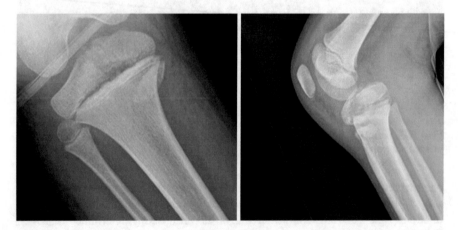

Figs. 28.9 and 28.10 AP, lateral of the right tibia and fibula. Note the posterior translation of the epiphysis and metaphysis of the proximal tibia on the lateral view. This is a subtle finding, but this pattern is very high risk for neurovascular injury

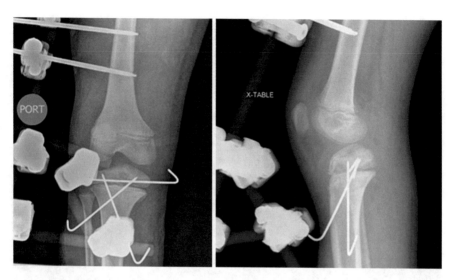

Figs. 28.11 and 28.12 Post-operative AP and lateral of the knee demonstrating pins and external fixation

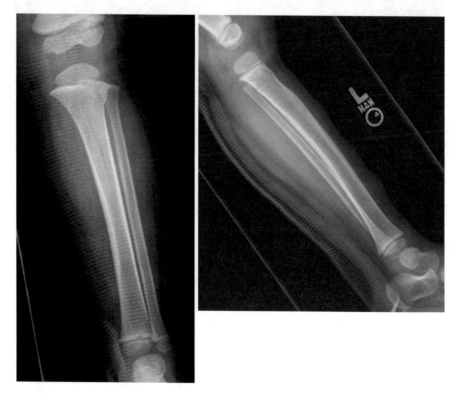

Figs. 28.13 and 28.14 AP, lateral of the left tibia demonstrating incomplete proximal tibia fracture with buckling of the lateral metaphyseal cortex and no other significant displacement

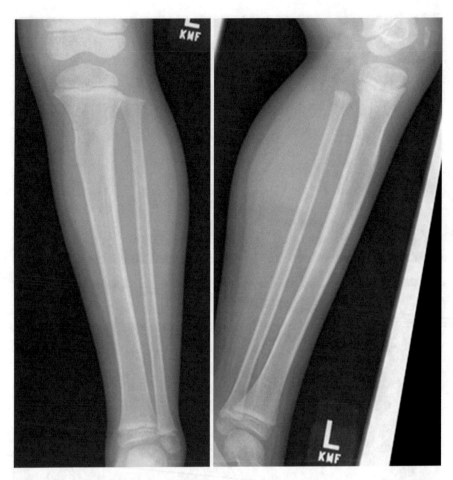

Figs. 28.15 and 28.16 Cozen's phenomenon showing development of valgus at the proximal tibial metaphysis fracture site, which is healed

follow-up after fracture healing but returned to clinic 17 months later with valgus appearance of the affected extremity that is continuing to be monitored annually (Figs. 28.15 and 28.16). The patient is asymptomatic currently. Cozen's phenomenon was discussed with the family at the very first orthopedic visit, and they have been attentive to follow-up requests.

Pearls and Pitfalls

Injuries to the proximal tibia physis or to the tibial tubercle should be handled in an expeditious manner and referred to a pediatric emergency department for further care, as they will require monitoring and likely surgical intervention. Missing one of these injuries can be detrimental, particularly a tibial physeal injury, which may not be easily noticeable on a radiograph. If there is a suspicion for an injury to the physis or to the tibial tubercle, referral to a hospital with orthopedic specialists is prudent.

Tibial spine/Segond Fracture injuries are not surgical emergencies but do require orthopedic specialist care. A patient can be placed into a knee immobilizer for comfort and instructed to follow-up in the office of a pediatric orthopedist. In the case of a tibial spine fracture, timely follow-up is ideally within a week. Segond fractures indicating ACL injury without spine fracture are best to follow up around 2 weeks after injury.

If a tibial spine fracture is seen on a radiograph, be wary of performing ACL testing on the knee (Lachman and anterior drawer testing), as these maneuvers may displace the fracture even more and preclude the ability to treat the injury non-operatively.

Chapter Summary

Proximal tibia injuries in the pediatric population are often a result of avulsion injuries, due to weakness at the level of the physis. These injuries mimic injuries that would be seen in an adult population: tibial tubercle fractures are akin to patellar tendon ruptures and tibial spine fractures are akin to ACL ruptures. If these injuries are non-displaced, they are often treated with closed reduction and a long-leg cast in extension. When displaced, they require reduction and fixation to align the bones to allow for appropriate healing. When a patient is found to have a proximal tibial physeal or a tibial tubercle avulsion injury, the patient should be monitored closely for vascular injury and compartment syndrome.

Helpful websites videos, etc.

http://www.wheelessonline.com/
  https://www.orthobullets.com/

Chart/table

Condition	Tibial tubercle fractures
Description	Fracture through the tibial tubercle physis; an avulsion injury of the extensor mechanism of the knee
Epidemiology	M > F, 14–16 years
Mechanism (common)	Indirect injury, likely jumping
History and exam findings	Knee pain, inability to straighten knee, palpable defect inferior to the tibial tubercle
Management	If minimally displaced, non-operative in long-leg cast. If displaced, closed versus open reduction and cannulated screw fixation

Condition	Tibial spine fracture and Segond fractures
Description	Tibial spine fracture is an avulsion of the ACL off the tibial plateau. Segond fracture is an avulsion of the ALL off of the lateral tibial plateau. A Segond fracture may indicate an occult ACL injury
Epidemiology	1/300,000 pediatric traumas, M = F, 8–14 years
Mechanism (common)	Indirect injury, a twisting injury to the knee, often with hyperextension Commonly associated with foot placed against ground, while on bicycle in younger patients
History and exam findings	Indirect injury, while pivoting or twisting about the knee. Significant knee swelling and positive Lachman testing or anterior drawer testing, due to incompetent ACL
Management	Non-operative management in long-leg cast, if non-displaced. Operative management with open reduction or arthroscopic reduction and internal fixation if displaced

Condition	Proximal tibial metaphyseal injury
Description	Fracture of the proximal metaphysis of the tibia
Epidemiology	3–6 years, F > M
Mechanism (common)	Hyperextension, varus/valgus injuries; trampoline injuries
History and exam findings	Pain, inability to bear weight. Tenderness over the fracture site
Management	Reduction and long-leg casting. Delayed valgus deformity is common (Cozen's phenomenon) and often resolves by 2–3 years of post-injury

Condition	Proximal tibial physeal injury
Description	Fracture of the proximal tibial physis
Epidemiology	Typically older than those affected by metaphyseal injury. Reported 10–16 years of peak age
Mechanism (common)	Varus/valgus and/or hyperextension injury Can be associated with high energy direct blow
History and exam findings	Significant swelling often present, concern for nerve or vascular injury even with normal pulse to palpation
Management	Usually operative, consider ABIs, neurovascular monitoring

References

1. Little RM, Milewski MD. Physeal fractures about the knee. Curr Rev Musculoskelet Med. 2016;9(4):478–86.
2. Guled U, Gopinathan NR, Goni VG, Rhh A, John R, Behera P. Proximal tibial and fibular physeal fractures causing popliteal artery injury and peroneal nerve injury: a case report and review of literature. Chin J Traumatol. 2015;18(4):238–40.
3. Mayer S, Albright JC, Stoneback JW. Pediatric knee dislocations and physeal fractures about the knee. J Am Acad Orthop Surg. 2015;23(9):571–80.
4. Herring JA. Growth and development. In: Herring JA, Adams RC, editors. Tachdjian's pediatric orthopaedics from the Texas Scottish Rite Hospital for Children. 5th ed. Philadelphia: Elsevier Saunders; 2014.
5. Schiller J, DeFroda S, Blood T. Lower extremity avulsion fractures in the pediatric and adolescent athlete. J Am Acad Orthop Surg. 2017;25(4):251–9.
6. Mubarak SJ, Kim JR, Edmonds EW, Pring ME, Bastrom TP. Classificaiton of proximal tibial fractures in children. J Child Orthop. 2009;3(3):191–7.
7. Shaikh H, Herbst E, Rahnemai-Azar AA, Bottene Villa Albers M, Naendrup JH, Masahl V, et al. The Segond fracture is an avulsion of the anterolateral complex. Am J Sports Med. 2017;45(10):2247–52.
8. Pretell-Mazzini J, Kelly DM, Sawyer JR, Esteban EM, Spence DD, Warner WC Jr, et al. Outcomes and complications of tibial tubercle fractures in pediatric patients: a systematic review. J Pediatr Orthop. 2016;36(5):440–6.
9. Gans I, Baldwin KD, Ganley TJ. Treatment and management outcomes of tibial eminence fractures in pediatric patients. Am J Sports Med. 2014;42(7):1743–50.
10. Herman MJ, Martinek MA, Abzug JM. Complications of tibial eminence and diaphyseal fracture sin children: prevention and treatment. J Am Acad Orthop Surg. 2014;22(11):730–41.
11. Pandya NL, Edmonds EW, Roocroft JH, Mubarak SJ. Tibial tubercle fractures: complications, classification and the need for intra-articular assessment. J Pediatr Orthop. 2012;32(8):749–59.
12. Scrimshire AB, Gawad M, Davies R, George H. Management and outcomes of isolated paediatrictibial spine fractures. Injury. 2018;49(2):437–42.
13. Frank JS, Gambacorta PL. Anterior cruciate ligament injuries in the skeletally immature athlete: diagnosis and management. J Am Acad Orthop Surg. 2013;21(2):78–87.
14. Egol KA, Koval KJ, Zuckerman JD. Pediatric fractures and dislocations. In: Egol KA, Koval KJ, Zuckerman JD, editors. Handbook of fractures. 4th ed. Philadelphia: Lippincott Williams & Wilkins; 2010.
15. Jackson DW, Cozen L. Genu valgum as a complication of proximal tibial metaphyseal fractures in children. J Bone Joint Surg Am. 1971;53(8):1571–8.
16. Coates R. Knock-knee deformity following upper tibial greenstick fractures. J Bone Joint Surg Br. 1977;59-B:516.
17. Tuten HR, Keeler KA, Gabos PG, Zoints LE, MacKenzie WG. Posttraumatic tibia valga in children. A long-term follow-up note. J Bone Joint Surg Am. 1999;81(6):799–810.
18. Morin M, Klatt J, Stevens PM. Cozen's deformity: resolved by guided growth. Strategies Trauma Limb Reconstr. 2018;13(2):87–93.
19. Weinberg DS, Scarcella NR, Napora JK, Vallier HA. Can vascular injury be appropriately assessed with physical exam after knee dislocation? Clin Orthop Relat Res. 2016;474(6):1453–8.
20. Dean EM, Rogers K, Thacker MM, Kruse RW. Inter-observer reliability of the ankle-brachial index in a pediatric setting. Del Med J. 2015;87(3):77–80.

Chapter 29
Meniscus Injury

Miranda Gordon-Zigel and Valerie E. Cothran

Anatomy and Normal Function

The meniscus is located between the femoral condyles and tibial plateaus. It acts to protect the articular cartilage by maintaining stability of the knee and transmitting forces across the knee joint. It also aids with proprioception. It is made primarily out of type I collagen bundles, which are circumferential and radially oriented to help to prevent tearing [1].

The medial meniscus is the larger of the two menisci; it is C-shaped, covers about 50% of the medial tibial plateau and has a larger posterior horn than anterior horn. It has bony attachments to the anterior and posterior horns at the meniscal root; peripherally, it has attachments to the joint capsule and to the deep fibers of the medial collateral ligament (Fig. 29.1). The medial meniscus provides anteroposterior stability to the knee [1].

The lateral meniscus is more circular in shape; it covers about 70% of the lateral tibial plateau and has similarly sized anterior and posterior horns. Anteriorly, it attaches next to the anterior cruciate ligament; "posteriorly it attaches behind the intercondylar eminence anterior to the attachment of the posterior horn of the medial meniscus" [1]. It also has attachments via the meniscofemoral ligaments, popliteo-meniscal fasciculi, and the ligament of Wrisberg, which travels posterior to the posterior cruciate ligament and attaches to the femur [1].

The medial meniscus has a stronger attachment to the joint capsule, which makes it less mobile and more susceptible to meniscocapsular separation and tears. The lateral meniscus is more mobile, because of weaker attachments. The meniscal blood supply comes via the medial and lateral geniculate arteries. At birth the entire

M. Gordon-Zigel · V. E. Cothran (✉)
Primary Care Sports Medicine, University of Maryland,
Department of Family and Community Medicine, Baltimore, MD, USA
e-mail: vcothran@som.umaryland.edu

© Springer Nature Switzerland AG 2021
N. Coleman (ed.), *Common Pediatric Knee Injuries*,
https://doi.org/10.1007/978-3-030-55870-3_29

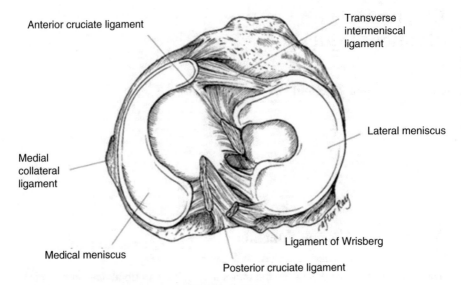

Fig. 29.1 Meniscal anatomy and relationship to important structures of the knee joint [1]

meniscus has a direct blood supply; however, this changes with age. By 9 months of age, the inner one-third of the meniscus is avascular. By 10 years of age, the blood supply is similar to that of the mature meniscus with an avascular inner third and vascular outer third. The direct vascular supply in the outer one-third is referred to as the red zone (Fig. 29.2). The white zone, the inner portion of the meniscus, is avascular and receives nutrition through synovial diffusion [3, 4].

Pathology and Dysfunction

Meniscal pathology in children and adolescents can occur in the setting of a morphologically normal or abnormal meniscus. Meniscal tears are classified according to their orientation (horizontal, radial, complex, root injury, bucket handle) and location (zone of the meniscus) [4].

Normal Meniscus

In a morphologically normal meniscus, the majority of meniscal injuries are traumatic (i.e., often occur during athletic activities), isolated, and peripherally located. Most traumatic meniscal injuries occur after the age of 12 [2].

Fig. 29.2 Classification of
meniscus according to
vascularization (red,
red–white, and white
zone) [2]

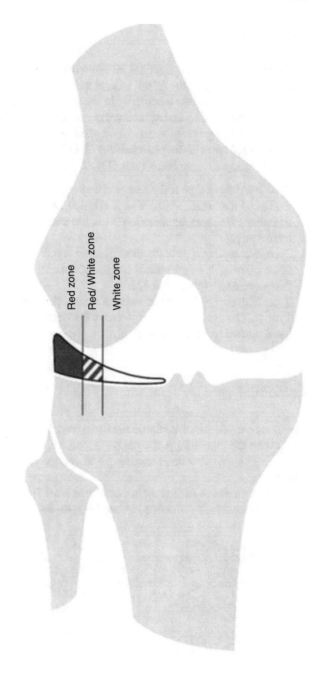

Red zone

Red/White zone

White zone

Discoid Meniscus

A discoid meniscus is a congenital variant with abnormal morphology and may create innate instability of the lateral meniscus. It is thicker and has poor tissue quality and instability. It has less vascularity in the periphery than a normal meniscus. Due to the abnormal vascularity, abnormal morphology, and attachments, discoid menisci are more prone to tears, which may be symptomatic or asymptomatic [5]. There are three types of discoid meniscus described by the Watanabe Classification – Wrisberg, complete, and incomplete (Fig. 29.3).

- Type I/Wrisberg type is the least common type. The meniscotibial attachment of the lateral meniscus is absent, so it is only fixed at the posterior meniscofemoral ligament (Wrisberg ligament). This is the most unstable variation of a discoid meniscus [2].
- Type II/complete type is the most common type. The meniscus covers the entire tibial plateau; it has a normal tibial attachment; and the meniscus is typically thickened and hypertrophic [2].
- Type III/incomplete type is more common than Type I but less common than Type II. The meniscus partially covers the tibial plateau and is thickened; it also has a normal tibial attachment [2].

Epidemiology

The exact prevalence of pediatric meniscal tears is unknown, although it has been rising with the increased participation in youth sports. Meniscal injuries are most common in sports that involve cutting and change of direction, as well as in contact sports.

Discoid meniscus is thought to occur in at least 3–6% of the US population, but the true incidence is difficult to know, because some may be asymptomatic. The

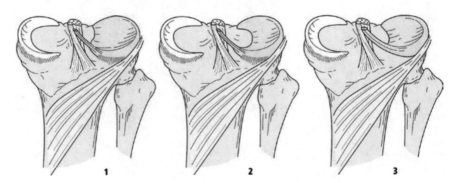

Fig. 29.3 Illustration of the Watanabe classification of discoid meniscus. 1 – complete type, 2 – incomplete type, 3 – Wrisberg type [2]

incidence also varies in different populations. In Europe, the incidence has been reported as 1.2–5.2%, whereas in East Asian countries it has been reported as 13–46% [2]. The incidence of discoid meniscus is similar between females and males.

Mechanism of Injury

In a morphologically normal meniscus, the usual mechanism of injury is a pivot-shift or rotational injury during athletic activity. In a discoid meniscus, the mechanism of injury may be similar to that of a normal meniscus, may be due to a lower impact injury, or may be without any injury mechanism.

Diagnosis (History/Exam Findings/Testing)

History

In the setting of an acute injury, the patient will complain of knee pain and may have a knee effusion following a pivot-shift injury or direct trauma to the knee. In addition to pain, he/she may complain of locking, catching, giving way, or a lack of full knee extension.

A discoid meniscus may be asymptomatic, if stable and untorn. A torn discoid meniscus may present with pain or instability, similar to that of a traumatic injury. An unstable discoid meniscus may be symptomatic even without a tear. In these cases, a patient may complain of intermittent snapping or popping, loss of full knee extension, knee pain, and/or a bulge at the lateral joint line, which can represent a subluxing lateral meniscus.

Physical Exam

On exam, tenderness in the medial or lateral joint lines can indicate a meniscal injury. There may not be a joint effusion. Special exam maneuvers can help to assess the meniscus. It is important to test the remainder of the stabilizing structures of the knee, as well, as a meniscal injury may happen in the setting of another injury, like an ACL tear.

The McMurray test is commonly used. "With the patient supine, the examiner brings the knee from full flexion to 90 degrees of flexion first with full tibial internal rotation and then with full tibial external rotation. A positive test produces a 'click' and reproduces the patient's painful sensation" [6]. The Thessaly test is more patient-controlled. "The patient stands with all weight on one extremity, holds onto a stationary item for support, then internally and externally rotates his or her knee and body while keeping one foot planted with the knee flexed at 5 degrees and then 20 degrees. Joint line pain with the maneuver indicates a possible meniscus tear" [6]. Some practitioners may also use the Apley grind test, during which a "strong external rotation force [is] applied to the knee while flexed at 90 degrees at rest, with distraction, and with compression. Joint-line pain with distraction is concerning for ligamentous injury. Joint-line pain with compression is concerning for meniscal pathology" [6]. Another patient-controlled test is the Squat test. The patient performs a full squat with the legs externally and then internally rotated. Posterior-medial joint line pain with squatting in external rotation suggests medial meniscal injury, and posterlior lateral joint line pain with internal rotation suggests lateral meniscal injury.

Imaging

Plain radiographs may show no findings; with more severe injuries, they can show squaring of the lateral femoral condyle, cupping of the lateral tibial plateau, and widening of the lateral joint space or hypoplastic lateral tibial spine [4]. Radiographs are also useful to rule out other injuries, such as fractures or osteochondritis dissecans [7].

Magnetic resonance imaging (MRI) can aid in the diagnosis. There are three typical types of MRI findings that can be seen in the setting of a discoid meniscus. These include anterior–posterior diffusely hypertrophic type (slab), anterior hypertrophy type, and posterior hypertrophy type [2]. MRI can also help to classify the location, direction, and type of tear, which helps to determine management.

Classification of Meniscal Tear Types

Meniscal tears are classified based on their location (red zone versus white zone) and their orientation (Fig. 29.4). Tear orientation is described as longitudinal (or vertical), horizontal, radial, oblique, or complex. Longitudinal tears are perpendicular to the tibial plateau and parallel to the long axis of the meniscus. Horizontal tears may be referred to as cleavage tears. They split the meniscus parallel to the tibial plateau, they are more common in older adults. Radial tears are perpendicular to both the tibial plateau and the long axis of the meniscus (looks like a spoke in the wheel of the meniscus).

In the pediatric population, tears of the medial meniscus are more common than those of the lateral meniscus. The classification of the tear is important in determining the treatment needed. Treatment options are non-operative (physical therapy and rest) and operative. Surgical treatment options include meniscal repair, partial

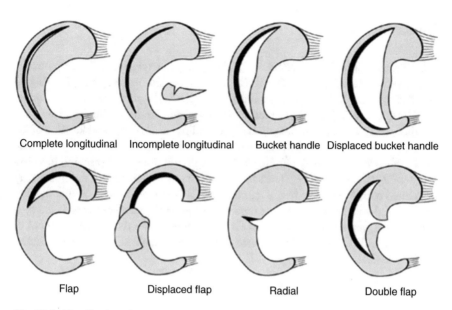

Complete longitudinal   Incomplete longitudinal   Bucket handle   Displaced bucket handle

Flap   Displaced flap   Radial   Double flap

Fig. 29.4 Classification of meniscal tear types [2]

or total menisectomy, and masterly neglect [7]. In the pediatric population, the main principle in operative management is to preserve as much meniscal tissue as possible to minimize the risk for early osteoarthritis. Tears that are smaller than 5 mm and are located in the avascular area are often stable and can be treated non-operatively. Larger tears and those that are unstable generally require surgical intervention. Often times it is difficult to determine the stability of a meniscal tear from imaging alone. In these cases, a diagnostic arthroscopy is performed to determine the stability of the lesion upon probing. Bucket-handle tears are particularly unstable, due to their propensity to flip over on themselves, causing a mechanical block, leading to the necessity for surgical intervention [7].

A bucket-handle meniscal tear is "an oblique or vertical tear that extends longitudinally throughout the meniscal body from the posterior horn to the anterior horn. The inner fragment can displace into the intercondylar notch causing mechanical symptoms" [8]. Bucket-handle tears usually occur as the result of a traumatic sports injury in a morphologically normal meniscus. It is a rare injury pattern in children younger than 10 years of age. Patients will present with pain, swelling, instability, and mechanical symptoms after a traumatic injury [8]. Due to the displacement that occurs with this tear pattern along with the loss of range of motion, these injuries are surgically repaired in a more expedited fashion, and it is important for these patients to be evaluated by a surgeon as soon as possible after the injury.

Tears in the attachment of the meniscus to the tibia or root tears result in impaired distribution of forces and meniscal extrusion. They most often occur in the posterior attachment of the lateral meniscus and are often occur in association with ACL tears [9].

Management

An asymptomatic discoid meniscus can be managed expectantly. If symptomatic, conservative management with physical therapy should be tried first. If conservative management fails, surgery is indicated to preserve the meniscus with saucerization (surgical reshaping of the meniscus) and repair. In the setting of a traumatic meniscal tear, surgery may be indicated, depending on the shape and location of the tear. Tears that are small and stable and that have good blood supply may not need repair; however, some may require surgical exploration (i.e., arthroscopy) to assess the stability of the lesion [7]. Tears that do not require repair or meniscectomy may be treated with a period of rest in a knee immobilizer and with non-weight bearing or protected weight bearing [7]. If repair is not possible, meniscectomy is the next step [4]. As meniscectomy has been found to increase the risk of development of early osteoarthritis, the preference is to maintain as much native meniscal tissue as is possible [10].

Demonstration Cases

Common Presentation

A 14-year-old girl presents with a swollen and painful knee after twisting it during a soccer game 2 days ago. She was running and, when pivoting to change direction, she felt pain in her knee. Later that night she noticed some swelling. Over the last couple of days, she has had swelling, pain, clicking, and decreased range of motion. She says that, for the last year or so, she has had some clicking in the knee, but it was never painful.

Her exam is significant for decreased range of motion in extension, a moderate knee effusion, tenderness to palpation over the lateral joint line, a negative Lachman, a negative anterior drawer and posterior drawer, no laxity with varus or valgus stress, and a positive McMurray.

She had an MRI of the knee performed without contrast, which showed a moderate joint effusion, a meniscus with discoid morphology with an acute lateral bucket-handle meniscal tear. Her ACL, PCL, MCL, and LCL were all intact.

She was put in a knee immobilizer and was given crutches and told to be non-weight bearing. She was taken to the operating room for a meniscal repair 1 week after her injury. She completed a course of postoperative physical therapy. After completing her physical therapy, she was able to return to playing soccer.

Uncommon Presentation

A 5-year-old boy presents with intermittent left lateral knee pain and popping. There was no known trauma. The patient was a health active 5-year-old without any past medical history. Mom and patient report two previous episodes of mild swelling of the left knee after prolonged activity, which resolved with rest.

His physical exam reveals a visible and audible pop at the left lateral joint line with full active flexion. This was minimally painful. There was no effusion. There was a similar, yet less noticeable, pop on the right.

MRI revealed bilateral lateral discoid menisci without meniscal tears. He was diagnosed with bilateral symptomatic discoid menisci with reproducible posterior subluxation during flexion. This was confirmed with direct visualization during arthroscopy. The patient underwent arthroscopic lateral discoid meniscus saucerization. He completed postoperative physical therapy and returned to full activity after 4 weeks.

Chapter Summary

Meniscal injuries in the pediatric population can occur in the setting of a morphologically normal meniscus or in a discoid meniscus. In the setting of a morphologically normal meniscus, injuries are generally related to a specific trauma that is most commonly athletics related. In the setting of a discoid meniscus, injuries can be traumatic or there can be symptomatic pathology directly related to the abnormal morphology.

Condition Table

Meniscal injury (Normal meniscus)	Normal meniscal injury
Description	Traumatic tear of meniscus
Epidemiology	True incidence of injury is unknown; however, it has been rising with the increase of participation in youth sports
Mechanism (common)	Pivot-shift injury, rotational injury, or direct trauma to the knee
History and exam findings	History – joint line pain, locking, catching, instability Exam – joint line tenderness; knee effusion; positive McMurray, Thessaly, Apley grind, or squat test
Management	Depends on the size and location of the tear Consider initial conservative management with physical therapy Surgical repair with conservative treatment failure or with severe tear

Meniscal injury (Discoid meniscus)	Discoid meniscal injury
Description	Abnormal morphology of meniscus allows for instability and easy tear
Epidemiology	Incidence ranges (based on geography – in Europe 1.2–5.2%, in United State 3–6%, in East Asian countries 13–46%). Similar incidence between males and females
Mechanism (common)	Pivot-shift injury, rotational injury, direct trauma to the knee, or may be an atraumatic injury
History and exam findings	History – joint line pain, locking, catching, instability Exam – joint line tenderness; knee effusion; positive McMurray, Thessaly, Apley grind, or squat test
Management	If asymptomatic, observe If symptomatic, consider repair

References

1. Torres SJ, Hsu JE, Mauck RL. Meniscal anatomy. In: Kelly IV J, editor. Meniscal injuries. New York: Springer; 2014.
2. Hirschmann MT, Friederich NF. Classification: discoid meniscus, traumatic lesions. In: Beaufils P, Verdonk R, editors. The meniscus. Berlin, Heidelberg: Springer; 2010.
3. Francavilla ML, Restrepo R, Zamora KW, Sarode V, Swirsky SM, Mintz D. Meniscal pathology in children: differences and similarities with the adult meniscus. Pediatr Radiol. 2014;44:910–25.
4. Kocher MS, Logan CA, Kramer DE. Discoid lateral meniscus in children: diagnosis, management and outcomes. J Am Acad Orthop Surg. 2017;25:736–43.
5. Chambers HG, Chambers RC. The natural history of meniscus tears. J Pediatr Orthop. 2019 Jul;39:S53–5.
6. McHale KJ, Park MJ, Tjoumakaris FP. Physical examination for meniscus tears. In: Kelly IV J, editor. Meniscal injuries. New York: Springer; 2014.
7. Lorbach O, Pape D, Seil R. Meniscus lesions in children-indications and results. In: Beaufils P, Verdonk R, editors. The meniscus. Berlin, Heidelberg: Springer; 2010.
8. Nooh A, Waly F, Abduljabbar FH, Janelle C. Bucket-handle meniscal tear in a 9-year-old girl: a case report and review of the literature. J Pediatr Orthop B. 2016;25:570–2.
9. Willimon SC, Christino M, Busch M, Perkins C. Meniscus root tears in children and adolescents. Orthop J Sports Med. 2019;7(3 Suppl):2325967119S00032. Published 2019 Mar 29. https://doi.org/10.1177/2325967119S00032.
10. Yang BW, Liotta ES, Paschos N. Outcomes of meniscus repair in children and adolescents. Curr Rev Musculoskelet Med. 2019;12:233–8.

Chapter 30
Osteochondritis Dissecans of the Knee (Femoral Condyle and Patella)

Kayla E. Daniel and Anastasia N. Fischer

Anatomy and Normal Function

The knee joint is composed of bones, cartilage, ligaments, and tendons. The bones and cartilage play an essential role in joint function, specifically at the osteochondral surface of the distal femur and patella. The osteochondral surface refers to the subchondral bone surface and articular cartilage. Cartilage is avascular and is metabolically supported by synovial fluid and subchondral bone. Articular cartilage functions to decrease friction and distributes loads to underlying subchondral bone.

Pathology and Dysfunction

Osteochondritis dissecans (OCD), also referred to as an osteochondral defect, is a localized alteration of subchondral bone structure with risk for instability and disruption of adjacent articular cartilage [1]. Softening of the overlying articular cartilage leads to early articular cartilage separation, then to partial detachment of the lesion, and finally to osteochondral separation with loose body formation. The exact etiology has been a subject of debate. Multiple theories exist for OCD pathophysiology, including disruption of the normal endochondral ossification, genetic factors,

K. E. Daniel
Department of Orthopaedic Surgery, Washington University School of Medicine, St. Louis, MO, USA

A. N. Fischer (✉)
Division of Sports Medicine, Nationwide Children's Hospital, Dublin, OH, USA

Department of Pediatrics, The Ohio State University College of Medicine, Columbus, OH, USA
e-mail: Anastasia.Fischer@nationwidechildrens.org

© Springer Nature Switzerland AG 2021
N. Coleman (ed.), *Common Pediatric Knee Injuries*,
https://doi.org/10.1007/978-3-030-55870-3_30

focal ischemia, and repetitive microtrauma, the most widely accepted theory [1–3]. The typical location for OCD lesions is on the lateral aspect of the medial femoral condyle [4]. This area is at risk for trauma, secondary to impingement against the tibial spine, thus supporting the theory of repetitive microtrauma as a primary etiology [3, 4]. Lesions at the medial femoral condyle account for 70–80% of knee OCD lesions, and 15–20% are found in the infero-central lateral condylar region. Patellar lesions are less common and account for 5–10% of knee OCD lesions. OCD lesions in the patella are frequently found at the inferior pole [5].

Epidemiology

Children ages 12–19 have three times greater risk in developing OCD lesions of the knee, compared to children ages 6–11. Males have a much higher incidence of OCD and approximately four times the risk of developing OCD lesions, as compared to age-matched females [6]. There is approximately a 29% incidence of bilateral knee OCD lesions. Female sex and younger age at presentation are risk factors for bilateral disease [3]. Risk for OCD lesions increases with year-round, high-level sports and specific sports involving repetitive force and high-frequency injuries of the knee. These activities include long-distance running, soccer, football, and basketball [1, 6].

Mechanism of Injury

There is no clear mechanism of injury for the development of OCD lesions. Based on the theory of repetitive microtrauma, OCD lesions can be classified as an overuse injury [3, 4]. OCD lesions of the knee are often found incidentally on radiographs, while the athlete is being evaluated for an unrelated injury or following a traumatic event [1].

Diagnosis

History – Most children present with chronic, vague, intermittent, achy, activity-related knee pain. In unstable lesions, children may experience catching, locking, or a popping sensation from a loose osteochondral fragment [1, 2]. OCD lesions may also be incidentally found in children presenting with other primary complaints.

Exam – Pain is often poorly localized. A knee effusion, crepitation, or antalgic externally rotated gait pattern may be observed [2]. Children may have a positive Wilson sign. A positive Wilson sign is the production of pain at the anteromedial aspect of the knee, when the knee is flexed to 90° and the tibia is then internally rotated while the knee is brought to 30 degrees of flexion [1].

Testing – Plain radiographs can localize and measure the lesion, describe the morphology, and determine the skeletal maturity of the child (Figs. 30.1 and 30.2). Four specific views are recommended, including anterior–posterior, lateral, merchant (or sunrise) view, and flexed tunnel view [1, 2]. Plain radiographs cannot sufficiently

Fig. 30.1 Medial femoral condyle OCD radiograph in a 13-year-old boy (with smaller lateral femoral condyle OCD lesion)

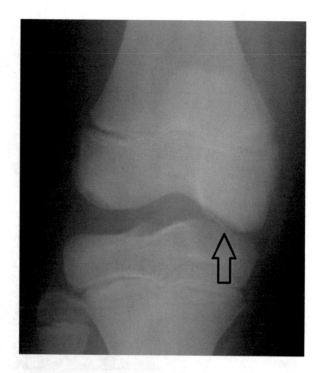

Fig. 30.2 Patellar OCD radiograph in a 14-year-old boy

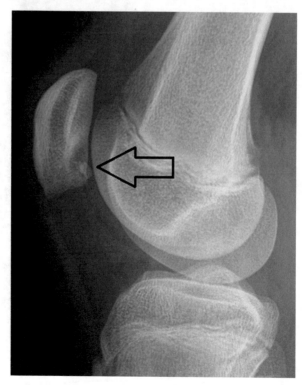

Fig. 30.3 Medial femoral
condyle OCD MRI in a
13-year-old boy (with
smaller lateral femoral
condyle OCD lesion)

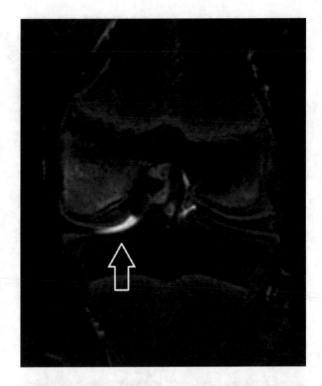

Fig. 30.4 Patellar OCD
MRI in a 14-year-old boy

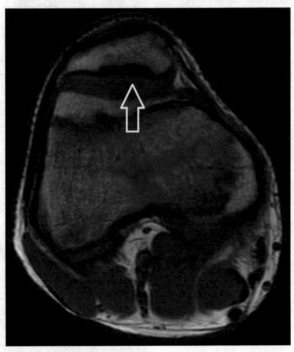

Table 30.1 MRI classification of juvenile osteochondritis dissecans [9]

Grade	MRI finding
Grade I	No break in articular cartilage. Thickening of articular cartilage
Grade II	Articular cartilage breached, low signal rim behind fragment indicating fibrous attachment
Grade III	Articular cartilage breached with high signal T2 changes behind fragment suggesting fluid behind the lesion
Grade IV	Loose body with defect of the articular surface

determine the stability of an OCD lesion. MRI is helpful in diagnosing, characterizing, and staging OCD lesions (Figs. 30.3 and 30.4). Several classification systems for OCD stability are based off of MRI imaging (Table 30.1), specifically looking at distinct fragments, high T-2 signal intensity between the parent and progeny bone, chondral disruption, and identifiable loose bodies [2, 4]. Ultrasound (US) can be used to screen and monitor OCD stages II–IV; however, US is limited in assessing OCD stage I, as well as defects localized to the intracondylar notch or the posterior lateral condyle [7]. While MRI remains the gold standard for diagnosing and monitoring OCD lesions, the gold standard for diagnosing stability of OCD lesions is arthroscopy [2, 7]. MRI predictability of high-grade, unstable lesions is less reliable. In addition, lesions that are in atypical locations, such as the lateral femoral condyle, often present as higher-grade lesions on arthroscopic evaluation [8].

Management

The skeletal maturity of the patient and stability of the fragment determine the treatment options for OCD lesions of the knee [1, 2]. In a skeletally immature patient with open physes and a stable lesion, the initial treatment is often non-operative management. Non-operative or conservative management may include anti-inflammatory medications, range-of-motion exercises, and stretching and strengthening exercises either at home or with a physical therapist [1]. A brace or cast with crutches may be recommended to immobilize and protect the joint. The purpose of conservative therapy is to eliminate pain and give the lesion time to heal [2]. Healing may take up to 6 months. Trends toward early intervention of chronic, stable lesions prior to conservative management are currently being explored. In a case series of multifocal OCD lesions only 25% healed with conservative management; stable lesions that underwent surgical management healed more reliably than unstable lesions [10]. If the lesion is unstable, or if the child fails to improve with conservative management, surgical treatment is then recommended. The specific surgical procedure depends on different factors, such as the size and shape of the lesion and the condition of the surrounding cartilage. Surgical treatment of patellar OCD lesions is uniquely challenging, due to the thickness of the lesion and the required surgical approach. Internal fixation is preferred over fragment excision and drilling, due to inferior functional results [11]. Regenerative surgical options, such as micro-fracture surgery, aim to stimulate natural cartilage healing and have recently become first-line therapies. Microfracture surgery promotes cartilage regeneration by expos-ing chondral lesions, through perforations, to mesenchymal stem cells from bone marrow. Microfracture surgery, in combination with the use of specific hydrogel scaffolding, improves the quality of chondrogenic differentiation to mimic the his-tological and biomechanical properties of native hyaline cartilage [6, 7, 12].

Demonstration Cases

Common Presentation

A 13-year-old male presents to the office with chronic, non-specific knee pain and reports intermittent swelling that is worse with activity. He recently had to sit out from gym class because of pain. His exam shows no joint effusion, no specific point tenderness, and no signs of ligamentous instability. Four view radiographs reveal subtle flattening and an indistinct radiolucency of the cortical surface on the medial femoral condyle. An MRI confirms the presence and stability of the OCD lesion. He is treated with conservative management and is removed from participation in sports, while healing. He completes physical therapy and is transitioned to home exercises. He is asymptomatic at his 6-month follow-up visit with reassuring radio-graphic changes and is cleared for return to play.

Uncommon Presentation

A 14-year-old male presents to the office with chronic, non-specific, activity-related knee pain that has acutely worsened. He reports that the pain is associated with inter-mittent swelling and states that his "knee is catching and locking in place." He limps into the exam room and is noted to have a small knee effusion but no additional signs of ligamentous instability. Four view radiographs reveal a well-circumcised frag-ment of bone with a lucent defect in the medial femoral condyle. An MRI confirms the presence of a stage IV, unstable, OCD lesion of the medial femoral condyle. He is referred to an orthopedic surgeon for surgical evaluation and treatment.

Pearls and Pitfalls
OCD lesions are often missed on anterior–posterior radiographs of the knee. Lateral, notch, and merchant views are recommended to identify OCDs on radiographs.

Open femoral physes are the best predictor for successful non-operative management. Lesions at the patella and lateral femoral condyle have poorer prognosis.

Chapter Summary

Osteochondritis dissecans is an alteration in the subchondral bone structure, often in the femur, with the risk for instability and disruption of the adjacent articular cartilage. Children may present with chronic, vague, activity-related knee pain. If the lesion is unstable, children may have mechanical symptoms, swelling, and gait abnormalities. OCD lesions are often initially diagnosed on radiographs and then confirmed, characterized, and staged with MRI. Depending on the stability of the lesion and patient characteristics, OCD lesions are either treated with conservative management non-operatively or with surgical intervention.

Suggested Website

https://www.nationwidechildrens.org/specialties/sports-medicine/sports-medicine-articles/osteochondritis-dissecans

Condition	Osteochondritis Dissecans
Description	Localized alteration in the surface of a joint involving pathology of articular cartilage and underlying bone
Epidemiology	Most common in children ages 12–19 Nearly four times more common in males
Mechanism (common)	No clear mechanism or etiology. May be associated with repetitive microtrauma
History and exam findings	Stable lesions: Chronic, non-specific, activity-related knee pain with normal exam Unstable lesions: Pain associated with knee catching and locking. Knee effusion and gait abnormality on exam
Management	Stable lesions are treated with non-operative conservative management Unstable lesions are treated surgically

References

1. Bauer KL. Osteochondral injuries of the knee in pediatric patients. J Knee Surg. 2018;31(5):382–91.
2. Grimm NL, et al. Osteochondritis dissecans of the knee: pathoanatomy, epidemiology, and diagnosis. Clin Sports Med. 2014;33(2):181–8.
3. Cooper T, et al. Prevalence of bilateral JOCD of the knee and associated risk factors. J Pediatr Orthop. 2015;35(5):507–10.

4. Carey JL, Grimm NL. Treatment algorithm for osteochondritis dissecans of the knee. Orthop Clin North Am. 2015;46(1):141–6.
5. Flynn JM, Kocher MS, Ganley TJ. Osteochondritis dissecans of the knee. J Pediatr Orthop. 2004;24(4):434–43.
6. Kessler JI, et al. The demographics and epidemiology of osteochondritis dissecans of the knee in children and adolescents. Am J Sports Med. 2014;42(2):320–6.
7. Jungesblut OD, et al. Validity of ultrasound compared with magnetic resonance imaging in evaluation of osteochondritis dissecans of the distal femur in children. Cartilage. 2019:1947603519828434.
8. Samora WP, et al. Juvenile osteochondritis dissecans of the knee: predictors of lesion stability. J Pediatr Orthop. 2012;32(1):1–4.
9. Dipaola JD, Nelson DW, Colville MR. Characterizing osteochondral lesions by magnetic resonance imaging. Arthroscopy. 1991;7(1):101–4.
10. Backes JR, et al. Multifocal juvenile osteochondritis dissecans of the knee: a case series. J Pediatr Orthop. 2014;34(4):453–8.
11. Barth J, et al. All-arthroscopic suture fixation of patellar osteochondritis dissecans. Arthrosc Tech. 2017;6(4):e1021–7.
12. Pipino G, et al. Microfractures and hydrogel scaffolds in the treatment of osteochondral knee defects: a clinical and histological evaluation. J Clin Orthop Trauma. 2019;10(1):67–75.

Chapter 31
Pediatric Athlete Development and Appropriate Sports Training

Nailah Coleman

Introduction

This book has reviewed a variety of pediatric knee injuries, both acute and chronic, including the unique mechanisms that contribute to those injuries. Unfortunately, there are system issues that also contribute to injuries in youth, be they athletes or not. Some youth may be overtraining, which can lead to overuse injuries (among other conditions); other youth may not be achieving even the daily recommended activity levels and, due to their low fitness and coordination, can sustain an acute injury with little activity.

Sports Specialization and Injury

Let's first begin with our youth sports enthusiasts, more specifically, those who are participating in sports at increased or excessive levels. Roughly 60 million youth participate in athletics annually [1], and that number has been increasing over time [2]. Although we appreciate that youth athletes are involved in activities that can improve their overall health and wellness, there are some youth, early sports specializers, who are at increased risk of injury and other conditions associated with overtraining.

Sports specialization can be traced back to Olympic athlete development programs, which were traditionally very intense and, in terms of medals, very successful [3]. Unfortunately, the lure of similar glory and knowledge of intense, but

N. Coleman (✉)
The Goldberg Center for Community Pediatric Health, Children's National Hospital, Washington, DC, USA
e-mail: ncoleman@childrensnational.org

© Springer Nature Switzerland AG 2021
N. Coleman (ed.), *Common Pediatric Knee Injuries*,
https://doi.org/10.1007/978-3-030-55870-3_31

successful, training regimens likely allows for continuation of the practice today [3]. An early display of talent can also lead to pressure for more intense training and early sports specialization [2].

Sports specialization has three general components: an athlete participates in one main sport; that participation extends for 8 or more months in the year; and the athlete has quit other sports in favor of that one main sport [1, 4]. Depending on whether he/she has achieved one, two, or three of those components, the youth athlete could be considered a low, moderate, or high sports specializer [4].

For the most part, early sports specialization does not necessarily result in elite athlete status, with the exception of athletes participating in sports who benefit from early preparation and foundational skills development, like gymnastics and figure skating [3]. In addition, those who do well early may not continue to excel and some may actually burn out of their sport [3]. From a numbers standpoint and given the limited number of elite positions available, not all youth athletes will progress to an elite or professional level, regardless of ability or lack thereof [5].

Why is there a concern about youth sports specialization? There is a proven link between training volume and injury risk. Although age-related volume recommendations have not been well studied, the general rule is to limit formal activity hours per week to age in years or less [1, 3, 4]. In addition, current recommendations support limiting intense training to 16 hours per week [1, 3, 4]. Those who exceed that maximum training volume display an increased injury rate [4]. In fact, a 2:1 ratio of organized to recreational sports participation is associated with an increased risk of overuse injury [3]. There is also an increased injury risk with year-round training [1, 4].

Training intensity levels also have a similar, and independent, association with injury. Increased intensity can lead to increased injury [4]. This may be related to a variety of factors. As it often limits participation in a variety of activities and can impact the development of important and diverse motor skills [3], participating in a single sport may not provide the appropriate mix of neuromuscular training to prevent injury [4]. The uninterrupted repetition of a small number of skills can lead to overuse [4]. Excessive training can also affect growth, such as with female gymnasts, although they can experience some catch-up growth after retiring [2].

Given the increased demands for training and competition [4], this singular focus on one activity may also impact long-term physical activity participation and enjoyment [3]. The stress and pressure to participate in one sport can lead not only to overuse injuries but also to burnout, depression, feeling out of control [1, 4, 6], isolation, fatigue, and mental health conditions (ex. depression, substance abuse, and eating disorders) [2]. Some attrition from sports participation can be linked to injury and fear of re-injury [4]. Unfortunately, post-injury recovery can lead to inactivity and obesity, further complicating a potential return to sport [6].

For those participating in youth sports, we should ensure programs are developmentally appropriate for the youth (physically, psychologically, mentally) and address any particular deficits the individual child may have [3]. We should also monitor youth athletes for signs of burnout [3, 6], including decreased appetite, fatigue, apathy, injury, poor sleep, and frequent colds [6], and for injury, particularly if they are exceeding the recommended training volumes [3, 6].

Training workloads for youth athlete development should focus on quality over quantity, allow time for rest within the training progression plan, focus on the athlete's development and not on the specific results desired, and ensure a pre-season conditioning program that allows for neuromotor skills development [6]. Pre-season conditioning programs can, thus, be designed to offer a variety of motor skills training [3]. Pre- and off-season training should provide non-sports-specific skill learning opportunities, especially for those sports that favor specialization (ex. gymnastics and figure skating) [6]. We should allow intensely training athletes time for recovery, especially for competitions that last several days [6].

As we want our youth to participate successfully in physical activities and as we want that participation to extend across the lifespan, there are things we can do to facilitate their participation. We should provide daily time and opportunities for free, unstructured play (directed by youth) and encourage sport sampling to support the development of a variety of skills for neuromotor development [3, 4]. Sport sampling allows for exposure to and learning of a variety of motor skills above and beyond the skills the child might inherently possess or find easy [3, 6]. A physical education (PE) program might provide youth with opportunities to learn the fundamental skills for a variety of sports [3, 6]. Unfortunately, current PE programs are inadequate or nonexistent [6].

The Physical Activity Spectrum

Moving from youth who participate, at times, excessively in physical activity to those who get very little, we will take some time to review the current youth physical activity recommendations. Everyone should be active throughout their lifetime [5]. Worldwide, it is currently recommended that all youth obtain at least 60 minutes or more per day of moderate to vigorous activity [6, 7] and strength- and bone-based activities three times weekly [6].

Unfortunately, worldwide children and adolescents are generally not meeting currently recommended activity levels [5, 6, 8], in part due to decreased opportunities for participation in physical activity and exercise [7]. There are also the system factors referenced earlier, including any or all of the following contributors: decreased (or no) active transportation, poor diet, poor sleep [6], limited (or no) recess/free play and PE [6, 8–10], too much sedentary time (on screens) [6, 10], and crime/fear for self [7].

In general, we tend to think of young athletes as meeting or exceeding the current youth physical activity recommendations. Unfortunately, participation in sport does not always guarantee one will meet the daily recommended amounts of physical activity [6, 10]. In fact, only 24% of athletes in sport meet current activity recommendations, in part due to a significant amount of practice time spent receiving instruction and waiting [9].

Physical inactivity is now the fourth leading risk factor for death due to noncommunicable disease worldwide [8, 10]. As physical activity is important for physical, emotional, social, and cognitive health [7], this daily deficiency requires correction. We need to ensure that youth across the physical activity continuum [9] meet the current physical activity level recommendations, be they highly inactive or overly intense/specialized [9]. As was noted earlier, the specialized youth are at increased risk of injury; however, the inactive youth, due to a lack of skills (or balance of skills), can also sustain an injury, acute or overuse [9].

Exercise Deficit Disorder and the Physical Inactivity Triad

Most people tend to think of children as constantly moving; however, this is increasingly an outdated phenomenon. The current peak physical activity in this generation tops off around age 6 [6, 9, 10], meaning they gradually decrease their physical activity levels after that age. In fact, 70% of youth drop out of all sports by age 14 [9]. This limitation in physical activity is leading to decreased fitness and muscle strength levels in youth [6, 10].

This decrease in fitness and inability to attain the recommended daily physical activity level recommendations can lead to the Physical Inactivity Triad (PIT), which is composed of exercise deficit disorder (EDD), low muscle strength/power, and physical illiteracy [8]. EDD is the medical condition of having a low level of physical activity (i.e., not meeting the current recommendations) [7, 10]. Physical illiteracy describes limited body knowledge and confidence with movement [8]. PIT leads to low fitness levels, limited (or no) participation in physical pursuits, and injury (when activity occurs) [8].

The worry about youth physical inactivity continues over their lifetime. Although it would be hopeful to think that adults, regardless of activity history, will achieve their recommended levels of physical activity daily, we know this is not the case. Physical activity behaviors from childhood tend to progress into adulthood [10].

As noted earlier, there is an increased risk of injury in those with low physical activity, especially if they have received no education to improve their fundamental movement skills. Overweight and obese youth tend to be less active kids. Although there may be an association with increased body fat in infancy (and potential developmental delay), these children lose interest in and the ability to participate in physical activity (if they already had the fundamental movement skills), leading them to evolve into less active adults [7]. Sustaining an injury then makes physical activity even less likely, creating a cycle of inability and unwillingness to participate and leading to excess weight and its negative health effects [10]. Compared to normal-weight children, the injury rate in overweight and obese youth is two times higher in sports and with general physical activity, due to a variety of factors, including decreased strength, low motor and postural control, and low tolerance for fatigue [6].

How can we help our inactive youth? It is important to reach youth early in their lifetime, so as to avoid the cycle of continued inactivity and the effects of physical inactivity lasting into adulthood [8]. We need to address their motor skill development and gross motor strength development before increasing their general physical activity levels to avoid injury, as well as discomfort and embarrassment [6]. We need to focus on improving their physical literacy by increasing opportunities for youth to improve their physical activity with fun activities [7]. Structured programs that target all children at risk (i.e., children not meeting physical activity recommendations, not just overweight/obese children) and work to improve physical literacy and fundamental movement skills, while being developmentally appropriate, should be easily accessible [8]. It is important that sports skill development be considered important for all youth [5].

Resistance training improves general fitness and neuromuscular health, leading to a stronger youth with better fundamental movement skills (ex. running, kicking, balance) and decreased risk of acute and overuse injury [2, 9]. Resistance training can be used as a way to introduce those fundamental movement skills [9] and can improve body confidence and well-being [2, 9]. Young girls, who have an increased risk of injury (particularly minority females), would benefit from focused training [9]. Those with fundamental movement skills tend to continue a lifetime of physical activity, including sports participation [9]. With a 68% decreased injury risk associated with resistance training, females seem to benefit from resistance training more than males [9].

We can also consider integrative neuromuscular training (or the like) for all children, as they develop fundamental movement skills, including in the off season for those in sports [3, 6]. Integrative Neuromuscular Training (INT), training designed to support the attainment of general motor and sport-specific skills in a developmentally appropriate manner [3, 6, 7], could be useful as part of a PE program or as a component of sports training or off-season conditioning. Overweight and obese children who participate in INT (or the like) have a decreased injury rate [6]. INT and resistance training can often serve as an easy/early win for overweight/obese youth [6], augmenting their body confidence. INT, with its simple moves and limited time requirement, can also help kids get past some of the barriers of limited skills and physical illiteracy [10].

Increasing physical activity opportunities for and levels in our youth requires all who interact with kids to be involved [8]. Healthcare providers should ask about play history and exercise habits and treat appropriately, if the child is not meeting guidelines [7]. Medical providers need to be able to seek payment for diagnosing and treating EDD [10]. We must connect medical providers to appropriately trained pediatric exercise specialists, who can design and implement a program to resolve the EDD for the child and family [7, 10]. These specialists will likely need better and more extensive training in this area [10]. Parents need to serve as physically active role models [7]. Schools and after school programs should offer quality programming that is developmentally appropriate and progressive [7].

How Can We Help Both Groups, Our Specializers and Our Low Movers?

We need to incorporate principles that focus on appropriate youth athlete and physical activity development. Everyone benefits from a baseline of fundamental movement skills, regardless of purpose, be it for fun or competition [9]. A program should be adapted to the needs of the youth, be enjoyable, and aim to develop those basic skills over time [5, 6], ensuring both motor competency and strength [5]. Regardless of apparent or lack of early ability, we should be open to all youth achieving higher levels of skills [5]. We should avoid a strict focus on training volume (ex. 10,000-hour rule) [5] and focus on training quality instead. The general progression of physical activity programming from child to adolescent should begin with skill development, move on to sports sampling, and then provide the choice for specialization and/or recreational participation [5].

According to current resistance training recommendations, a youth should start training when able to attend appropriately and maintain good posture and form, roughly around the age of 6 or 7. Youth would also benefit from the incorporation of INT in their program. All exercises should be supervised. A typical resistance training session should include 6–8 exercises of 8–15 reps and 2–3 sets per exercise [2, 9], avoiding maximum weight reps, which are unsafe for the growth plates (just like powerlifting) [2]. There should be no more than 2–3 sessions per week, and they should not occur on consecutive days [2]. Their training program should include times for free play [2, 9]. Exercises should include the large muscle groups with agonists and antagonists addressed in each session [2].

Youth aerobic training recommendations are much less defined. Aerobic activities should match the youth's current level of development and ability. The athlete should select the activity; it is up to the adults to ensure he/she has an appropriate training program, environment, equipment, and technique to participate safely and as long as he/she so chooses [2]. As such, it is essential to improve the education and training of those providing these programs at schools [6]. As medical providers, we can advocate for such youth training programs (PE and sports) for preseason and in-season training and for general health and wellness [9].

Summary

Regardless of the level of activity, above or below the current recommendations, youth can sustain acute and chronic sports injuries. As these injuries can lead to attrition from sports and to the consequences of physical inactivity and overweight/obesity, we need to advocate for appropriate youth physical activity programming that is designed to support the child's development, physically, psychologically, and mentally. Successful youth physical activity development will be evident with a sustained progression to continued, healthy physical activity in adulthood.

References

1. Post EG, Trigsted SM, Riekena JW, Hetzel S, McGuine TA, Brooks MA, Bell DR. The association of sport specialization and training volume with injury history in youth athletes. Am J Sports Med. 2017;45(6):1405–12.
2. Logsdon VK. Training the prepubertal and pubertal athlete. Curr Sports Med Rep. 2007;6(3):183–9.
3. Myer GD, Jayanthi N, DiFiori JP, Faigenbaum AD, Kiefer AW, Logerstedt D, Micheli LJ. Sports specialization, part II: alternative solutions to early sport specialization in youth athletes. Sports Health. 2016;8(1):65–73.
4. Myer GD, Jayanthi N, Difiori JP, Faigenbaum AD, Kiefer AW, Logerstedt D, Micheli LJ. Sport specialization, part I: does early sports specialization increase negative outcomes and reduce the opportunity for success in young athletes? Sports Health. 2015;7(5):437–42.
5. Lloyd RS, Oliver JL, Faigenbaum AD, Howard R, De Ste Croix MBA, Williams CA, Best TM, Alvar BA, Micheli LJ, Thomas DP, Hatfield DL, Cronin JB, Myer GD. Long-term athletic development: part 1: a pathway for all youth. J Strength Cond Res. 2015;29(5):1439–50.
6. Lloyd RS, Oliver JL, Faigenbaum AD, Howard R, De Ste Croix MBA, Williams CA, Best TM, Alvar BA, Micheli LJ, Thomas DP, Hatfield DL, Cronin JB, Myer GD. Long-term athletic development: part 2: barriers to success and potential solutions. J Strength Cond Res. 2015;29(5):1451–64.
7. Faigenbaum AD, Myer GD. Exercise deficit disorder in youth: play now or pay later. Curr Sports Med Rep. 2012;11(4):196–200.
8. Faigenbaum AD, Rebullido TR, MacDonald JP. Pediatric inactivity triad: a risky PIT. Curr Sports Med Rep. 2018;17(2):45–7.
9. Zwolski C, Quatman-Yates C, Paterno MV. Resistance training in youth: laying the foundation for injury prevention and physical literacy. Sports Health. 2017;9(5):436–43.
10. Myer GD, Faigenbaum AD, Stracciolini A, Hewett TE, Micheli LJ, Best TM. Exercise deficit disorder in youth: a paradigm shift toward disease prevention and comprehensive care. Curr Sports Med Rep. 2013;12(4):248–55.

Chapter 32
Community Outreach – Education

Kyle Yost

Sports medicine and primary care providers have many roles and responsibilities. These may include educating the public on preventative health issues and taking care of athletes both on and off the field. Additionally, providers strive to contribute to the communities they serve through community outreach. As this outreach has proven difficult for providers, The American Academy of Pediatrics (AAP), American Academy of Family Physicians (AAFP), and other medical academies have called for more community involvement among physicians. Although the Accreditation Council for Graduate Medical Education has required physicians-in-training to be involved in community health and education for several years, the number of physicians engaging in community health has declined. In a study performed by Minkovitz et al., only 39.9% of pediatricians were involved in community health in 2010 compared to 45.1% in 2004 [1]. In 2010, fewer physicians reported formal training at any time, but more reported training in residency, leading researchers to conclude that, with more formal training, physicians are more likely to engage in the community outreach [1].

A big challenge many providers face, in regard to community outreach, is how to incorporate this into their practice. Another challenge is how to assess the needs of the individual patient, as well as those of the community [2]. One way is to develop a more comprehensive screening protocol that includes a more extensive social history. The Institute of Medicine recommends implementing the 12 "psychosocial vital signs": alcohol, tobacco use and exposure, race and ethnicity, residential address, depression, education, census-tract median income, financial resource strain, intimate partner violence, physical activity, stress, social connections and social isolation [3]. These "vital" signs allow physicians to get a better understanding of the essential factors affecting their patients' health.

K. Yost (✉)
Department of Family and Community Medicine, University of Maryland School of Medicine, Baltimore, MD, USA

© Springer Nature Switzerland AG 2021
N. Coleman (ed.), *Common Pediatric Knee Injuries*,
https://doi.org/10.1007/978-3-030-55870-3_32

Community data, such as economy, demography, and epidemiology, are tools to aid a provider's understanding of the physical and social barriers their patients endure [4]. Knowing this information will supply a primary care provider with the knowledge to treat his/her patients in the environment in which they live [5]. This makes it easier for providers to engage their patients in the community and provide optimal care.

Most children spend the majority of their day outside the home at school programs, childcare facilities, community recreational centers, etc. Providers can utilize these resources to impact their patients. A provider can become involved with a local school to integrate care. Providing care at a school-based clinic enhances access to care by limiting the need for transportation [6]. This also gives the provider an opportunity to see the children interact in their social environment and links children to a medical home [7].

In order to provide better care for patients, providers need to be comfortable with an interdisciplinary team approach. Primary care providers are the point guard for the medical team of their patients. They coordinate care between themselves and other specialists, such as Social Work, Nutrition, Psychiatry, etc. The primary care provider will direct care with specialists, the patient, and their loved ones, to promote maximal health outcomes [8].

Another way a provider can engage in community education is during the pre-participation physical evaluation (PPE). Consensus guidelines recommend the PPE be performed yearly in the primary care provider's office [9]. Local regulatory agencies may require different intervals for the exam. In general, PPEs are necessary for all new athletes and at least every other year for returning athletes. A PPE should be performed 6 weeks ahead of the start of the season, which would allow time for potential follow-up tests and other specialist visits before the season starts. A PPE should consist of a comprehensive history and physical exam. The history should include questions about personal health history, such as elevated blood pressure, exertional dyspnea, chest pain, prior history of an arrhythmia, prior cardiac problems, syncope or near syncope, asthma or exertional bronchospasm, concussion, spinal injuries, stingers, hematologic disorders, absence or loss of a paired organ (or its function), musculoskeletal injuries, and heat illness; and a family history of sudden cardiac death less than 50 years old, disability from heart disease in a family member less than 50 years old, relatives with known cardiac conditions (ex. hypertrophic cardiomyopathy, dilated cardiomyopathy, Marfans disease, long QT syndrome, or other arrhythmias). If the athlete is female, the history should include questions about her menstrual cycle: has she ever had a menstrual period; how old was she, when she had her first menstrual period; and how many periods has she had in past year. Providers can also take this time to ask more sensitive questions about alcohol, drug, and supplement use; concern for anxiety or depression; stress at school or at home; and risk-taking behaviors. The physical exam should consist of blood pressure measurement, visual acuity assessment, auscultation of heart and lungs, palpation of radial and femoral pulses, and a focused orthopedic exam, including a duck walk and other functional maneuvers. Auscultation of the heart should be performed dynamically with the patient standing, as well as lying supine and performing a Valsalva maneuver [9]. The updated, standard PPE forms can be found at https://www.aap.org/en-us/advocacy-and-policy/aap-health-initiatives/Pages/PPE.aspx.

Sports medicine providers also have a great opportunity to educate the community by working with a sports team. The athletic environment is often less threatening than the medical office, which allows the physician to develop relationships with and gain the trust of the athletes. With this trust, an athlete is more likely to be engaged and willing to participate in educational programs. The pre-season is an optimal time for the team physician to have meetings with players and their families [10]. The educational sessions can be on a plethora of topics from mental health, sexual health, injury prevention, nutrition, banned substances, etc. Other opportunities for education may arise during athlete follow-ups with the clinician.

One other way to get providers involved in communities is at the base of a medical provider education: school. Once community engagement is part of the curriculum, just like Pathology, this will provide clinicians with a foundation, upon which they can build from school to training and beyond. Additional community outreach requirements in training programs would give learners better access to providers, who are regularly engaged in community outreach and who can serve as a mentor. This could result in increased numbers of community-based providers, programs, and resources, which could have a demonstrable effect on community health outcomes [11, 12].

Providers can also have a role as advocates for their community. One way is becoming a state legislative contact. This will allow a provider to develop connections outside the community and stay involved and make an impact on a broader level [13]. Another way a provider can be an advocate is by public speaking, helping to raise awareness about health issues affecting the community. When the community understands more about the issue, they can participate in its prevention and eradication. Another powerful method of advocacy is writing and publishing (ex. op-ed articles). Various forms of publication can help raise public awareness and contribute to community engagement and change for the better. Being an advocate for your community is a vital aspect of being involved in your community.

Providers have multiple ways in which they can engage their community and impact their patients' health. By implementing the above concepts, medical caregivers can get closer to achieving the aim of a healthier population in their community.

References

1. Minkovitz CS, Grason H, Solomon BS, Kuo AA, Oconnor KG. Pediatricians involvement in community child health from 2004 to 2010. Pediatrics. 2013;132(6):997–1005.
2. Minkovitz CS. Pediatricians' involvement in community child health from 1989 to 2004. Archives of Pediatrics & Adolescent Medicine. American Medical Association; 2008.
3. Ewing R. How "psychosocial vital signs" in electronic medical records can improve medical care and public health. [Internet]. 2014 [cited 2019 Sep 23]. Available from: https://drexel.edu/now/archive/2014/november/psychosocial-vital-signs/.

4. Rushton FE Jr, American Academy of Pediatrics Committee on Community Health Services. The pediatricians role in community pediatrics. Pediatrics. 1999;103(6):1304–6.
5. 5 ways pediatricians can partner with community development to help their patients [Internet]. Build Healthy Places Network. 2017 [cited 2019Jun29]. Available from: https://www.build-healthyplaces.org/whats-new/5-ways-pediatricians-can-partner-with-community-development-to-help-their-patients/.
6. American Academy of Pediatrics. Committee on School Health. School health centers and other integrated school health services. Committee on School Health. Pediatrics. 2001;107(1):198–201.
7. Abramson JH, Kark SL. Community oriented primary care: meaning and scope. In: Community oriented primary care: new directions for health services delivery. Institute of Medicine. Washington, D. C.: National Academies Press (US); 1983. Available from: https://www.ncbi.nlm.nih.gov/books/NBK234632/.
8. Motivating Collaborations: The Convergence of Public Health and Community Development [Internet]. Build Healthy Places Network. 2019 [cited 2019 Sep 23]. Available from: https://buildhealthyplaces.org/whats-new/motivating-collaborations-the-convergence-of-public-health-and-community-development/.
9. Bernhardt DT, Roberts WO. PPE: preparticipation physical evaluation. Itasca: American Academy of Pediatrics; 2019.
10. Hoffman S, Marci E. The preparticipation physical evaluation. In: Bahr R, Blair S, Cook J, Crossley K, McConnell J, McCrory P, Noakes T, editors. Clinical sports medicine. 4th ed. New York: McGraw-Hill; 2014. p. 1176–84.
11. Palfrey JS. Transforming child health care. Pediatrics. 2013;132(6):1123–4.
12. Community Outreach and Activities [Internet]. Community outreach and activities - Medical Student Education - Department of Family Medicine - University of Rochester Medical Center. [cited 2019 Jul 24]. Available from: https://www.urmc.rochester.edu/family-medicine/medical-student/community-outreach.aspx.
13. State Legislative Handbook. American Medical Society for Sports Medicine. In: AMSSM. Accessed from https://www.amssm.org/Legislat_Handbk.php on 22 Oct 2019.

Index

© Springer Nature Switzerland AG 2021
N. Coleman (ed.), *Common Pediatric Knee Injuries*,
https://doi.org/10.1007/978-3-030-55870-3